MW00844424

Plant Medicine in Practice

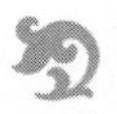

Using the Teachings of John Bastyr

Plant Medicine in Practice

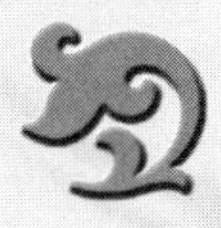

Using the Teachings of John Bastyr

William A. Mitchell, Jr., ND
Naturopathic Physician
Seattle, Washington

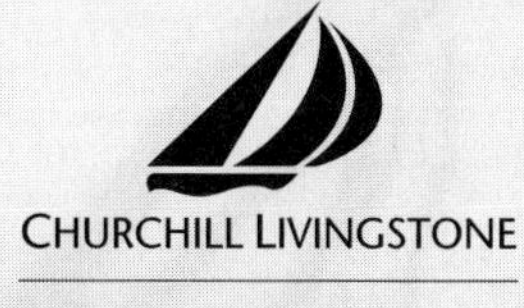

CHURCHILL LIVINGSTONE
An Imprint of Elsevier Science

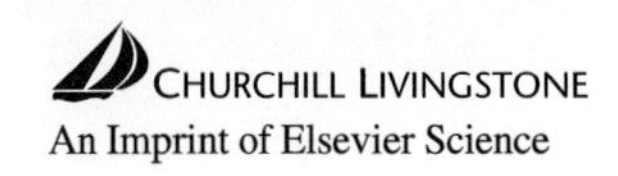

CHURCHILL LIVINGSTONE
An Imprint of Elsevier Science

Robert Stevenson House
1-3 Baxter's Place
Leith Walk
Edinburgh EH1 3AF

PLANT MEDICINE IN PRACTICE ISBN 0-443-07238-8

NOTICE

Complementary and alternative medicine is an ever-changing field. Standard safety precautions must be followed, but as new research and clinical experience broaden our knowledge, changes in treatment and drug therapy may become necessary or appropriate. Readers are advised to check the most current product information provided by the manufacturer of each drug to be administered to verify the recommended dose, the method and duration of administration, and contraindications. It is the responsibility of the licensed prescriber, relying on experience and knowledge of the patient, to determine dosages and the best treatment for each individual patient. Neither the publisher nor the editors assume any liability for any injury and/or damage to persons or property arising from this publication.

Publishing Director: Linda Duncan
Publishing Manager: Inta Ozols
Associate Developmental Editor: Melissa Kuster Deutsch
Project Manager: Peggy Fagen
Designer: Teresa Breckwoldt
Cover Design: Studio Montage

Printed in the United States of America

First published 2003
Reprinted 2003

Preface

I quizzed Dr. Bastyr when I was a student at the National College of Medicine on a complex case and presented all the the laboratory tests that had been run, all the medicines we had tried, and my frustration that the patient was not improving. He listened patiently and after a brief pause said, "I think this patient needs more water, William." With increased hydration, over several weeks, the patient completely recovered.

This book is about the use of plant medicine as Dr. Bastyr taught and practiced. It will frustrate those who are used to encyclopedic coverage of herbs, sticklers for botany and botanical description, and scientists who want chemical diagrams and evidence-based medicines, tried and tested by numerous double-blind placebo-controlled studies.

Doctors who cure patients with glasses of water, the healing power of nature, exercise, relatively inexpensive but effective plant extracts, and other sensible therapies probably will be of more interest to those practitioners who appreciate the relevance and usefulness of the medicines of those who came before us.

Certainly Dr. Bastyr had—and modern naturopathic physicians have—a knowledge of the prescription drugs and a respectful appreciation of diagnostic technical advances. Indeed, we know allopathic drugs very well because our patients often come in using these drugs and we need to know drug-plant and drug-nutrition interactions. In fact, many of the patent drugs are modeled after natural ones. Dr. Bastyr never taught his students to be divisive or to dislike or disregard the accomplishments and thinking of the modern allopathic community. He encouraged the scientific pursuit of natural medicine. The current institutions of naturopathic medical education are heavily involved in scientific research. He taught and encouraged naturopathic physicians to appreciate and study historical traditional medicine that has been evolving its therapeutics for countless ages and offers a wealth of timeless information.

What this work tries to do is to present the plant medicines formatted as Dr. Bastyr presented them in the lectures, by physiologic systems. I further selected my choices as to what I said about each remedy based on two criteria: First, I chose Dr. Bastyr's highlights—that is, the action and use of the medicines that he more clearly had experience with himself—and second, as often as possible, I wrote about the uses of the plants as I observed them to work in my own practice of 26 years. Where I have little experience with a plant, I try to indicate those limitations.

Dr. Bastyr was a master of medicine. He delivered over 800 babies, did surgery in his early years in a hospital setting, memorized most of the homeopathic *Materia Medicas*, and skillfully prescribed botanical medicines in many forms. He also understood nutritional medicine and kept up to date on nutritional breakthroughs. He was a master at adjusting the spine, using hydrotherapy and electrotherapies such as galvanic and diathermy, and certainly could perform any office procedure such as bladder irrigation or sigmoidoscopy. The list could go on.

Yet with all his knowledge and experience, one would find him in the front row taking notes at all of the educational seminars and conventions that were offered regionally and nationally in naturopathic medicine.

This book is offered to those who would like a glimpse at botanical medicine as practiced in the eclectic Euro-American tradition. Throughout the text, I offer suggestions on the use of the medicines and doses as I have seen them work personally. In my practice, I use plant medicines with almost every patient. I have been doing this for the last 26 years. This has afforded me the opportunity to watch and record progress of a large number of patients using natural medicine over time. The reader will find some more modern use of the plants laced in throughout the text. These additions reflect the eclectic process wherein new therapies are integrated with the old.

I remember Dr. Bastyr being asked what to use to treat a patient with a particular illness; his response was, "Use whatever works." He wasn't being glib. He was demonstrating the eclectic mind.

Dr. Bastyr practiced for many years (until the end of his practice) in a converted three-story house on 10th Ave E. just south of Broadway in the capitol hill district of Seattle. Walking into his office was like walking into grandma's living room. The smells that delighted the senses would be from whatever poultice or muscle rub or potion that highlighted that particular day. He charged $10 for an office call even into the late 1980s.

When one walked in to see him, the healing began immediately. Dr. Bastyr was what pure goodness would look like if it could walk on two legs. I believe, I suppose, somewhere deep within the best part of myself, that John Bastyr did not need any medicines to heal people. He himself was the medicine. If what we need most as patients, in this day of sterile medical madness, is someone guided by truth and light to take our hands and tell us that we are going to be fine, then I would give you Dr. John Bastyr.

After practicing medicine for over 50 years, Dr. Bastyr passed away in 1995. He was 83 years old. This book is about his work. It is for him because I and so many others dearly loved him. He never wrote, but he must never be forgotten.

William A. Mitchell, Jr., ND
November 2002

ABOUT THE AUTHOR

William A. Mitchell, Jr., ND, graduated from the University of Washington in 1971. He then attended the National College of Naturopathic Medicine from 1972 to 1976 at the Seattle campus. He has practiced naturopathic medicine in the Seattle area for the past 22 years and still maintains an active full-time schedule of patients. In 1978 he co-founded Bastyr University along with Les Griffith, ND, Joseph Pizzorno, ND, and Shiela Quinn.

Dr. Mitchell has four children and now two grandchildren. He enjoys hiking in the Cascades, visiting his kids, playing with his grandchildren, and teaching yoga, which he has been doing for the last 6 years.

This is Dr. Mitchell's third major book. He wrote the first, *Naturopathic Applications of the Botanical Remedies*, in 1983. His second book was entitled *Foundations of Natural Therapeutics: Biochemical Apologetics of Naturopathic Medicine*, which he wrote in 1997.

Besides maintaining an active practice in Seattle, Dr. Mitchell teaches Advanced Naturopathic Therapeutics at Bastyr University.

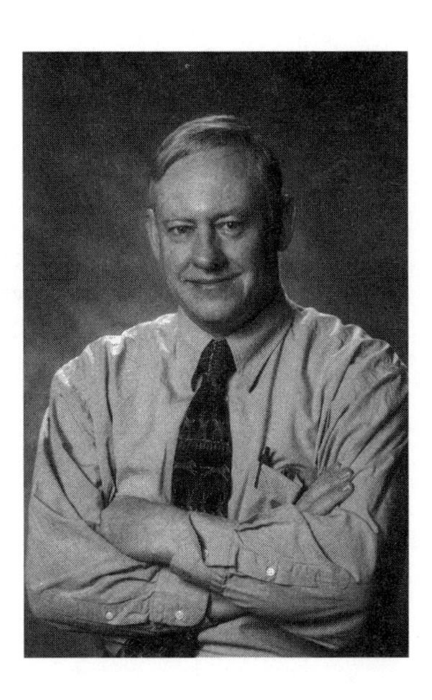

ACKNOWLEDGMENTS

It gives me great pleasure to thank a number of people without whose help this work would not have been possible. Alphabetically, they are as follows;

Thanks to Dr. John Bastyr, who selflessly shared his knowledge and experience with his students. In the practice of naturopathic medicine, he was, simply, the best of the best.

Thanks to Maria Bell, ND, who was the primary editor for the project up to the last two rewrites. Moreover, of singular importance was her insistence that this work have a well-defined central focus. Thematic cohesion is not my strong suit. Without her initial guidance, this book would have told you far less about Dr. Bastyr's use of the medicines.

Thanks to Leah Mitchell, ND candidate, Bastyr University class of 2005. Leah did the final two full editings of the manuscript, a labor that involved many many days of diligent work. She made sure that the final text was clear and that we stayed with the fundamental mission of the book. Leah also made sure that the writing accurately stated the clinical ideas and information. Yes, Leah is my daughter. (I have four brilliant and wonderful fully-grown children—Rachel, Saul, Leah, and Noah—all of whom I love to spend time with. Leah is the third in age. I also now have two grandchildren, David and Regan. They all immeasurably enrich my life.)

Thanks to Joseph Pizzorno, Jr., ND, for so many things. We are united by our work originally in founding Bastyr University. The four co-founders were Joe, myself, Les Griffith, ND, and Shiela Quinn. Dr. Pizzorno introduced me to Churchill/Livingstone through his own publishing agent and put in a good word about the potential usefulness and historical relevance of the manuscript.

Thanks to Dirk Powell, ND, a classmate and mountain climbing buddy of mine at the National College of Naturopathic Medicine, Seattle campus, in the early 1970s. He heard the same lectures from Dr. Bastyr I did and also did some clinical preceptoring with Dr. Bastyr at his office. Dr. Powell read an early formative manuscript and offered comments and information that we had learned in class. To this day, whenever I talk to Dirk, it seems that we dig up more memories of those wonderful years when we had the privilege of being taught by Dr. Bastyr and some of the other truly great masters of naturopathic medicine.

This book is dedicated to John Bastyr, ND,
whose lectures on botanical medicine stimulated my
interest in the exploration and usage of plant medicinals.

Contents

Note About the Text

Doses given in this work are for adults. In calculating the child's dose, one may follow Clark's rule. It reads as follows:

$$\frac{\textbf{Weight of the child in pounds}}{\textbf{150 pounds (average adult weight)}} = \textbf{Percent of adult dose}$$

CHAPTER

1

ADAPTOGENS

CHAPTER • OUTLINE

Eleutherococcus senticosus
Ascorbic acid
Pantothenic acid
Ganoderma lucidum
Carotenes
Curcuma longa
Placebo
Procyanidolic polymers and other fruit bioflavonoid compounds
Camellia sinensis

Dr. Bastyr spoke about the category of adaptogens without ever using that specific term because the term *adaptogen* was not in common use in the 1970s. It is a term that has gained popularity since the time of his death. Adaptogens are materials that enhance our ability to cope with the physiological stress that we encounter when dealing with toxins in the environment or with stress from life itself. The numerous toxic materials that we must interact with daily have stimulated us to explore the pathophysiological consequences of these materials on the tissues and systems of our bodies. Adaptogenic medicine may be thought of as a specialty of naturopathic medicine. One task of naturopathic medicine has always been to help patients adapt to a changing environment. Adaptogens are finding an especially important niche in our armamentarium because we are exposed to so many toxins in our current environment. The topic of adaptogens is vast, and the field is exciting. The list of plants I have chosen here is small; however, I hope that it may be helpful to those patients who are having a particularly difficult time adjusting to the environment or convalescing from disease.

Eleutherococcus senticosus

COMMON NAME ■ Siberian ginseng

The medicine is made from the root. This plant is a shrub that grows to about 2 meters in height. It is native to northern China and the eastern reaches of Russia. Given the brutal weather conditions in which it survives, it is no wonder it is ranked among the world's great adaptogens.

Siberian ginseng contains eleutherosides, which are triterpine saponins. The ability of Siberian ginseng to exert an immunomodulatory effect has been demonstrated by researchers.[1] This effect appears to be caused in part by the eleutherosides contained in the plant. In addition, Siberian ginseng contains other steroid-like compounds such as glycosides of syringaresinol and daucosterol, which may have some activity in the endocrine system. Clearly, scientific research needs to be done to further explore the actions of these constituents.

Siberian ginseng increases T-helper cells and the activity of natural killer cells. It stimulates the adrenal cortex, which enhances one's capacity to work.[2] The adaptogenic aspects of Siberian ginseng have been studied in Russia.[3,4] I use Siberian ginseng as an adaptogen for various abnormalities in one's sense of well-being. These abnormalities can include nervous exhaustion, depression, and disease, especially flu. I have found that convalescence from both disease and surgery occurs more rapidly when one uses this plant.

The general dose of Siberian ginseng that I give is 6 mg of the powdered root per kilogram of body weight twice daily. If a tincture is used, the general dose is 90 drops twice daily. In addition, I have two favorite mixtures involving Siberian ginseng. I use the first mixture to help rebuild the nervous system after disease or injury. It contains one part Siberian ginseng and two parts *Avena sativa.* I give this mixture in doses of 30 drops in a little water four times daily. I use the second formula to increase general energy. It contains two parts Siberian ginseng tincture together with one part *Glycyrrhiza glabra typica* fluid extract and one part *Panax quinquifolium* tincture. The dose of this mixture is 60 drops daily.

I occasionally take a squirt of Siberian ginseng tincture in the midafternoon on long workdays as a gentle, but fairly effective, pick-me-up. It then has a curious calming aftereffect. I have found that most tonics are enhanced by adding a little Siberian ginseng. I make a tasty tea that can be taken as a calmative. It contains 30 drops of Siberian ginseng tincture and $\frac{1}{2}$ teaspoon of glycine in a cup of hot water. Glycine is a sweet-tasting amino acid that calms the midbrain by binding to the locus ceruleus and decreasing the output of norepinephrine in that part of the brain. This tea calms rather than sedates the brain.

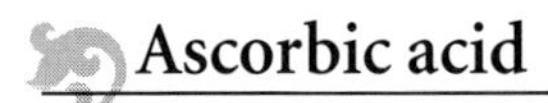

Ascorbic acid

COMMON NAME ■ Vitamin C

Vitamin C is a good adaptogen even though it is not a botanical medicine. It is, however, made out of sugar by plants, a task that human beings cannot perform. Vitamin C must be obtained from our diets because we cannot make it in our bodies. We lack the enzyme L-gluconolactone oxidase, which converts sugar to vitamin C.

Vitamin C has been shown to increase rat survival time when the animal is put in a tank of cold water and allowed to swim to the point of exhaustion.[5] Although this clearly demonstrates the use of adaptogenic materials, I think it is an unfortunate method.

Vitamin C helps us to adapt to daily stress. We know that vitamin C is needed to make dopamine-β-monoxygenase, which is involved in the conversion of dopamine to its hydroxylated derivatives and ultimately to catecholamines. A number of my colleagues, who are well acquainted with vitamin C, have reported that they notice a decrease in frequency and duration of acute illness during flu season when they use divided doses of vitamin C. I recall Dr. Jerry Martinez, one of my teachers at the National College of Naturopathic Medicine (NCNM), telling me that 1000 mg of vitamin C given every other hour knocked out sinusitis in his patients. I have used vitamin C in doses of 1000 mg per hour to clear up acute mastitis. When using vitamin C as an adaptogen, I prescribe doses of 1000 mg twice daily. Using vitamin C together with 400 mg of quercetin twice daily creates a tremendous antioxidant effect.[6] I remember sitting in Dr. Bastyr's class at NCNM in 1974 and hearing him say that if we gave children vitamin C and cod liver oil daily, the incidence of childhood colds and flu would decrease by 75%. I have found this to be true in my practice.

Pantothenic acid

Because pantothenic acid is incorporated into coenzyme A, which functions in two-carbon unit metabolism, acetylation and other acylation reactions depend on its presence as a cofactor. The release of energy from carbohydrates and the degradation and metabolism of fatty acids also involve pantothenic acid.[7] Individuals who are deficient in pantothenic acid are more susceptible to stress.[8]

I use pantothenic acid to help relieve "burning feet syndrome," increase antibody production, and increase both body heat and energy. I have found that it is especially useful for patients who complain of cold hands and feet. For this condition, I prescribe 1000 mg at lunchtime. It works!

In my practice, I can recall numerous cases in which the use of high doses of pantothenic acid resulted in the elimination of multiple warts on the hands.

Perhaps this has something to do with a change in the temperature of the extremities. I have found that a trial period of 3 weeks is sufficient for verrucae. If this remedy has not worked within 3 weeks, then it is not the remedy of choice. Long-term use of any concentrated nutrient, including pantothenic acid, should be monitored by a physician. My use of pantothenic acid as part of a protocol to combat depression will be discussed later.

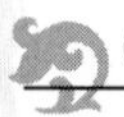

Ganoderma lucidum

COMMON NAME ■ Reishi mushroom

Ganoderma lucidum belongs to a group of plants known as wood fungi. It contains two polysaccharides known as ganodermic A and ganodermic B acids that seem to enhance the activity of the immune system. The adaptogenic effects of *Ganoderma* occur as a result of a number of effects on the body. It enhances self-improving mechanisms on the central nervous system, improves heart function and efficiency, tonifies the parasympathetic nervous system, enhances macrophage and polymorphonuclear leukocytes, and exhibits antihistamine activity.

In addition, *Ganoderma* contains ganodermic acid S. This compound has been examined in great detail for its ability to inhibit platelet aggregation. The median lethal dose for *Ganoderma* is greater than 5000 mg/kg, rendering this plant quite safe to use. I prescribe 1800 mg of the powdered material twice daily.

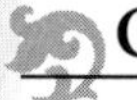

Carotenes

Foods containing carotenoids include yams, squash, carrots, greens, sweet potatoes, pumpkins, paprika, and cayenne. All green vegetables, as well as the aerial portions of almost all herbs, contain some amount of carotenes. I include carotenes in the list of adaptogens because they directly decrease the inflammatory effects on body tissues that are caused by the body's reaction to inhaled or ingested environmental substances. I recommend that my patients eat diets rich in carotenes. I believe that this is beneficial for almost everyone.

To some extent, the ingestion of carotene-rich plants protects the skin from exposure to the photon energy of the sun. Carotenes specifically quench singlet oxygen, thus decreasing free-radical damage. They also help to keep the body from overreacting to pollution in the environment. By pollution, I mean any toxic materials that we come in contact with frequently, such as pesticides, ozone both in the atmosphere and from copy machines, food additives, and industrial or workplace chemicals. Carotenes also help to decrease thymic involution.[6] This prolongs the thymus gland's role in the body's immunity. Carotenes also help with night vision adaptation.

I have found that three carrots or a yam daily is sufficient to provide adequate carotenes. Sometimes ingesting whole foods is the best way to obtain the desired nutrients. Carotene capsules often contain *trans*- rather than *cis*-carotenoids. *Trans*-carotenoids are not effective antioxidants.

Curcuma longa

COMMON NAME ■ Turmeric

Other species of turmeric that also contain the active ingredient curcumin are *Curcuma domestica*, *Curcuma aromatica Salisb*, and *Curcuma zedoaria*. I have chosen to add *Curcuma* to the list of adaptogens because of the wide range of therapeutic benefits afforded by this helpful plant.

Curcumin is an excellent antioxidant, antithrombic,[9] antimutagenic in smokers,[10] hypocholesterolemic agent,[11] and mild hypoglycemic agent. In addition, research performed on mice has demonstrated its ability to inhibit the initiation and promotion steps in certain types of cancer. Curcumin inhibits tumor initiation by 7,12-dimethyl-benz[a]anthracene and tumor promotion by 12-O-tetradecanoylphorbol-13-acetate in CD-1 mice.[12] It also inhibits cyclooxygenase- and lipoxygenase-dependent metabolism of arachidonic acid to prostaglandins and hydroxyeicosatetraenoic acids. Curcumin enhances interleukin-4, thus acting as an immunomodulator.

Given *Curcuma's* broad scope of action on many human and animal models and systems, it may be wise to consider taking curcumin, one of *Curcuma*'s principal active ingredients, as an adaptogen. I recommend that patients take curcumin capsules when they are going to be in an airplane due to the proinflammatory air quality. As an antioxidant and antimutagenic, curcumin helps to protect smokers from the harmful effects of cigarette smoke; however, this therapy should not be construed as a reason to keep smoking.

Placebo

A placebo embraces the desired effect. Dr. Bastyr mentioned that the placebo effect is extremely powerful. The strongest adaptogens are created by the body, using all of the organizational skills available. The wisdom of the body directs the marshalling of forces to adjust to changing conditions. Tantamount to achieving this effect is the belief that the body is capable of doing what is necessary.

Rudolph Fritz Weiss, MD, states that the "Placebo releases soul forces in man, creating mental concepts that also have a somatic effect."[13] Any medicine chosen has a direct effect and a placebo effect, which is contingent on the patients' belief in the doctor, in themselves, and in the medicine.

I use the placebo effect in my practice. However, I do not use pure placebos such as small sugar pills. Rather, I will give an herbal combination that is most likely tonifying to the patient. By tonifying I am referring to increasing the vital force in the body as a whole, or any specific system in the body. It is a term that naturopaths use frequently when we speak of improving the functional integrity of human systems. I name the tonifying remedy something like "Bob's strengthening and centering adaptogen." I list all of the ingredients on the label. I tell Bob that the medicine has a healing effect whose full power and potential are unknown but that every time he takes 10 drops directly on the tongue, he will feel the healing properties of the plants working within him. I tell him to breathe deeply and relax for 1 minute to allow the plant properties to be absorbed into the body and help to direct the healing traffic. I tell Bob that I am interested in what he discovers in the ensuing weeks and to report back to me with any exciting or significant news.

I have engaged the botanical and placebo effect in this exercise. I have created the expectation of change and movement toward wellness. Never tell patients that the medicine is going to do something specific such as cure their cancer once and for all. Keep the placebo effect directed at the general vital force of the body. Then let the body do what no doctor can. Know that healing is a mystical as well as a scientific endeavor.

Procyanidolic polymers and other fruit bioflavonoid compounds

There really is no common name for the procyanidolic polymers. The term *procyanidolic polymers* is used to embrace a large number of molecules derived from berries and their seeds, as well as the seeds of other fruit. Sometimes one will come across the term *procyanidolic oligomers.* The term *oligomer* refers to a polymer consisting of two, three, or four monomers. At any rate, I like to think of the procyanidolic compounds as berry bioflavonoids. Included in this category are proanthocyanidin dimers, trimers, and other polymers of flavanoids.

The blueberry anthocyanins consist of bioflavonoids bound to sugar groups. The hawthorn berry proanthocyanidin is an example of a dimer consisting of two flavans linked together. The vitexin-4-rhamnoside is also from hawthorn berry and consists of a basic bioflavonoid skeleton attached to two different kinds of sugars. The variety and complexity escalate from there. There are thousands of permutations of polyphenolic compounds linked in various ways to other molecules in nature. Many of them function as antioxidants[14] and stabilizers of collagenous connective tissue. Others are attracted to different human systems.

The adaptogenic function of these procyanidolic polymers is in their ability to function as potent antioxidants, especially in connective tissue. They also serve to inhibit damaging molecules such as xanthine oxidase, hyaluronidase, elastase, and collagenase, all of which are enzymes that can break down connective tissue. The ingestion of large quantities of berries will provide these various protective molecules. They help significantly to prevent heart and arterial disease, increase energy, and protect connective tissue, especially as we age.[15] They help us to adapt to the environment. Every patient in my office is given bioflavonoids, especially the anthocyanidins from berries.

Camellia sinensis

COMMON NAME ■ Green tea

The adaptogenic capacity of green tea epigallocatechin and other flavonoid compounds found in this plant has been studied extensively. In fact, in experimental studies the antioxidant qualities of green tea seem to outperform both vitamin C and vitamin E.[16] Of equal or greater interest to me is the discovery that green tea polyphenols significantly increase the activity of detoxifying enzymes, including glutathione peroxidase, glutathione reductase, glutathione transferases, catalase, and quinone reductase. The activity of these enzymes has been observed in the tissue of the small intestine, lungs, and liver.[17]

What is particularly exciting about this information is that these enzyme systems, which are necessary for detoxification, help us to cope with daily exposure to the ever-expanding levels of toxins in our environment. *Drink green tea!* I recommend starting each morning with a cup of green tea. Although green tea does contain 30-40 mg of caffeine per cup, I have rarely seen it adversely over-stimulate a patient. A little sugar may be added to combat the slight bitterness of the tea. Do not use milk with the green tea, as it tends to bind the flavonoids, making them less available to the body.

CHAPTER

2

ALTERATIVES

CHAPTER • OUTLINE

Echinacea angustifolia
Baptisia tinctoria
Berberis aquifolium
Berberis vulgaris
Solanum dulcamara
Polemonium reptans
Sambucus nigra
Taraxacum officinale
Pterocaulon pucnostachyum
Parthenocissus quinquefolia
Lanthus glandulosa
Medicago sativa
Phytonadione
Glycine max

The term *alterative* is a rather antiquated term. It was frequently used by eclectic physicians and thus, in the old materia medicas, one will come across this term quite frequently. Alteratives are remedies that normalize a pathological condition. They may also be defined as medicinal materials that reestablish healthy function in various systems of the body. A true alterative reestablishes normal function whether the systems in question are hyperactive or hypoactive. For example, *Medicago sativa* is a phytoestrogenic plant that lessens the effects of excessive estrogen in the human body. It does this by means of competitive inhibition of the strong estrogens by milder estrogens. On the other hand, if the body was deficient in estrogen, *Medicago* would add a phytoestrogen effect to the estrogen-deficient system.

Rather than belaboring the definition of alteratives and the questionably important distinctions relative to selecting them, I have selected the following 14 remedies. The first 10 might be called the "classic alteratives" simply because they have been defined as such in older works in botanical medicine, such as those of Kutz-Cheraux, Felter, and Ellingwood. Dr. Bastyr taught us the alterative effects of these botanicals when I was a student at National College of Naturopathic Medicine in Seattle. At the end of this section, I have listed several additional alterative remedies. I have chosen to include these because they offer such biochemically elegant examples of the alterative principle. Alteratives were fundamental to Dr. Bastyr's practice, and they are fundamental to mine; I use them daily.

Because the alterative action of plants is often not clearly defined, my discussion of the classic alteratives will give primarily an overview of the general action of the plant as a whole. Its alterative action will often be unclear. I apologize for this obscurity.

Echinacea angustifolia

COMMON NAME ■ Purple coneflower

The root and aerial parts are used to make medicine. *Echinacea*'s action has been described as antibiotic, alterative, and tonic. Eclectic practitioners and herbalists have used topical applications for throat irritations, tonsillitis, and other infections. Internally, Dr. Bastyr used the tincture for septicemia, pyuria, and gangrene. Use large amounts of *Echinacea* for these conditions. I suggest 1 teaspoon of tincture six times daily. I recommend mixing *Echinacea* with *Hydrastis* for the treatment of gangrene. When treating gangrene, I would suggest the use of large amounts of flavonoids in addition to *Echinacea.* A thousand milligrams of anthocyanins made from concentrated mixed berries taken five times daily is a good starting dose. Blueberry and bilberry concentrates are especially effective, although elderberry is another great anthocyanin for this purpose. A number of my patients have had gangrenous ulcers of the feet and lower legs. They have done well with large doses of the berry anthocyanins taken internally, and with alternating hot and cold hydrotherapy applications to the affected area.

Dr. Bastyr spoke highly of *Echinacea* for treating many infections, for deficiencies of immune function, and for general coughs and colds. However, the dose he suggested was much smaller than the dose we use today. This was true of most of the other eclectic physicians as well. For them, a typical dose was 10 to 30 drops three times daily.

To treat infections, Dr. Bastyr thought that *Baptisia* mixes well with *Echinacea.* He said to combine one part *Baptisia* with five parts *Echinacea* and give 60 drops of the combination three times daily. The eclectics used *Echinacea* for septic blood conditions including snake, spider, and dog bites. For decubitus ulcers, Dr. Bastyr used diluted *Echinacea* topically. *Echinacea* can also be used after vaccinations to decrease the side effects on the body. Dr. Bastyr taught us to use *Thuja* 200X homeopathically for this purpose. The dose of *Echinacea* as an alterative is 60 drops of tincture four times daily or 1 level teaspoon per cup of water as a tea two to three times daily.

Echinacea contains the immunostimulatory polysaccharide inulin. This molecule enhances immune function.[18] *Echinacea* inhibits hyaluronidase, which can result in a decrease in the spread of viruses.[19] It stimulates complement, as do most inulin-containing plants. Complement is a sequence of proteins that combine on the surface of pathogens, causing their rupture. When faced with hypocomplementemia, I mix equal parts of *Echinacea* and *Arctium lappa*. The dose that I give is 120 drops of the mixture four times daily to stimulate complement. Use caution when giving *Echinacea* in allergy conditions; it can worsen the symptoms.

Other constituents in *Echinacea* include two caffeic acid esters, echinacoside and cynarin.[20] The exact function of these constituents in human health is uncertain, although caffeic acid and other polyhydroxylated compounds are often good antioxidants and can be hepatoprotective. For a further discussion of constituents, consult the *Textbook of Natural Medicine* by Pizzorno and Murray.[19]

Baptisia tinctoria

COMMON NAME ■ Wild indigo

The roots and leaves are used to make medicine. Eclectic physicians have described *Baptisia* as an alterative circulatory stimulant, antiseptic, laxative, and tonic. *Baptisia* contains an array of quinolizidine alkaloids, including cytisine, anagyrine, sparteine isoflavonoids, and formononetin.[21] Cytisine is a toxic principle, which may account for *Baptisia*'s antimicrobial properties and may also contribute to its emetic qualities when taken in large doses. Sparteine may have cardiovascular effects and has been categorized as oxytocic.[21] Formononetin, which occurs in *Baptisia*, is the major estrogenic factor in clover species such as *Trifolium subterraneum* and *Trifolium pratense*.[22,23]

I use 5 drops of *Baptisia* tincture three times daily as an alterative, especially in infectious diseases. Dr. Bastyr lectured extensively about *Baptisia*. This was clearly a remedy that he used frequently in combination with other remedies, especially *Echinacea*, *Phytolacca*, and *Sanguinaria*. I remember telling Dr. Bastyr that I had mixed *Baptisia* with *Echinacea* and *Hydrastis* to make a cold and flu remedy. He told me that adding the *Baptisia* was a good idea and that it would probably help to increase the effectiveness of the remedy.

Baptisia is an important medicine in most septic and degenerative diseases manifesting in ulcerations and eruptions.[24] I mix the tinctures of *Baptisia* and *Melissa officinalis* together to help fight herpetic infections. The proportions are one part *Baptisia* to three parts *Melissa.* The dose is 30 drops three times daily.

According to the eclectics, *Baptisia* works well with *Echinacea* for typhoid fever. Dr. Bastyr said that it is also a good remedy for dysentery and *Proteus* species infections. I use *Baptisia* as an ingredient in formulas for bacterial enteritis or colitis. My formula for treating colitis is one part of the tincture of *Baptisia* mixed with three parts *Hydrastis* tincture, three parts *Ulmus fulva* fluid extract, and one part *Zingiber* tincture. I prescribe 60 drops three times daily.

Baptisia's stimulant effects are directed at the cardiac and respiratory centers. In large doses, it is an emetocathartic. However, because of its cardiac and respiratory actions, I would not suggest using it this way. In smaller doses, it stimulates metabolism.

Berberis aquifolium

COMMON NAME ■ Oregon grape root

This plant is more currently referred to as *Mahonia aquifolium.* The root is used to make medicine. Dr. Bastyr described *Berberis* as a good alterative for syphilitic constitutions. *Berberis* has also been used as a digestive stimulant in hypopancreatism. I use *Berberis* for skin conditions such as acne. This may seem like a curious acne medicine, but 30 drops three times daily has been effective, especially when combined with other therapies. For example, I use *Berberis* together with 50 mg of zinc daily. It is also beneficial to encourage adequate hydration. For this purpose, I recommend at least six glasses of water daily. Dr. Bastyr taught that *Berberis* could be used to treat pityriasis rosea, herpes, and psoriasis. These conditions were considered by the elder eclectics to be disorders of the blood or of the internal metabolism. *Berberis* is a tonic to the intestines and kidneys.

Berberis contains berberine alkaloids as does *Hydrastis.* I remember Cascade Anderson-Geller, a great herbalist now living in the Pacific Northwest, saying that *Berberis* is a poor person's goldenseal (*Hydrastis canadensis*); however, *Hydrastis* has a stronger action than *Berberis.* In serious infection such as strep throat, *Hydrastis* is preferred because it tends to be more effective; *Berberis* is useful as a gargle for sore throat. I use a little mild saltwater with 15 drops of *Berberis* as a gargle.

Berberis vulgaris

COMMON NAME ■ Barberry

The root is used to make medicine. *Berberis vulgaris* contains berberine, as does *Berberis aquifolium.* It also contains at least two other bitter alkaloidal principles, oxycanthine and berbamine. As with most alteratives, *Berberis vulgaris* helps the patient to overcome pathological conditions by toning, improving metabolic processes, aiding elimination, and improving other body functions. *Berberis vulgaris* is a tonic to the spleen. I have treated splenomegaly successfully using a combination of four parts *Ceanothus americanus* and one part *Berberis vulgaris.* The dose that I prescribe is 30 drops of the tincture mixture twice daily. *Berberis vulgaris* has been used by the eclectics to treat cholecystitis and cholelithiasis. Most of the alkaloidal principles in barberry are antimicrobial. Further investigation will undoubtedly clarify which organisms are the most affected. Dr. Bastyr taught that the dose of *Berberis vulgaris* as an alterative is 1 to 3 mL of tincture three times daily.

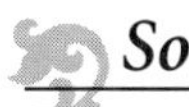

Solanum dulcamara

COMMON NAMES ■ Woody nightshade, Bittersweet

The whole herb is used to make medicine. Dr. Bastyr said that this plant is used for acute coryza, or discharge from the nose, and in vesicular disorders to help resolve the rash. He said that eclectic physicians used *Solanum* for bronchial asthma at a dose of 10 drops of tincture three times daily. If an adverse reaction occurs, the dose should be decreased. Dr. Dirk Powell, a classmate and friend of mine, remembers Dr. Bastyr using *Solanum* to treat psoriasis and eczema. He also recalls Dr. Bastyr saying that *Solanum* is useful in rheumatic afflictions that are agitated by cold, wet conditions. In addition, Dr. Powell recalls Dr. Bastyr using *Solanum* for acrocyanosis.

I have tried this plant myself. It has a sweet taste and an immediate effect on the brain, although that effect is hard to define. It can be felt in the forehead around the eyes. Interestingly, the fruit of *Solanum* contains an alkaloid called solasodine, which is a starting material for steroidal drugs. The antiinflammatory property of this plant may be the result of its effects on antiinflammatory steroids in the body.

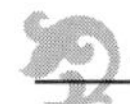

Polemonium reptans

COMMON NAME ■ Abscess root

The root is used to make medicine. This plant is diaphoretic, astringent, alterative, and expectorant. Dr. Bastyr taught its use for febrile inflammatory disease, colds, and bronchial and lung complaints. He told us to have our patients drink extra water when taking this remedy because *Polemonium* produces copious perspiration. He said that the standard tea should be taken in wineglass doses, together with extra water to avoid dehydration.

Sambucus nigra

COMMON NAMES ■ Black elder, Elderberry

The flowers, fruit, and inner bark are used to make medicine. *Sambucus* contains flavonoids, flavone glycosides, and phenolic acids, including quercetin, kaempferol, isoquercitrin, rutin, pectin, and *p*-coumaric acid. I have wildcrafted this plant with Dirk Powell, ND. I use only the buds and flowers to make a tincture. Wildcrafting refers to gathering plants in their natural environment and using them to make herbal preparations.

Sambucus has been used as an alterative, a diuretic, a diaphoretic, and an antiflu medicine. A strong purgative can be made from the bark of the young tree. Dr. Bastyr said that the tincture could be used topically for weeping eczema such as that seen in poison oak, poison ivy, or poison sumac. I use *Sambucus* in a potent upper respiratory remedy that seldom fails. The formula contains one part each of the fluid extracts of *Sambucus, Glycerrhiza, Grindelia, Tussilago,* and *Berberis aquifolium*, together with one-half part *Lomatium* tincture. The dose is 90 drops of the mixture four times daily.

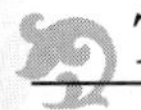

Taraxacum officinale

COMMON NAME ■ Dandelion

The whole plant may be used to make medicine. I have included *Taraxacum* with the alteratives because of its broad tonic effects. It benefits digestion and liver function and is generally high in vitamins, minerals, and some amino acids. The leaves are very nutritious. They are loaded with minerals, including magnesium, zinc, and manganese. The vitamin A content is exceptional. The root benefits the liver, and the leaves, which are diuretic, help both the liver and the kidneys.

Among Native American tribes, *Taraxacum* has been used as a laxative, a stomach tonic, and a diuretic. It is possible that the tonic, energizing effect of *Taraxacum* is the result of the monohydroxy triterpene, taraxasterol. *Taraxacum* also contains choline, inulin, and glutamic acid. Dr. Bastyr talked about *Taraxacum* mostly as a liver remedy rather than as an alterative. *Taraxacum* is both a cholagogue and a choleretic and is therefore an especially effective liver detoxifying medicine. I use 30 drops of tincture three times daily as an alterative and liver tonic. This remedy has served me well when mixed with other plants. A favorite naturopathic liver combination includes equal parts of *Taraxacum, Chelidonium,* and *Chionanthus.* The dose is 40 drops of the tincture mixture three times daily.

Pterocaulon pucnostachyum

COMMON NAME ■ Black root

Do not confuse this plant with *Leptandra virginica*, which has also been called black root. The root is used to make medicine. When used as an alterative, *Pterocaulon* root was made into a standard tea and consumed in wineglass doses twice daily. A "wineglass dose" is the dose given in a lot of folk medicine books. I take that dose to be about 4 ounces of liquid. I have no personal experience with this plant. I have included it for historical purposes.

Parthenocissus quinquefolia

COMMON NAME ■ American ivy

The bark and twigs are used to make medicine. *Parthenocissus* is an alterative. It is also a diaphoretic, an astringent, a tonic, and a mild expectorant. Dr. Bastyr mentioned its usefulness in treating colds and persistent nagging respiratory disorders. His dose was 10 to 20 drops of tincture four times daily, or 2 tablespoons of the standard tea every 2 hours.

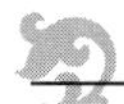

Lanthus glandulosa

COMMON NAME ■ Chinese sumac

Dr. Dirk Powell recalls Dr. Bastyr including *Lanthus* as an alterative. Dr. Powell reports that Dr. Bastyr used *Lanthus* to treat pharyngitis, tonsillitis, scarlet fever, excoriating discharges from the nose or mouth, and low-grade fevers with weakness. The dose Dr. Bastyr gave was up to 20 drops of the tincture twice daily.

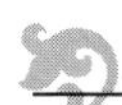

Medicago sativa

COMMON NAME ■ Alfalfa

The whole flowering plant and germinating seeds are used to make medicine. *Medicago* is a terrific example of an alterative, specifically an endocrinological alterative. *Medicago* contains a host of active constituents. The leaves and berries contain carotenoids, including lutein, and isoflavonoids, including formononetin, genistein, and daidzein. *Medicago* also contains triterpene saponins such as sojasapogenols and hederagenin; several coumarins such as lucernol, sativol, and trifoliol; and the triterpenes stigmasterol and spinasterol.[25]

During the past 22 years, I have used *Medicago* extensively as an alterative for female patients. *Medicago* contains phytoestrogens, which are useful in either hypoestrogen or hyperestrogen conditions. The phytoestrogens are weaker than estradiol and, in competing with estradiol for estrogen receptor sites, modify the effect of estradiol. At the same time, these phytoestrogens are strong enough to have an estrogen effect in hypoestrogenism and therefore help to decrease the effects of estrogen deficiency on the body. The dose given by Dr. Ed Madison is $\frac{1}{4}$ teaspoon of the solid extract daily.

Bruneton, in his textbook entitled *Pharmacognosy, Phytochemistry and Medicinal Plants*,[26] notes that blood cholesterol levels are lowered in animals given *Medicago*. He says that this cholesterol-lowering effect is clearly linked to the presence of saponins.

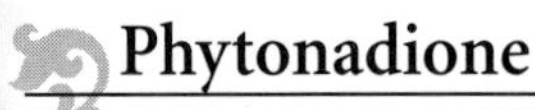

Phytonadione

COMMON NAME ■ Vitamin K

I have included vitamin K as another example of an alterative medicinal effect. Vitamin K occurs in most dark green, leafy, edible plants such as chard and kale. It helps in the blood-clotting process and so is used for patients whose blood-clotting time is too slow. On the other hand, vitamin K participates in fibrinolysis by means of its maturation of protein S and therefore participates in the dissolution of clots for patients who have excess blood clotting. The function of vitamin K in the body is to mature the calcium-managing proteins. Specifically, the function of vitamin K is to add a carboxyl group to the end-chain glutamic acid in a peptide so that the peptide chain ends with a gamma-carboxyl glutamic acid. Gamma-carboxyl glutamic acid is able to latch onto calcium to manage it. The dose that I recommend is 2 to 5 mg daily.

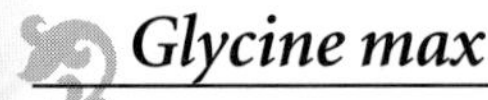

Glycine max

COMMON NAME ■ Soybean

Look for this plant also under the name *Glycine soja*. The beans are used to make medicine. Soy products may be thought of as alteratives for menopause. For women, menopause is a natural stage of life; however, some women experience more severe menopausal symptoms, including excessive osteoporosis, hot flash activity, or depression. Eating tofu, soybeans, tempe, soy cheese, or soy milk has modified these excessive symptoms in some of my patients.

Of interest lately is ipriflavone, which is an isoflavone synthesized from the soy isoflavone daidzein. An impressive amount of literature is turning up suggesting ipriflavone as a promising flavone in the prevention of osteoporosis. Ipriflavone would appear to be an osteoporotic alterative. It will be worth our attention to follow the promising use of ipriflavone in the modification and treatment of other metabolic diseases affecting bones such as Paget's disease.[27]

Soybeans are rich in the isoflavones genistein and daidzein, both of which are promising in the prevention of breast cancer. Currently, breast cancer is so widespread that anything that is promising in the prevention of this terrible disease must be of interest to the practitioner.

CHAPTER

3

ANODYNES

CHAPTER • OUTLINE

Dioscorea villosa
Citrullus colocynthis
Zingiber officinale
Mentha piperita
Monarda punctata
Filipendula ulmaria
Foeniculum vulgare
Jasminum lanceolatum
Salvia multiorrhiza
Atropa belladonna
Aconitum napellus
Piscidia erythrina
Collinsonia canadensis
Nicotiana tobacum
Gaultheria procumbens
Bryonia alba
Ananas comosus
Tanacetum parthenium

Anodynes are remedies that relieve pain. Dr. Bastyr used many of the anodynes in homeopathic doses for pain relief. He usually used 3X homeopathic potency preparations for acute pain and higher potencies for deeper pain. In addition, he applied many of these remedies as topical poultices for local pain relief.

Dioscorea villosa

COMMON NAME ■ Wild yam

The root is used for medicine. *Dioscorea* is an antispasmodic and an anodyne. For years I have used *Dioscorea* for muscle pain. *Dioscorea* is also useful in treating abdominal pain in children. Dr. Bastyr said that it could help relieve cramp-like pains in the uterus.

According to Dr. Bastyr, *Dioscorea* could be used to relieve the pain of bilious colic. It relieves spasm in the circular muscles of the gastrointestinal tract. Dr. Dirk Powell, my classmate and friend, recalls Dr. Bastyr giving the following instructions for using *Dioscorea* for gastrointestinal pain and spasm: Give 20 drops of *Dioscorea* tincture in a cup of hot water to be taken in frequent, small sips. The remedy should be stopped if there is no relief within 2 hours. In addition, Dr. Powell recalls him saying that the same dose of *Dioscorea* in cold water could be used for menstrual cramps. Dr. Bastyr also said that *Dioscorea* is beneficial for dysmenorrhea caused by ovarian neuralgia. Use 45 drops of tincture in a cup of water four times daily.

Dr. Bastyr also used *Dioscorea* for gallbladder colic. He said that if it does not work within 20 minutes, it is not the preferred remedy. The dose of the tincture is 20 drops.

My son Noah is a body builder and tells me that when he takes a particular muscle-strengthening product containing *Dioscorea*, he has better endurance and more productive workouts.

The reader is encouraged to obtain the tape of Wade Boyle speaking about eclectic medicine. In the tape, he speaks elegantly of *Dioscorea.* The tape is available from Gaia Herbs. Wade Boyle was one of the very promising young naturopathic/eclectic physicians during the 1980s. Unfortunately, he died in his 40s and the world was deprived of his penetrating insights into the use of plant medicines. I was fortunate to have had several lengthy conversations with this great naturopathic physician about plant medicines.

There is an important point that I think should be made here. The commercial interests adopted *Dioscorea* several years ago and tried to push it off as a natural answer to hormone replacement therapy. Some of the resulting products contained added, laboratory-derived hormones in the formula. I feel that the confusion that results from the misrepresentation of plants is an abuse of science-based natural medicine. The plants are extremely complicated, and trying to learn the intricacies of their interaction with our bodies and minds is an ongoing search that requires sensitivity, testing, and a strong sense of truth in medicine. *Dioscorea* does contain a steroidlike molecule, diosgenin, which may be able to be used by the body to enhance hormone activity.

Citrullus colocynthis

COMMON NAME ■ Bitter apple

The fruit pulp is used to make medicine. *CAUTION: Please note that $1\frac{1}{2}$ teaspoons of the powder will cause death by severe gastroenteritis.* Even 5 drops of tinture function as a hydrogogue cathartic. Colocynthin, the active ingredient in *C. colocynthis*, accounts for the cathartic effect.

Small doses of *colocynthis* are antispasmodic and anodynal. *Colocynthis* is useful for acute cutting pains in the abdomen. Dr. Bastyr specifically told us to use a 3X homeopathic potency for children who tend to pull up their legs into a fetal position to obtain pain relief. He said that this remedy works very rapidly. I have used *colocynthus* to treat menstrual cramps, orchalgia, ovarian cysts, and rheumatoid neuralgia. Viscera supplied by splanchnic nerves seem to respond quite well to *colocynthis.* I use *colocynthis* in the homeopathic preparation, generally in a 3X or 6X potency. When using *colocynthus* as an anodyne, Dr. Bastyr said that 5 drops of tincture can be mixed in 2 ounces of water. This mixture is taken in doses of 1 teaspoon every 1 to 3 hours.

Zingiber officinalis

COMMON NAME ■ Ginger

The root is used to make medicine. The pungent principles in *Zingiber* are zingerone, gingerols, and shogaols. Shogaol, which is an active constituent, inhibits the release of substance P, a neurotransmitter associated with carrying pain impulses. Dr. Bastyr taught that *Zingiber* helps with cramps preceding menses. In addition, I have had a number of patients who have experienced a decrease in frequency and duration of headaches, even cluster and migraine headaches, which may be the result of the blood dispersion and vascular normalization effects of *Zingiber.* A dose of 5 to 40 drops of tincture is given several times daily. The standard ginger tea is also useful. Dr. Dirk Powell recalls Dr. Bastyr clarifying the point that ginger is used for conditions in which there is pain without inflammation.

Mentha piperita

COMMON NAMES ■ Peppermint, Balm mint

Peppermint is in the mint family, *Labiatae.* Most of the same active ingredients in peppermint can be found in *Mentha arvensis.* The leaves are used to make medicine. Peppermint is an anodyne and an antispasmodic. Herbalists use a strong tea to relieve headaches. A Qi Gung master once told me to rub mint oil on the temples, in the front of the ears, and on the angle of the jaw. Then rub the oil briskly on the back of the neck paraspinally. This usually gets rid of headaches instantly.

Classically, peppermint tea has been used as an anodyne in colic and gastrodynia, and it is soothing to the stomach. A combination of spearmint, horehound, and fennel can be given for colic and cramps. Combine the herbs in equal parts and give 30 drops of tincture two to three times daily.

The oil of peppermint is useful in digestive tract spasms such as those seen in spastic colitis or tight, spastic sphincters. By relieving spasms, pain is decreased. I learned from one of Dr. Alan Gaby's lectures that enteric-coated peppermint oil capsules have been used to lessen gastric and intestinal spasms. The dose is 300 mg three times daily. Patients with bilious symptoms caused by gallstones will benefit from peppermint.

Peppermint oil capsules have recently been "discovered" to be a wonderful remedy for spasms of the intestines and sphincters. The modern dose is the same dose that Dr. Bastyr recommended 25 years ago. It is interesting how mainstream medicine often "discovers" treatments that have been used by naturopaths for decades. For example, the miracle cure of the 1950s was aspirin. As a matter of fact, the saying, "Take two aspirin and call me in the morning" is American banter. European herbalists used willow bark tea to treat fevers hundreds of years before aspirin was discovered. Aspirin is a derivative of willow bark.

Monarda punctata

COMMON NAME ■ Horsemint

The whole herb is used to make medicine. *Monarda* oil contains about 20% thymol. *Monarda* is listed as an emmenagogue and a mild stimulant. Dr. Bastyr said that, as an anodyne, it is used in a similar manner to peppermint. Herbalists use *Monarda* oil mixed with olive oil and other oils topically as a muscle rub for sore and aching muscles. Kuts-Cheraux, an MD/ND who practiced medicine in the 50s, mentions it as a "favored old domestic remedy for functional gastric upsets. Much like peppermint and spearmint, it stimulates gastric secretions and circulation, relieving gastrodynia and its associated nausea."[28] Dr. Bastyr said that the dose is 10 to 40 drops of tincture, or 2 to 6 minims of the oil, twice daily. Dirk Powell noted that Dr. Bastyr also said that *Monarda* could be used to control vomiting. For this purpose, he said to take *Monarda* on the tongue.

Filipendula ulmaria

COMMON NAMES ■ Meadowsweet, Queen of the meadow

The dried aerial parts are used to make medicine. *Filipendula* is a good anodyne in that it contains salicylaldehyde and ethyl and methyl salicylates. As such it is anodynal and antiinflammatory. In addition, *Filipendula* contains flavonol glycosides, including spiraeoside, rutin, hyperin, and a kaempferol glucoside. These bioflavonoids tend to be good antiinflammatories. *Filipendula* is also a stomachic. Dr. Bastyr said that it is used for atonic dyspepsia with heartburn and hyperacidity. It is also useful in cases of peptic ulcer because of its astringency. In my practice, I have found that *Filipendula* warms and tones the stomach, so it is no wonder that it has been described in the herbal texts as a digestive aid. It is thought to protect and soothe the mucous membranes of the entire gastrointestinal tract. The dose is about 2 mL of tincture three times daily.

In addition, *Filipendula* is an antirheumatic, astringent, and febrifuge. I use it primarily as an antirheumatic remedy at a dose of 120 drops of tincture three times daily. The cut herb can be used to make tea as well. I have found that 2 teaspoons several times daily can afford some relief from arthralgias and myalgias. Dr. Bastyr said that *Filipendula* is useful in treating acute catarrhal cystitis.

Foeniculum vulgare

COMMON NAME ■ Fennel

The roots and seeds are used to make medicine. *Foeniculus* is a carminative, an anodyne, a galactagogue, a diuretic, and a diaphoretic. Dr. Bastyr taught that *Foeniculus* could be used to help relieve abdominal cramps and flatulence. He said to use 10 to 30 drops four times daily. I suggest using 30 drops four times daily.

Dr. Bastyr said that a decoction of the seeds could be used as an effective eyewash to treat conjunctivitis and to prevent viral blepharitis. This preparation must be made and used immediately because boiling the herb sterilizes the tea. Obviously, the mixture must be allowed to cool to a comfortable temperature before application to the eye.

Dr. Bastyr said that *Foeniculus* improves memory in addition to its use as an anodyne. In my practice, I have found that *Foeniculus* does improve the mental capacity of patients.

Jasminum lanceolatum

COMMON NAME ■ Jasmine

The oil is obtained from the flowers. Eclectically, it has been listed as an anodyne. I include it because it is in my notes on anodynes from Dr. Bastyr's class, but I know nothing about its use as an anodyne. Massage practitioners have told me that they add the essential oil to massage oils as an antidepressant because the odor is uplifting and heavenly. The odor comes from the *cis*-ketone of jasmone.

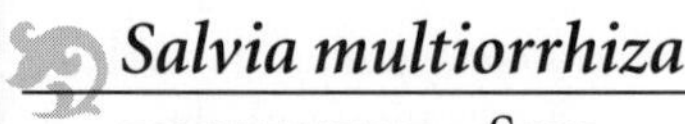

Salvia multiorrhiza

COMMON NAME ■ Sage

The whole plant is used to make medicine. I read about a Chinese doctor who practiced medicine at the Shanghai hospital. He said that *Salvia* relieves the pain of coronary thrombosis. The dose of the tincture is 20 drops four times daily. It is known that the orthoquinones, tanshinones I and VI, and cryptotanshinone prevent the complications of myocardial ischemia on the isolated rat heart. In China, tanshinone II A, solubilized by sulfonation, has undergone successful clinical trials for the treatment of angina pectoris.[26]

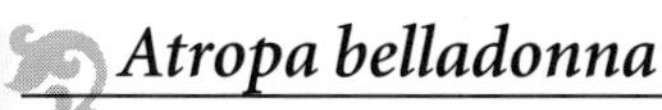

Atropa belladonna

COMMON NAME ■ Deadly nightshade

The root and leaves are used to make medicine. The main active ingredient in belladonna is atropine, which is an anticholinergic. I have used belladonna specifically for relief of headache and as a general anodyne. I use the homeopathic remedy at a potency of 3X to 6X for relief of headache. In addition, I use belladonna to relieve most types of body pains, especially pain involving the head. This includes the temporary relief of toothache. Dr. Bastyr said to take a 3X or 6X homeopathic preparation sublingually every 15 minutes until a dentist can be found. Use a tincture of the root in liniments for topical applications in cases of neuralgic pains. I start with 10 drops of the tincture twice daily to relieve intestinal cramping and pain.

Dr. Powell added several comments from Dr. Bastyr on this remedy. First, Dr. Bastyr said that belladonna is contraindicated in glaucoma. Second, he used belladonna especially for lumbago, or back pain in general, as a plaster.

Aconitum napellus

COMMON NAMES ■ Aconite, Monkshood

The root and leaves are used to make medicine. *CAUTION: Aconite is poisonous.* Therefore its usefulness is primarily limited to external applications and homeopathic remedies. Dr. Powell noted that Dr. Bastyr contraindicated *Aconitum* in asthenia. One of the active ingredients in *Aconitum* is aconitine. I have used *Aconitum* in three different ways. Homeopathically, I use a 3X potency as an anodyne and febrifuge in early-stage fevers. Dr. Bastyr almost always used *Aconitum* homeopathically. For the past 15 years, I have been using a specific tincture mixture that consistently relieves earache in about 15 seconds. The formula consists of one part *Aconitum*, three parts *Hydrastis*, and four parts *Verbascum*. I give 4 drops of this mixture in the ear up to four times daily as needed to relieve pain. I have found that this formula is extremely effective.

Aconitum is antibacterial, especially against the coccal groups. The eclectics used a dilution of *Aconitum* to treat sore throats. It was diluted 1:10 with boric acid and sprayed in the throat for acute tonsillitis. One may also use *Aconitum* in liniments for external use. In cases of neuralgia, use *Aconitum* tincture at a dose level of 1 drop three times daily.

Finally, I have used *Aconitum* for patients who are experiencing tremendous fear. The dose that I use is a 200X potency, given once and repeated over time if necessary. This will often decrease the fearfulness of the patient.

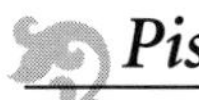

Piscidia erythrina

COMMON NAME ■ Jamaican dogwood

The root bark is used to make medicine. *Piscidia* has been used naturopathically for distress after bone fracture. The dose that I recommend is 60 drops of tincture four times daily. This remedy may be used for facial, brachial, and sciatic neuralgia. For these conditions, I use 90 drops of the tincture three to four times daily. In addition, I use *Piscidia* to relieve menstrual cramping. One of *Piscidia*'s active ingredients is piscidic acid, which may account for its analgesic effect. I give one capsule every 2 to 3 hours until the menstrual cramps are gone. This is the best plant that I know of for menstrual cramp relief. The results are consistent. Dr. Ed Madison, a classmate of mine, reintroduced me to *Piscidia* in 1986. It is from him that I learned of its excellent effects in relieving menstrual cramps.

Dr. Bastyr's uses for this remedy, as noted by Dr. Powell, include arthritis, spasmodic cough, bronchitis, dysmenorrhea, neuralgia, rigid os, and toothache. He said that in rigid os, it will not interfere with contractions. He applied it locally for toothache.

Collinsonia canadensis

COMMON NAME ■ Stone root

The whole plant is used to make medicine. The tannic acid content accounts for part of the astringent property of *Collinsonia*. *Collinsonia* is an anodyne. Dr. Bastyr used *Collinsonia* enemas for proctological problems such as proctitis, hemorrhoids, and mild fissures. He said to use 60 drops of tincture to a cup of water to make an enema solution and that this would relieve the soreness. Dr. Bastyr also talked about *Collinsonia* suppositories in his lectures. The suppositories can be used at bedtime for these same conditions.

Dr. Powell recalls a patient that Dr. Bastyr mentioned who was an opera singer with a sore throat and voice problems. Dr. Bastyr prescribed *Collinsonia* in an atomizer for this patient to spray in the throat. This treatment was successful for this patient.

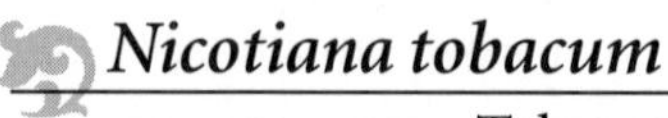

Nicotiana tobacum

COMMON NAME ■ Tobacco

The leaves are used to make medicine. Dr. Bastyr said that chewed *Nicotiana* leaves could be put on wasp and bee stings to relieve the stinging pain. In addition, he said that the powdered leaves could be mixed with *Lobelia* and lanolin to make a paste. He said to apply this paste to painful thrombic hemorrhoids. Interestingly, *Nicotiana* and *Lobelia* contain alkaloids that have similar actions on the body. Because of this similarity, *Lobelia* can be taken to help break a patient of the tobacco habit. For this purpose, I prescribe 5 drops of tincture three times daily.

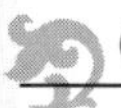

Gaultheria procumbens

COMMON NAME ■ Wintergreen

The dried leaves are used to make medicine. *Gaultheria* contains salicylates, which account for the anodynal and febrifuge effects of the plant. The eclectics applied *Gaultheria* oil to muscles as a topical application for myalgia. For toothache, apply *Gaultheria* topically against the gum. I use clove for this purpose because I have found it to be a better tooth and gum anodyne. For headache and fever, Dr. Bastyr said to drink a standard infusion of *Gaultheria* tea at a dose of 1 cup per hour until relief is attained.

Bryonia alba

COMMON NAME ■ White bryony

CAUTION: This is a toxic plant. Even five or six berries of this plant will cause abdominal distress in children. The stomach should be pumped and activated charcoal given. The root is used to make medicine. *Bryonia* contains cucurbitacin glycosides, including bryoside and cucurbitacin.[26] Use *Bryonia* as an anodyne in rheumatic pains and inflammations of the serous membranes, such as those seen in the pleura, pericardium, and fascia. Pneumonitis and synovitis respond to *Bryonia* as well. Like thousands of other practitioners, I have used it to treat any "itis" with characteristic pain.

I usually use *Bryonia* homeopathically, as taught by Dr. Bastyr. The homeopathic dose is a 3X or 6X potency given sublingually three times daily for rheumatic pains. Higher potencies of *Bryonia*, such as 12X, 30X, or 200X, can be used for more chronic, deeper pain. Dr. Bastyr said that several drops of tincture could be taken in a glass of hot water twice daily for rheumatic aches and pains in adults.

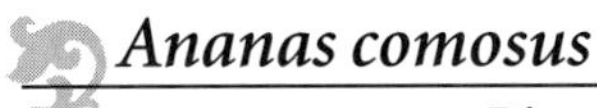

Ananas comosus

COMMON NAME ■ Pineapple

Bromelain is extracted from the pineapple plant. Bromelain blocks kinin formation, which decreases inflammation and therefore the pain resulting from injury. The dose that I prescribe is 1000 mg of bromelain twice daily. I have used bromelain on wounds as a debriding agent, usually mixed with powdered goldenseal. This combination both cleans and disinfects suppurative wounds.

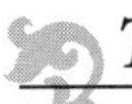

Tanacetum chrysanthemum parthenium

COMMON NAME ■ Feverfew

CAUTION: Do not use this remedy during pregnancy because it causes uterine contractions. The leaves are used for medicine. The active ingredient is a sesquiterpene lactone, parthenolide. *Tanacetum* is used to relieve painful menstrual periods. The tincture dose that I prescribe for this purpose is 30 drops twice daily. I use *Tanacetum* to treat migraine headaches. I prescribe 600 mg in capsule form at the first sign of a migraine. This dose is repeated every hour up to three doses.

CHAPTER

4

ANTHELMINTHICS

CHAPTER · OUTLINE

Artemesia cina
Artemesia annua
Spigelia marilandica
Dryopteris filix-mas
Convolvulus scammonia
Mallotus phillipensis
Berayera anthelmenthica
Punica granatum
Tanacetum vulgare
Althaea officinalis
Sempervivum tectorum
Quassia excelsa
Inula helenium
Opuntia species
Chenopodium ambrosioides
Ananas comosus
Juglans cinerea
Matricaria matricarioides

Anthelminthics are agents that are destructive to worms. Dr. Bastyr presented 16 such agents from the botanical world. I have had some clinical experience using most of them. Killing parasites and worms can be tricky business; diagnosing them can be even trickier. You may have to test and retest a number of times. Worms and their eggs and yeast organisms can usually be diagnosed in stool samples. However, flagellate and nonflagellate monocellular organisms are difficult to diagnose this way. I consider the presence of persistent diarrhea and/or intestinal discomfort after normal stool findings from laboratory tests to be red flags that these hard-to-diagnose monocellular organisms may be present. Scrapings of mucus from mucous membranes of the intestinal wall may have to be taken and sent to a laboratory familiar with such organisms to obtain an accurate diagnosis. If this is impossible, remember that *Artemesia annua* kills most of these organisms.

With all worm problems, prevention must always take precedence. Cleanliness is important. Patients should be reminded to wash their hands after handling vegetables, especially vegetables picked from the garden. When hiking, where the hands come in contact with the ground or contact is made with ground water, the hands should be washed before touching food. Dr. Bastyr commented that when children come in from play, a habit should be made of having the child wash his or her hands immediately. Most children handle food with their hands as much as with utensils. One of Dr. Bastyr's favorite cliches was "Cleanliness is next to Godliness."

Artemesia cina

COMMON NAME ■ Wormseed

The flowers are used to make medicine. *CAUTION: My classmate Dr. Powell said that Dr. Bastyr contraindicated* Artemesia *in pyrexia, or elevation of the body temperature. Artemesia* is an anthelminthic and a gastrointestinal bitter. Naturopaths and herbalists use *Artemesia* to treat *Ascaris lumbricoides.* Dr. Bastyr said to use it in small, persistent doses of $\frac{1}{2}$ to 1 grain. The active constituent is santonin, which is irritating to mucous membranes and can also result in headaches, dizziness, and visual disturbances. The remedy is therefore given for no more than a week at a time. The patient can be fasted on pineapple and pumpkin seeds and of course water. After a 1-week rest, repeat the *Artemesia* for 5 more days to kill newly hatched worms. Dr. Bastyr used the homeopathic remedy called *cina* 3X. Three pellets were given three times daily to kill worms. This was repeated for 1 week.

Artemesia annua

COMMON NAME ■ Sweet wormwood

This is an effective killer of monocellular flagellated and nonflagellated parasites. The dose that I give is 500 mg of the powdered herb twice daily for 10 days. This therapy is remarkably effective as gauged by the elimination of abdominal symptoms, decreased bloating, a feeling of well-being, and a return to normal stool patterns.

I prefer *Artemesia annua* to all other species of *Artemesia.* Of interest is the sesquiterpene lactone, artemisinin, an ingredient in *Artemesia annua* known as quinghao, which has been included in traditional Chinese medicine as an antimalarial for more than 2000 years.

Spigelia marilandica

COMMON NAME ■ Pinkroot

The dried rhizomes and roots are used to make medicine. *CAUTION: The seeds are toxic.* In fact, they were used by the Kuna Indians to execute criminals.[29] *Spigelia* contains isoquinoline, choline, benzoylcholine, 3,3-dimethylacryloylcholine, and actinidine.[30] Dr. Bastyr said to give children with intestinal worms 15 to 30 drops of tincture in the morning and at bedtime. *Ascaris lumbricoides* worms are particularly susceptible to treatment with *Spigelia.* He said to wait a few days and then give a laxative such as a large dose of vitamin C. I have used *Spigelia* often in the treatment of intestinal parasites. I mix *Spigelia* and *Artemesia* tinctures in equal proportions and give a dose of 30 drops of the mixture three times daily for 3 days. This is followed by a 3-day rest. The remedy is then repeated at the same dose for an additional 3 days.

In addition to its action as an anthelminthic, *Spigelia* is also useful as a heart remedy for functional palpitations. The dose recommended by Dr. Bastyr was 1 dram of tincture in a cup of water. He said to then give 15 drops every half-hour until the palpitations stop.

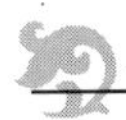

Dryopteris filix-mas

COMMON NAME ■ Male fern

The rhizomes are used for medicine. One may also use *Dryopteris marginalis. Dryopteris* is a taeniafuge and an anthelminthic. The active taenicidal ingredients are derivatives of the phenolic compound phloroglucinol. For tapeworm expulsion, Dr. Bastyr taught us to use 1 to 2 drams of tincture on an empty stomach in the morning. This was to be followed with a laxative that evening and the following morning if necessary. He said that the patient should fast on pineapple, flax seeds, and pumpkin seeds for 2 days, making sure to chew the seeds and nuts thoroughly and drink plenty of water.

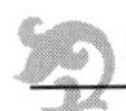

Convolvulus scammonia

COMMON NAMES ■ Bindweed, Scammony

Convolvulus jalapa is also used. The root is used to make medicine. This remedy is a vermifuge and a cathartic. It contains ergot alkaloids and ether-soluble resin glycosides called scammonic acid A. Dose the tincture of *Convolvulus* at 30 to 60 drops. This will cause purgation or emptying of the bowel. Some of the eclectics felt this was a good purge for rheumatism.[31] Use 3 to 12 grains of the powder for this purpose. Because this herb is a drastic cathartic, I give 500 mg of magnesium to decrease cramping. Three hundred milligrams of powdered *Piscidia* may also be given with *Convolvulus* to help decrease abdominal cramping. I have little personal experience with *Convolvulus.*

Mallotus phillipensis

COMMON NAMES ■ Spoonwood, Kamala

The glands and hairs covering the fruit are used to make medicine. *Mallotus* contains the anthelminthic phloroglucinol derivatives, rottlerin and isorottlerin. It is a vermifuge that is effective against tapeworms. Dr. Bastyr said that the dose of tincture is 30 to 60 drops twice daily for 3 days.

Berayera anthelmenthica

COMMON NAME ■ Kousso

The herb and unripe fruit are used to make medicine. In the treatment of tapeworms, Dr. Bastyr said that the patient should fast for 24 hours before taking *Berayera.* This is presumably done so that food will not inactivate the medicinal constituents. He said to have the patient take 5 drams of the macerated flowers in a cup of water and drink the solution in two or three doses. Drink extra water. *Berayera* is not a laxative; therefore, the administration of a laxative afterward may be necessary. I recommend 5000 mg of vitamin C every 2 hours to ensure cleansing of the bowel. Begin this laxative the day after the *Berayera* is given.

Punica granatum

COMMON NAME ■ Pomegranate

The dried root bark is used to make medicine. This plant is astringent and cathartic. Dr. Bastyr said that *Punica* was excellent for the expulsion of cestodes, or tapeworms. One of the active ingredients specific for this purpose is pelletierine, which is a piperidine alkaloid. Another constituent is the homotropane, pseudopelletierine.

Dr. Bastyr said to make a decoction by adding 2 ounces of the fresh root bark to 1 quart of water. Let it stand for 24 hours, then boil it down to

1 pint. He said to have the patient fast all day while taking this decoction in doses of 2 tablespoons every hour. This process should be repeated after several days.

Historically, besides using the bark as medicine, it was also was used in tanning and dyeing. The pomegranate seeds are demulcent.

Tanacetum vulgare

COMMON NAMES ■ Tansy, Bitter buttons, Bachelor's buttons

The dried leaves and flowering top are used to make medicine. This plant is antifungal and anthelminthic. *Tanacetum* contains a number of sesquiterpene lactones, which may account for its anthelminthic properties. Large doses may be used over a shorter period as a vermifuge against roundworms and pinworms. The original dose given by Dr. Bastyr was 1 ounce of the leaves and flowering tops infused in a pint of water and taken in cupful doses night and morning by the fasting patient. As an anthelminthic, the tincture of *Tanacetum* can also be given. The dose is 25 drops three times daily for 3 days. I mix *Tanacetum* with *Artemesia annua* as a general deparasitizing formula. This combination kills most worms and many of the flagellated and nonflagellated monocellular parasites. I mix *Tanacetum* and *Artemesia* in equal portions and prescribe the resulting tincture in doses of 60 drops three times daily for 3 to 5 days.

Althaea officinalis

COMMON NAME ■ Marshmallow

Do not confuse this with *Althaea rosea*, or common hollyhock. The whole plant is used to make medicine. *Althaea officinalis* is both demulcent and a vermifuge. I use it for its demulcent effects when using other stronger vermifuges. Dr. Bastyr said to use a handful of leaves per half-pint of water. Take 3 tablespoons of the resulting tea four times daily.

Sempervivum tectorum

COMMON NAME ■ Houseleek

The fresh leaves are used medicinally. This plant is an astringent, a vulnerary, and a vermifuge. As a vermifuge, Dr. Bastyr said to use 40 drops of *Sempervivum* tincture four times daily. Fast for 3 days while taking the tincture. According to herbalists, *Sempervivum* has historically been used externally for rashes, erysipelas, warts, stings, and burns. However, I prefer tea tree ointment for burns because it is far more effective.

Quassia excelsa

COMMON NAME ■ Bitterwood

Some sources may call this plant *Quassia amara* and *Picrasma excelsa.* Use an infusion of the wood and bark. *Quassia* contains two terpenoid compounds, quassin and neoquassin, which account for part of the anthelminthic properties. The plant also contains scopoletin, which may conceivably affect the nervous system of parasites.

Eclectic and herbal writings have identified *Quassia* as effective against *Ascaris lumbricoides*, pinworms, and threadworms. As an anthelminthic, Dr. Bastyr said that 10 to 30 drops of tincture could be given three times daily for 2 days. *Quassia* has a laxative effect. He said that a strong infusion of *Quassia* could be used as an enema to treat pinworms. He also taught us that a garlic oil capsule could be inserted rectally to help kill pinworms. Our concern as students was that this would be too harsh. Surprisingly, he said that it wasn't.

Inula helenium

COMMON NAME ■ Elecampane

The root is used to make medicine. *Inula* contains the lactone alantolactone, which is classified as an anthelminthic against nematodes. *Inula* is less toxic than santonin and is a faster anthelminthic. Dr. Bastyr said that ascaris were killed in 20 hours by using a 0.05% solution of *Inula*, whereas a 0.1% solution of santonin took 48 hours. To make a decoction, he said to take 1 ounce of the root per pint of boiling water and let it steep for 20 minutes. Strain the resulting mixture and take 4 fluid ounces three times daily.

Opuntia species

COMMON NAME ■ Prickly pear

The flowers are used to make medicine. *Opuntia* is specific for amebic dysentery. Dr. Bastyr said to use a handful of flowers to a pint of water. He told us to boil this mixture and drink 1 cup in the morning and evening. I recommend using *Opuntia* together with *Artemesia annua.* Take the *Opuntia* tea together with 500-mg capsules of powdered *Artemesia* twice daily. Continue this combined therapy for 7 days.

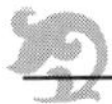

Chenopodium ambrosioides

COMMON NAME ■ Wormseed

The seeds are used medicinally. Either the oil or an infusion of the seed may be used. *CAUTION: This remedy is toxic and should be used with care.* Dr. Bastyr recommended its use only for patients more than 6 years of age. For these patients, he recommended 3 to 5 drops of the oil three times daily for 2 days. He said that they could also take a third of a teaspoonful of seeds mixed with honey twice daily. He said to follow this with a good laxative. Wait 5 days before repeating the treatment if further treatment is warranted. Kuts-Cheraux has mentioned its effectiveness against *Ancylostoma,*[28] which is a genus of nematode parasites. These parasites are commonly called hookworm.

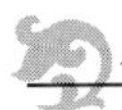

Ananas comosus

COMMON NAME ■ Pineapple

Bromelain from pineapple and papain from papayas are taken internally for *Trichuris trichiura,* or whipworms, ascaris, tapeworms, and pinworms. Bromelain is obtained from the stems of pineapple. I give the patient two 200-mg capsules of bromelain four times daily while the patient is fasting on water and pumpkin seeds. I continue this dose for 3 days. I have found that this often works for hard-to-treat parasites. This particular program can be used in conjunction with other vermifuges.

During his lecture on pineapple, Dr. Bastyr also happened to mention papaya. He said that eating fresh papaya yields no useful enzymatic activity. Neither does chewing the tasty candy-like papaya tablets seen in health food stores. However, he said that papain, which is obtained from the latex of the rind of unripe green papayas, is useful for severe constipation and obstipation.

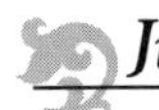

Juglans cinerea

COMMON NAMES ■ White walnut, Butternut

The inner bark is used for medicine. *Juglans* has a folk history of use for worms. Four or five pills of *Juglans* were taken at night for this purpose.[32] Other writers, such as Hulda Clark, speak of the anthelminthic properties of walnut, in particular the "green" walnut extract. Walnut turns dark as soon as it is worked, so I'm not sure what she actually meant by green walnut.

I have very infrequently used walnut in a concoction for worms, usually mixed with *Spigelia* or *Artemesia*. If anyone out there really has some experience with walnut of any kind for the treatment of worms or parasites and a case or two to share, please contact me.

Matricaria matricarioides

COMMON NAMES ■ Pineapple weed, Pineapple mayweed

Look for this plant also under the names *M. discoidea* and *M. suaveolens*. The little pineapple-like tops are used to make medicine. Rudolf Weiss, in his book *Herbal Medicine*,[13] says that this plant is an anthelminthic. He says that it is a good herb to treat threadworms, roundworms, and even whipworms, or *Trichuris trichiura*. When I think of pineapple weed, I think of a brave little plant growing up through the cracks in a field of inhospitable cement. It wants to be with us urban dwellers. As an adaptogen, 20 drops of the tincture is used twice daily.

CHAPTER

5

ANTIBACTERIALS/ ANTIMICROBIALS

CHAPTER • OUTLINE

Aconitum napellus
Valeriana officinalis
Scutellaria lateriflora
Paeonia moutan
Anthemis nobilis
Cinchona ledgeriana
Eucalyptus globulus
Allium sativum
Leptotania dissectum
Eupatorium perfoliatum
Inula helenium
Echinacea angustifolia
Berberis aquifolium
Arctium lappa
Trifolium pratense
Arctostaphylos uva-ursi
Tanacetum vulgare
Plantago lanceolata
Hydrastis canadensis
Ligusticum porteri
Artemisia tridentata
Arbutus menziesii
Vaccinium macrocarpon
Peumus boldus

Antibacterials and antimicrobials are plants that kill or inhibit the growth of microorganisms. This section covers bacterial, rickettsial, and fungal organisms. The chapter originally covered primarily antibacterials, which remains the focus of this section; however, a number of plants that inhibit or kill yeast and other fungal organisms have been added. This section promises to grow and will eventually be divided into a number of sections specific to the various families of organisms affected.

Aconitum napellus

COMMON NAMES ■ Aconite, Monkshood

The root and leaves are used to make medicine. *CAUTION: Aconite is poisonous, therefore its usefulness is primarily limited to external applications and homeopathic remedies.* Dr. Dirk Powell noted that Dr. Bastyr contraindicated *Aconitum* in asthenia. The active constituent in *Aconitum* is aconitine, which is a diterpenoid alkaloid. *Aconitum* has antibacterial activity against intestinal and coccal groups. The tincture may be used topically. Aconite is an important component of the ear remedy that I compounded years ago. The tincture remedy consists of one part *Aconitum*, four parts *Hydrastis*, and four parts *Verbascum*. These drops are put in the ear for earache and work within seconds. Dr. Bastyr said that the diluted tinctures may be used to spray the throat or used in the ears as mentioned above, but the total internal dose of aconite should never exceed 5 drops of tincture per day. In reports of accidental aconite poisoning, the alkaloid aconitine usually caused death by means of respiratory paralysis, although death can result from cardiac arrest in diastole. Dr. Bastyr said to use aconite homeopathically for patients who are experiencing fearfulness. I have found this to be very useful with my patients. Very fearful patients often respond well to 200X potency.

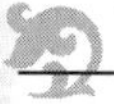

Valeriana officinalis

COMMON NAME ■ Valerian

The root is used medicinally. The constituents, valerine and chatinine, form crystalline salts that are effective against gram-positive bacteria. Valerian also contains several epoxy-iridoid esters called valepotriates. As an antibacterial, I recommend 20 drops of the fluid extract four times daily. This is slightly more than Dr. Bastyr's original dose of 15 drops four times daily.

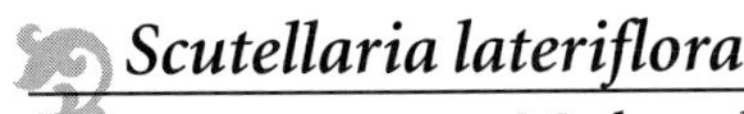

Scutellaria lateriflora

COMMON NAMES ■ Madweed, Skullcap

Use the whole plant to make medicine. The constituent wogonin, a flavone, inhibits *Vibrio cholerae.* The dose that I recommend is 30 drops of the tincture four times daily.

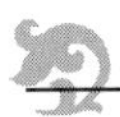

Paeonia moutan

COMMON NAME ■ Peony

Paeonia lactiflora may also be used. The fresh underground parts and the dried ripe seeds are used to make medicine. Peony completely inhibits the growth of *Escherichea coli* and *Bacillus subtilis* at a dilution of 1:1500, and inhibits the growth of *Staphylococcus aureus* and *Streptococcus faecalis* at a 1:2000 dilution in vitro. I cannot remember a reference for this, but I do remember being impressed by the information. There has been little research done on peony, but given the recent concern over *Staphylococcus,* it may be worth revisiting this remarkable plant. I was given 50-year-old peony roots that had to be removed from a housing project. I still have the tincture that I made from them. Occasionally, I mix this tincture with *Hydrastis* for local application to festering wounds.

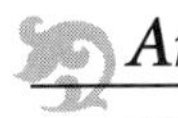

Anthemis nobilis

COMMON NAME ■ Roman chamomile

Chamomile is a member of the sunflower family, *Compositae.* The flower heads are used to make medicine. Chamomile is often thought of solely as a calmative, but it is also an effective antibacterial. It is inhibitory to gram-positive and gram-negative bacteria. It also inhibits the erythrocyte lysotoxin effects produced by *Staphylococcus.*

I use a chamomile salve for skin infections. I usually mix it with tea tree ointment. For internal infections such as enteric infections, I prescribe 25 drops *Anthemis* fluid extract four times daily.

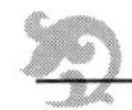

Cinchona ledgeriana

COMMON NAME ■ Peruvian bark

The parenchyma cells of the middle layers of the bark are used to produce medicine. *Cinchona* contains over 20 closely related alkaloids,[33] chief among these are quinine, quinidine, and cinchonidine. A 1:20,000 dilution in water can kill *Plasmodium* species, which is the organism that causes malaria. Dr. Bastyr said that a dose of 5 to 20 drops of tincture is used. Given the resistance of *Plasmodium* species to quinine, this may no longer be accurate. Dr. Bastyr said that the original dose of *Cinchona* was 1 gram. In class, we asked Dr. Bastyr if he had treated any malaria patients. He said that we might be surprised to find some patients walk through our doors who have contracted malaria on vacation. He had treated a number of such cases.

Cinchona is a cardiac depressant. As an aside, I recall Dr. Bastyr saying that a homeopathic dose can be used to treat tinnitus.

Eucalyptus globulus

COMMON NAME ■ Eucalyptus

The leaves and inner bark are used to make medicine. The active ingredient in eucalyptus oil is cineole, or eucalyptol. Eucalyptus is antistaphylococcal. An aqueous extract is useful against many gram-positive and gram-negative bacteria. Historically, 1 to 5 drops of the oil of eucalyptus was given twice daily for 3 days.

Eucalyptus may be added to vaporizers for the treatment of asthma or as a general air disinfectant during flu epidemics. Eucalyptus leaf wax contains several interesting antioxidants called beta-diketones. One is *n*-tritriacontan-16,18-dione and the other is 4-hydroxytritriacontan-16,18-dione.[34] Both of these are more potent antioxidants than curcumin. Of some interest is that Osawa et al. reported that *n*-tritriacontan-16,18-dione strongly inhibited hepatic and pancreatic carcinogenesis.[35]

Allium sativum

COMMON NAME ■ Garlic

The whole bulb is used for medicine. In low concentrations, garlic is bacteriostatic against *Mycobacterium tuberculosis* and in higher concentrations, it is bacteriocidal. Two antibacterial ingredients in garlic are allicin and alliin. Albert Schweitzer used garlic primarily to treat tuberculosis in Africa. He also used garlic to treat many other conditions as well, especially infections. Garlic has been used to treat typhus and *Escherichia coli* infections. It is effective against many gram-positive and gram-negative bacteria. Garlic oil may be put in the ear for viral or bacterial otitis media. In my practice I have used garlic frequently to treat a wide variety of infections. Two capsules of garlic four times daily is a great adjunctive treatment along with other antibacterials. I have found garlic to be antibacterial and antiviral. It should not be missed as an excellent remedy for colds and flu. Dr. Bastyr told us to add garlic to our diets.

Leptotania dissectum

COMMON NAME ■ Lomatium

The resin from the root is used to make medicine. This plant is effective against gram-positive bacteria at a 1:100,000 dilution. It is effective against gram-negative bacteria at a 1:10,000 dilution. It is effective against *Shigella, Salmonella typhi, Pseudomonas, E. coli, Staphylococcus aureus, Streptococcus pyogenes,* and *Streptococcus viridens.* It is partially effective against *Neisseria gonorrhoeae* and *Mycobacterium tuberculosis.* I use this plant in bacterial or viral respiratory pathology. I add lomatium to my upper respiratory formula. Dr. Dirk Powell recalls Dr. Bastyr using lomatium with *Eupatorium perfoliatum* to treat flu. He used 10 drops of tincture every 2 hours.

Lomatium is also a good urinary tract medicine. For urinary tract infections, add one part of lomatium tincture to four parts of *Chimaphila* or other indicated botanicals. I use a dose of 90 drops of the tincture formula four times daily. Max Barlow, author of *From the Shepherd's Purse,* taught me to appreciate lomatium.[36] He has thoroughly researched this plant and should be consulted for further information.

Dr. Bastyr used to wildcraft lomatium. He would obtain it from his favorite wild patch on the eastern slopes of the Cascade Mountains. He kept the whereabouts secret; however, based on a couple of clues, Dr. Dirk Powell and I discovered the location of his patch. It is actually quite a big patch. In his honor we will keep its location secret. Dr. Powell recalls that Dr. Bastyr brought a lomatium root to class to teach us how to make tinctures. We used 95% alcohol.

Eupatorium perfoliatum

COMMON NAME ■ Boneset

The top of the plant and leaves are used to make medicine. In 1951, Bishop and MacDonald presented a paper in the *Canadian Journal of Botany* showing *Eupatorium's* antibacterial action against *Staphylococcus aureus* and *Escherichia coli.* I have used *Eupatorium* against urethritis and cystitis following infection by *E. coli.* These urinary tract infections occur frequently. I prescribe 30 drops of tincture in a glass of water four times daily for this purpose. In naturopathic medicine, *Eupatorium* is usually combined with other botanicals to treat infections.

Eupatorium contains the bioflavonoid eupatorin. This molecule is both a hydroxyflavone and a methoxyflavone. Hydroxybioflavonoids are usually antioxidants and tend to decrease inflammatory reactions. Methoxybioflavonoids tend to stimulate hepatic detoxification systems.

Inula helenium

COMMON NAME ■ Elecampane

The rhizome is used to make medicine. *Inula* is an antiseptic and bactericidal. My good friend and premier herbalist David Hoffmann mentions in his books the use of *Inula* for tuberculosis, because it kills the tubercle bacillus. I have only treated half a dozen cases of tuberculosis over my 22 years of practice and therefore am no expert in this area. However, I have used *Inula* in all of the tuberculosis patients whom I have seen within the last 10 years.

Inula's main use is as an antitussive in bronchitis. As an antibacterial, I recommend 60 drops of tincture three times daily. I use *Inula* in croupy coughs in children. I mix it with equal parts of *Glycerrhiza* and *Grindelia.* I prescribe 30 drops of the tincture mixture three times daily. Historically, *Inula* has been used successfully as a respiratory remedy for its expectorant and tonic qualities.

When Dr. Bastyr talked about elecampane, he highlighted its use as a respiratory remedy and an immune stimulant. *Inula*'s high inulin content accounts for its ability to increase complement. A stimulation of T-cell activity is also seen. *Inula* is also used to treat rashes of the labia and inner thigh.

Inula contains two sesquiterpene lactones, alantolactone and isolantolactone, which are antifungals. At concentrations of 10 micrograms per milliliter they inhibit the growth of *Microsporum cookei, Trichophyton menyanthes*, and *Trichophyton roseum.*[26]

Echinacea angustifolia

COMMON NAME ■ Purple coneflower

Echinacea is a member of the sunflower family, *Compositae.* The root is used to make medicine. An intravenous injection of *Echinacea* increases properdin and enhances phagocytosis in inflammatory reactions. Properdin is a highly basic serum protein believed to be a factor in endogenous immunity against bacterial and viral diseases. Additional immunity is afforded by *Echinacea's* caffeic acid content, which exerts bacteriostatic and bactericidal actions.

Echinacea stimulates fibroblasts to form a tissue barrier against local bacterial proliferation. It slows the spread of bacteria by decreasing hyaluronidase, which is an enzyme secreted by the bacteria to digest the host's connective tissue.

Echinacea can be used locally or systemically. It has been used in traditional herbal medicine for septicemia, blood poisoning, enteritis, stomatitis, and ulcers. Dr. Bastyr said that it has a good historical track record against snake and insect bites and is one of our best enteric antiseptics. For salpingitis, I use 90 drops of the tincture five times daily or $\frac{1}{2}$ teaspoon of the powder six times daily.

For suspected flu and colds, Dr. Bastyr used 30 drops of tincture hourly until the patient was asymptomatic. I use as much as 60 drops hourly, as I have found this larger dose to be more effective. Dr. Bastyr taught us that one of the fundamental combinations for colds and flu was four parts *Echinacea*, four parts *Hydrastis*, and one part *Phytolacca*. On a number of occasions when I had an opportunity to talk to him outside of class, he also spoke highly of adding *Baptisia* to this formula.

Berberis aquifolium

COMMON NAME ■ Oregon grape root

Also look for this plant under the name *Mahonia aquifolium*. The root is used to obtain medicine. *Berberis* is an antibacterial that acts similarly to *Hydrastis*. Dr. Bastyr said that *Hydrastis* and *Berberis* were in function basically the same, although he said that *Hydrastis* was slightly stronger as an antibacterial. Other plants that are similar in action because of their berberine content are *Mahonia repens, Mahonia bealei*, and *Mahonia fremontii*. Besides containing berberine and hydrastine, *Berberis* contains other isoquinoline alkaloids, including berbamine and oxycanthine.

Berberis works well in gastrointestinal and genitourinary tract infections. I also include *Berberis* in my upper respiratory formula. The dose that I recommend for these infections is 90 drops of the tincture three times daily. *Hydrastis* is stronger, but it is also much more expensive. *Berberis* is bitter and tends to tonify the system, especially the digestive system.

Arctium lappa

COMMON NAME ■ Burdock root

The root is used to make medicine. Dr. Bastyr commented on the fact that *Arctium* contains inulin, which is immunostimulatory. It also contains lignans, polyacetylenes, and various organic acids such as acetic and isovaleric acids. These organic acids stimulate the immune and detoxifying systems of the body. *Arctium* functions as an antimicrobial by stimulating the immune system. It is useful against *Staphylococcal* pathogens. One can use large doses of either *Arctium* powder or the tincture. I have more experience with the tincture and fluid extract. I recommend a dose of 30 drops of fluid extract, or 120 drops of tincture, four times daily. This plant is emollient to the tissues of the gastrointestinal tract.

Trifolium pratense

COMMON NAME ■ Red clover

The flower heads are used to make medicine. *Trifolium* has antibacterial activity against gram-positive bacteria, *Staphylococcus aureus, Micrococcus luteus,*

Micrococcus lysodeikticus, and *Bacillus megaterium*. Herbalists have used *Trifolium* for hundreds of years as a skin remedy to treat conditions such as eczema and psoriasis. Its effectiveness as a skin remedy results in part from its antibacterial properties, and in part from its hormonelike effects. I prescribe 40 drops of tincture six times daily. I like to mix *Trifolium* with *Berberis aquifolium* for eczematous skin problems. I mix two parts *Trifolium* with one part *Berberis* and give 40 drops of the tincture mixture three times daily in a large glass of water.

Trifolium contains coumarins such as coumasterol and coumarin, which are anticoagulants. In addition, it contains a number of the endocrine active flavonoids found in soy and other phytoestrogenic plants. Two such active ingredients are the isoflavones daidzein and genistein.

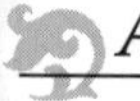

Arctostaphylos uva-ursi

COMMON NAMES ■ Bearberry, Upland cranberry

In Russia, researchers have demonstrated that the arbutin in *A. uva-ursi* is active against *Candida albicans*, *Staphylococcus aureus*, and *Escherichia coli*. *Uva-ursi* also contains the related compound methylarbutin, which is similar in action to arbutin. I suggest 60 drops of *uva-ursi* tincture five times daily, or $\frac{1}{4}$ teaspoon of the solid extract three times daily. I mix equal parts of *uva-ursi*, *Chimaphila*, and *Usnea* for the treatment of urinary tract infections. The dose I prescribe is 90 drops of the tincture formula four times daily in a cup of hot water. *Uva-ursi* exerts its urinary antiseptic effects as it is excreted.

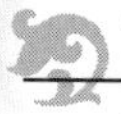

Tanacetum vulgare

COMMON NAMES ■ Tansy, Bitter buttons, Bachelor's buttons

Tansy is a member of the sunflower family, *Compositae*. The flowering herb is used for medicine. Tansy contains a number of sesquiterpene lactones such as parthenolide, artemorin, and matricarin. It also contains volatile oils and flavonoids, notably quercetin and apigenin. Tansy inhibits gram-positive bacteria and also kills protozoa. As an antibacterial, Dr. Bastyr used a dose of 10 drops of tincture three times daily. Tansy leaves may be stripped from the plant and put in a bag to keep away flying insects.[36]

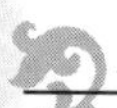

Plantago lanceolata

COMMON NAME ■ Plantain

The leaves are used for medicine. An ethanol extract of plantain is effective against *Staphylococcus aureus*, *Streptococcus pyogenes*, and *Bacillus subtilis*.

Plantain contains the flavonoids apigenin and scutellarin. It also contains iridoids and various plant acids including benzoic, fumaric, and oleanolic acids.

To alleviate sore throat and red, irritated mucous membranes, infuse a tablespoon of the dried herb in a cup of hot water for 15 minutes. Sip the tea over a half-hour period. The tincture dose is 60 drops four times daily. Dr. Bastyr used to add plantain to cough remedies, as do many other herbalists to whom I have spoken. It is excellent, and its mucilaginous content makes it soothing to the mucous membranes.

Dr. Bastyr talked about making a poultice of plantain to apply to wounds. Herbalists frequently talk about using plantain in the same way. I combine it with chickweed for this purpose.

Hydrastis canadensis

COMMON NAMES ■ Goldenseal root, Yellow root

Hydrastis is a member of the buttercup family, *Ranunculaceae.* The active constituents in *Hydrastis* are hydrastine and berberine. Additionally, hydrastinine is present as an oxidation product of hydrastine. The berberine alkaloids in *Hydrastis* are antibiotic. These alkaloids are active against syphilis (*Treponema pallidum*), gonorrhea (*Neisseria gonorrhoeae*), yeast (*Candida albicans*), pneumonia (*Diplococcus pneumoniae*), diarrhea-causing organisms (*Entamoeba histolytica, Vibrio cholerae,* and *Salmonella typhi*), chlamydia, and *Pseudomonas* species. This famous plant contains antimicrobial alkaloids that are effective against many staphylococcal and streptococcal organisms as well. *Hydrastis* has also been used historically by eclectic physicians against *Neisseria* and *Treponema.*

The list actually goes on and on depending on the source of information. For example, *Hydrastis* kills group A streptococci very effectively. This is partly the result of the ability of berberine to cause streptococci to lose lipoteichoic acid, which is an important substance responsible for the adhesion of streptococci to host tissues.[38] Even when treating streptococcal infections with antibiotics, I include *Hydrastis* in the treatment program specifically for this reason.

I have used powdered *Hydrastis* applied topically for thrush in children. Its active constituent, berberine, which is considered an antibiotic, also kills yeast. Most antibiotics cause yeast infections. For bacterial sepsis, I prescribe 60 drops of tincture internally four times daily. Capsules may be used. The dose is 2 capsules three times daily. The tincture of *Hydrastis* is used in the ears for otitis media. *Hydrastis* tincture is also used locally for throat infections. I have found that a dose of 10 drops held briefly in the throat eight times daily is usually effective. For trachoma, use a 0.2% solution of berberine. This kills *Chlamydia trachomatis.*[39]

In my practice, I give 1 capsule of powered *Hydrastis* three times daily at the first sign of colds or flu. By the way, I don't remember Dr. Bastyr talking about flu shots. I don't believe flu shots were given at that time, thus increasing our reliance on *Hydrastis* and other antimicrobials. I only suggest flu shots for people whose immune systems are compromised or for the elderly. This is because I believe that normal, healthy people are better off going through the process of fighting these diseases with their own immune systems. This improves the immune system's ability to respond to organisms. Furthermore, I believe that during the febrile stage of acute disease, cancer cells and other toxins are destroyed.

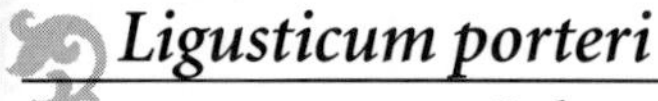

Ligusticum porteri

COMMON NAME ■ Osha

The root is used to make medicine. *Ligusticum* is antimicrobial and antispasmodic. The antimicrobial activity of *Ligusticum* is the result of furanocoumarins and monoterpenes. The tincture is applied topically as a local antiseptic. *Ligusticum* enhances the immune system. As an antibacterial, I combine equal parts of *Ligusticum* with *Echinacea* and *Astragalus* and give 30 drops of tincture four times daily.

Artemesia tridentata

COMMON NAME ■ Big sagebrush

Use the dried leaves to make medicine. *Artemesia* is most effective against gram-positive organisms. I use it against *Pneumococcus* and *Plasmodium* organisms. It makes a good flu remedy. Use 30 drops of the tincture twice daily for the flu.

Artemesia contains some very effective bioflavonoid antioxidants such as quercetin, apigenin, and kaempferol. Apigenin is a polyhydroxyflavone that is in the same class as quercetin. Both of these flavones are widespread in herbal medicines. Like quercetin, apigenin is antiinflammatory especially against allergy-induced inflammation.

Arbutus menziesii

COMMON NAME ■ Madrone

The dried leaves are used for medicine. Herbalists tell me that madrone can be used for bladder and upper respiratory infections. The leaves are decocted into tea and taken in doses of 1 cup three times daily. Dr. Bastyr did not talk about this remedy. I have added it because I have been experimenting with it for bladder infections. I don't have enough experience yet to be able to recommend it, but so far it looks promising.

Vaccinium macrocarpon

COMMON NAME ■ Cranberry

The berries are used to make medicine. Cranberry is a useful urinary tract antibacterial. Drinking the juice prevents adherence of certain bacteria to the wall of the bladder. *Escherichia coli,* which is a common infecting agent in cystitis, is particularly vulnerable to cranberry juice or capsules of powdered cranberry. The dose of capsulated cranberry varies. I have prescribed 500 mg three times daily for 5 days and found this to be an effective dose. The patient should drink plenty of water during therapy. I use other urinary antiseptics such as *Hydrastis* and *Chimaphila* in combination with cranberry. I have patients put 30 drops of *Hydrastis* and 60 drops of *Chimaphila* into 1 cup of cranberry juice and drink 3 cups of this mixture daily.

Peumus boldus

COMMON NAME ■ Boldo

Peumus boldus is a member of the *Monimaceae* family. The leaves are used to make medicine. I don't remember Dr. Bastyr speaking about this remedy as an antibacterial. I have added this remedy because I use it so frequently and am so fond of it. I use it principally as a cholagogue. I have included it in the antibacterial section for reasons listed below. The oil derived from the leaves has demonstrated in vitro antimicrobial activity against *Staphylococcus aureus, Streptococcus pyogenes, Enterococcus faecalis, Micrococcus* species, *Bacillus subtilis, Escherichia coli, Salmonella* species, *Shigella sonnei, Morganella morganii, Acinetobacter baumannii, Pseudomonas aeruginosa,* and *Candida.*

The list of constituents in the oil of the boldo leaves includes alpha-thujene, alpha-pinene, camphene, beta-pinene, sabinene, 3-carene, myrcene, alpha-phellandrene, alpha-terpinene, *p*-cymene, terpinolene, 1,8-cineol, linalool oxide, trans-sabinene hydrate, campholenal, camphor, linalool + cis-sabinene hydrate, pinocarvone, bornyl acetate, terpinen-4-ol, myrtenal, trans-pinocarveol, neral, cyptone, alpha-terpineol, borneol, ascaridol, geranial, carvone, myrtenol, cumin aldehyde, trans-carveol, thymol, carvacol, beta-caryophyllene, alpha-humulene, bicyclogermacrene, oxygenated sesquiterpenes, caryophyllene oxide, 6E-nerolidol, farnesol, and others.[40] These constituents are presented to give the reader an appreciation of the complexity of a "simple" leaf of a plant.

Understand that for many plants, the list of constituents will often be as long or longer. The study of plant medicine is really in its infancy. How to use the oil of the *Peumus* leaves as an antimicrobial remains to be discovered. Exactly what constituents provide protection against exactly which microbes remains to be determined. It should be noted, however, that research has shown that *Staphylococcus aureus* and *Streptococcus pyogenes* are very sensitive to boldo. Given that *Staphylococcus aureus* has demonstrated resistance to even the strongest antibiotics in recent years, the study of the plant constituents that may be effective against these organisms is of interest. These botanical medicines may save lives that would otherwise be lost because of rampant and uncontrollable infections.

CHAPTER

6

ANTICANCER AGENTS

CHAPTER • OUTLINE

Viola odorata
Allium sativum
Amygdalus persica
Croton tiglium
Colchicum autumnale
Aristolochia serpentaria
Echinacea angustifolia
Sanguinaria canadensis
Vinca rosea
Hydrastis canadensis
Flavonoids
Tangerine
Coenzyme Q_{10}
Pinus species
Taxus brevifolia
Brassica oleracea
Camptotheca acuminata
Camellia sinensis
Rosmarinus officinalis
Languas galanga
Glycyrrhiza glabra typica
Viscum album
Hypericum perforatum
Trifolium pratense
Tabebuia impetigonosa
Ceanothus americanus

The anticancer agents are plants that have been cited in herbal literature and research for their use in the fight against cancer. Research money for carefully controlled studies has not been available to the natural healing community. This is gradually changing as patients and physicians, frustrated with the toxic nature of current chemotherapeutic agents and techniques, are becoming more interested in natural remedies. If chemotherapy worked more consistently, the outcry for better treatments would not be as loud.

Anticancer agents include both preventive and aggressive plant medicines. The currently respected multistage model of chemical carcinogenesis divides it into three stages: initiation, promotion, and progression. Cancer prevention includes the use of therapies and medicines that inhibit the initiation and promotion stages of cancer development. Cancer treatment involves both the use of plant medicines and the enhancement of the immune system to fight cancer.

There are many plants that show promise as cancer fighters. Some plants work directly against the cancer, some protect the body by preventing rapid metastasis, some support organ- and tissue-specific areas, and some increase the vital force of the body so that it can fight more effectively. This brief treatment barely skims the surface of the vast and exciting body of knowledge emerging about the effects of plant medicines on cancer.

I treat cancer as part of the health care team, which includes an oncologist and other therapists appropriate to the case. Natural therapies and approaches combined with the best allopathic medicine are frequently successful. Patients given this approach often tolerate chemotherapy with fewer side effects, thus allowing them to receive the total intended dose of chemotherapeutic agents.

Dr. Bastyr never made any claims that he cured cancer. He said that sometimes all you can do is help the patient to feel better when they have the disease. However, after Dr. Bastyr's death a good number of his patients who had been diagnosed with cancer came to me at my office. Often they commented: "Dr. Bastyr saved my life!"

I have added a number of remedies to this section that Dr. Bastyr did not discuss. However, they are remedies worth our consideration based on current literature and my personal experience with them as anticancer agents.

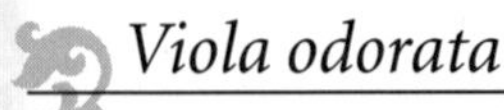

Viola odorata

COMMON NAME ■ Sweet violet

The whole plant is used to make medicine. Sweet violet is an antineoplastic agent. I have used it primarily with breast or alimentary canal cancers. It can be used after the cancer is extirpated to help prevent metastasis. Further discussion of the aforementioned can be found in the *British Herbal Compendium*.[20] The volatile oil of violet contains the monocyclic sesquiterpenoid, zingiberene. I have just begun to work with *Viola* as a cancer remedy.

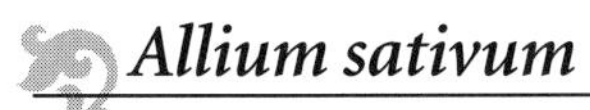

Allium sativum

COMMON NAME ■ Garlic

The whole bulb is used to make medicine. It is thought that the allicin in garlic tends to attenuate cancer cells and that garlic builds resistance against tumor cells. I speculate that this may be the result of garlic's ability to decrease viral and bacterial loads in the body and therefore decrease the strain on the immune system caused by those pathogens. Scientists report that they have discovered the existence of oncoviruses that turn on the cancer switch in some cells. If they are correct, garlic might weaken or kill those viruses, thus preventing the formation of cancer cells.

I recommend 5 cloves of garlic daily to help prevent recurrence of the cancer or development of a new cancer after chemotherapy or radiation, or 5 cloves three times daily for the concurrent treatment of active cancer. *Allium* contains two antithrombotic principles, Z-ajoene and E-ajoene.[41] The ajoenes also inhibit lipoxygenase,[26] making *Allium* an antiinflammatory agent.

Amygdalus persica

COMMON NAME ■ Peach tree

The twigs and leaves are used to make medicine. Look for this plant under the name *Prunus persica* also. Laetrile, or vitamin B_{17}, is derived from the peach tree. Laetrile is used interchangeably with amygdalin, which is a cyanogenic glycoside.

Dr. Bastyr taught us to use this plant material when it is fresh if possible. In the 1970s, reports circulated that laetrile was being used in some cases to treat cancer successfully. I have never used laetrile personally; however, Dr. Bastyr told us that he had seen it used, and that in some cases it seemed to work. If it truly cures cancer, one hopes it would be used routinely by oncologists. I am aware that research has been done but has shown no replicable results. I know of some patients who have tried laetrile and it has not been successful. What often happens with so-called cures is that the patient will become excited by what appears to be improvement, only to be disappointed later by recurrence of the cancer, which is then unresponsive to the wonder cure. Nevertheless, laetrile may indeed be worth revisiting by those interested in exploring it. Herbalists recommend a dose of 2 tablespoons of twigs and leaves chopped up and brewed as a tea. Let the tea sit in the water for 5 hours before consuming.

Croton tiglium

COMMON NAME ■ Croton seed

The medicine is obtained from the oil of the seed. Some early work at the University of Virginia showed some activity of croton oil against leukemia in mice. I cannot remember the exact reference. The problem with croton oil is administration. Dr. Bastyr cautioned us that croton is a drastic hydrogogue cathartic and purgative and is probably too toxic to administer. The cathartic property is the result of the hydrolysis of the C-20 acyl group from the phorbol triester. I have included this remedy for historical purposes but would recommend using other anticancer agents. I have never used croton oil to treat cancer.

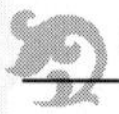

Colchicum autumnale

COMMON NAMES ■ Autumn crocus, Meadow saffron

The whole plant is used to make medicine. *Colchicum* is being explored as an antileukemic drug for children with acute lymphoblastic leukemia because it is antimitotic. A safe trial dose for a 10-year-old is 5 drops of the tincture twice daily. Higher doses can be used as the patient demonstrates tolerance.

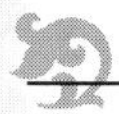

Aristolochia serpentaria

COMMON NAME ■ Virginia snakeroot

The root of the plant is used to make medicine. *Aristolochia* is reported by some sources to have anticancer activity.[42] As an antitumor remedy, this plant needs more investigation followed by carefully controlled trials. The specific tumor-inhibiting compound is aristolochic acid. The therapeutic dose is unknown. Dr. Bastyr suggested 20 drops of tincture three times daily. *Aristolochia*'s stimulating effect can also boost the energy in depressed or exhausted conditions of the nervous system.[43] Currently, *Aristolochia* is hard to come by. I can't seem to find it.

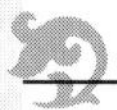

Echinacea angustifolia

COMMON NAME ■ Purple coneflower

The whole plant is used to make medicine. *Echinacea* inhibits some forms of tumor cells. Voaden and Jacobson, writing in the *Journal of Medical Chemistry,* reported that the lipid-soluble component of *Echinacea angustifolia* and *Echinacea pallida,* 1,8-pentadecadiene, stimulates macrophages to greater cytotoxic activity against tumor cells.[44] I use *Echinacea* as a general immune system aid to treat cancer. The minimum dose that I suggest for an adult is 90 drops four times daily. I usually combine three parts *Echinacea* tincture with one part *Astragalus* tincture and give 120 drops four times daily to improve immune function during the treatment of cancer.

Sanguinaria canadensis

COMMON NAMES ■ Blood root, Red puccoon

The whole plant, including the root, is used to make medicine. Several alkaloids in *Sanguinaria* have been shown to exert a notable therapeutic action on Ehrlich ascites sarcoma in mice and to exert a significant necrotizing effect on sarcoma 37 in mice. It can be applied topically to fight melanoma. *Sanguinaria* is a main ingredient in the famous red puccoon salve, which was put on tumors to draw the tumors out to the surface so that they could be expelled. Dr. Robert Carroll, who taught us nutrition at National College of Neuropathic Medicine, spoke about this salve but called it the black salve. Dr. Bastyr also mentioned the black salve, and he used it on breast cancer tumors. This salve can be applied to raw, exposed tumors because it seems to penetrate to the deeper layers of the tumor. I have used the *Sanguinaria* salve on several occasions with good results. The patients can feel the salve working. They report a tingling or mild burning effect locally. I have actually treated a patient with a suppurative breast cancer using this salve together with other herbal medicines. This patient refused allopathic treatment and wanted only natural, traditional earth medicine. The tumor suppurated and eventually the body healed itself. The cancer destroyed the breast itself, and when the wound healed all that was left was the chest wall with scar tissue and skin on it. It looked remarkably like the breast had been removed surgically.

The ingredients in the original salve were ½ tablespoon flour, 1 tablespoon chloride of zinc, 1 tablespoon powdered *Sanguinaria*, and 1 tablespoon black antimony, or trisulfide.

To make the salve, mix the flour, powdered *Sanguinaria*, and black antimony. Then spread the chloride of zinc over the top of the powdered mixture and let it stand for 24 hours or until the zinc melts. Mix this with a wooden spoon until it becomes a salve. It may take 3 or 4 days of stirring occasionally each day to really get a good consistency to the salve. Spread the mixture on the affected area for 3 nights. The chloride of zinc accounts for the burning sensation the patient feels when the salve is applied. Leave the pack on until the cancer falls out. To help the wound heal, I apply a mixture of chickweed and tea tree ointment. This salve comes to us courtesy of Mrs. Nettie Waggoner, who died in the 1980s. She had the instructions in a jar that was discovered by her niece and passed on through the family.

Two potent alkaloids contained in *Sanguinaria* are chelerythrine and sanguinarine. Sanguinarine possesses antimicrobial, antifungal, and antiinflammatory properties. Sanguinarine chloride binds selectively to dental plaque, inhibiting 98% of bacterial growth.[26,45] As an antimicrobial, the dose for *Sanguinaria* is 10 drops of the tincture three times daily.

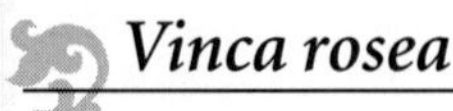

Vinca rosea

COMMON NAME ■ Periwinkle

The whole flowering plant is used to make medicine. This plant is probably more correctly known as *Catharanthus roseus.* In 1958, Professor Nobel found that the crude material has some carcinostatic activity against transplantable mammary adenocarcinoma in mice and against transplantable sarcoma in rats. Dr. Bastyr talked about the *Vinca* tincture for cancer; however, I don't remember very much about his comments.

Vinca is loaded with over 50 different types of alkaloids. The alkaloids with antineoplastic activity belong to a class of dimeric indole-dihydroindole derivatives. Vinblastine sulfate and vincristine sulfate are two alkaloids now used by the medical profession in the treatment of cancer, especially Hodgkin's disease and choriocarcinoma. *Vinca* alkaloids bind to tubulin, a dimeric protein found in the cytoplasm of cells. When the alkaloids are bound to tubulin, the process of assembly and dissolution of the mitotic spindle is inhibited, therefore exerting a cytotoxic effect. For an adult, I start with 20 drops of *Vinca* tincture three times daily.

Hydrastis canadensis

COMMON NAME ■ Goldenseal

The root is used to make medicine. I have used *Hydrastis* to help increase the white blood cell count in leukopenia secondary to chemotherapy. I have no idea why this particular application of *Hydrastis* sometimes works. The dose that I prescribe is one 500-mg capsule four times daily.

Flavonoids

Flavonoids with a free hydroxl group at the 3-ring position have anti-oncovirus activity. I remember Ed Madison, ND, discussing this in one of his lectures at Bastyr University. I include this information for historical purposes. Ed Madison was almost always right. Given this, I would encourage further investigation. I use 1 tablespoon of concentrated flavonoid extract twice daily for patients with cancer. In addition, anthocyanadins from berries improve the integrity of the capillary mesh, which may slow metastasis. I use these flavonoids for all my cancer patients.

Tangerine

Tangerines contain a bioflavonoid called tangeritin, which is the only bioflavonoid found to increase the functional integrity of E-cadherin, a cell-to-cell adhesive protein that helps to prevent metastasis of epithelial cancers. The epithelial tissues are the origin of 80% of cancers. Tangeritin is an exciting nutrient to add to the list of cancer therapies. It has been shown that E-cadherin is dysfunctional or deficient in nearly all tissue samples taken from cancer patients. Simply eating a few tangerines each day may help. I recommend this for all of my cancer patients. Much of the bioflavonoid is found in the white part of the tangerine rind, and therefore eating some of the rind is important. I tell my patients to buy tangerines when they can and then peel and freeze the rind for use during the off season.

Coenzyme Q_{10}

COMMON NAME ■ Ubiquinone

Coenzyme Q_{10} (CoQ_{10}) is a polyisoprenic fatty supplement that shows some exciting possibilities in the regression of breast cancer tumors.[46] I have been using ubiquinone for patients with breast cancer since early 1998. I started using it after hearing Alan Gaby, MD, lecture about it at the American Association of Naturopathic Physicians convention. The recommended dose is 100 mg three times daily in the treatment of breast cancer. CoQ_{10} enhances the immune system and increases the vital force.

Pinus species

COMMON NAME ■ Pine

There are many pine tree varieties. Two common species from which medicine such as turpentine is derived are *Pinus sylvestris* and *Pinus palustris.* The branches and needles are used to make medicine. Pine trees contain chiefly monoterpenoid hydrocarbons including alpha-pinenes, beta-pinenes, and camphene. Pine trees also contain a group of flavonoids called pycnogenol, which have been touted by some herbal enthusiasts as having carcinostatic effects.

Pine tea is rich in these flavonoids that strengthen connective tissue and help prevent the spread of cancer. It is a powerful drink that improves the function of the immune system. I instruct the patient to break off about 6 inches from the end of a small branch of the pine tree and chop everything including bark and needles into a pot containing 4 cups of water. This mixture is gently boiled for 15 minutes and then allowed to stand for 3 hours. It is then reheated and sipped throughout the day.

Taxus brevifolia

COMMON NAME ■ Pacific yew tree

The medicine is obtained from the bark of the yew tree. This antileukemic and antitumor agent works by inhibiting the tubulin disassembly process in the cell. It effectively inhibits mitosis. The specific active principle is taxol. A standard tea brewed from the bark of the yew tree will not yield an effective dose. To obtain a dose that is strong enough, the taxol is removed from the bark and concentrated. Taxol has considerable side effects; however, modern science is working to create taxanes that will be more effective than straight taxol and will have fewer side effects.

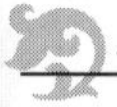

Brassica oleracea van *italica*

COMMON NAME ■ Broccoli

The edible vegetable is used. Broccoli contains sulforaphanes, which inhibit tumor growth. The broccoli sprouts contain more sulforaphanes than the broccoli florets.[47] It is difficult to determine an exact dose. I generally suggest that my patients consume $\frac{1}{4}$ pound of broccoli daily as cancer therapy.

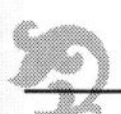

Camptotheca acuminata

COMMON NAME ■ Camptothecin

Camptothecins are promising antileukemic and antitumor agents. They are derived from the stem wood of this Chinese tree. One of the active ingredients is camptothecin. This is an extremely promising agent and is currently being researched and used in clinical trials by the medical profession. I am co-treating a number of patients who have been prescribed this medicine by their allopathic physicians. Although I am very interested in this remedy, I have not used it clinically.

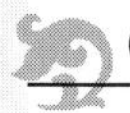

Camellia sinensis

COMMON NAME ■ Green tea

You may also find this plant listed under the name *Thea sinensis.* The leaves are used to make medicine. Much has been learned about this remedy since Dr. Bastyr's days. The following information is relatively new.

The difference between green tea and black tea is that green tea is produced by preventing the oxidation of the leaf polyphenols known as catechins. The enzymatic oxidation of the polyphenols occurs in the production of black tea.

The oral administration of green tea inhibits cancers induced by a number of chemicals. Administration of (-)epigallocatechin-3-gallate inhibits N-ethyl-N′-nitro-N-nitrosoguanidine–induced duodenal tumors in mice.[48] Lung tumors in mice that were induced by 4-(methyl-N-nitrosamino)-1-(3-pyridyl)-1-butanone were inhibited by the same polyphenol.[49]

Oral administration of green tea inhibits N-nitrosodiethylamine–induced tumors of the forestomach and lungs in mice.[50] Green tea also inhibits esophageal tumors in rats induced by N-nitrosomethylbenzylamine.

A number of studies have shown the inhibitory effect of green tea on cancers induced on the skin of mice. In these cases tumor promotion is inhibited. An example is the inhibition of 12-O-tetradecanoylphorbol-13-acetate–induced tumorigenesis in SKH-1 mouse skin.[51-54] Another study showed that green tea polyphenols inhibited azoxymethane-induced colon carcinogenesis in rats.[55] Green tea has been well studied. The above is only a small list of research currently being conducted in vivo on animal models. Green tea is the drink that I recommend for patients with lung, skin, or alimentary tract cancers. I also have patients who are exposed to chemically compromised environments drink green tea daily as a preventive and protective strategy. I prescribe 2 cups of the tea per day.

Both the initiation and the promotion of tumors may be decreased by drinking green tea. I have patients drink several cups per day. Capsules of caffeine-free green tea are also available. I give 3 capsules two to three times daily, especially if a tumor has been diagnosed. I like to remind patients that catechins reduce the formation of peroxides in lipids far more effectively than vitamin E.[56]

Rosmarinus officinalis

COMMON NAME ■ Rosemary

The upper aerial parts are used to make medicine. Rosemary presents us with an interesting study in constituents and their actions. Some of the constituents of rosemary are antioxidants, including carnosic acid and carnosol. The antioxidant capacity of rosemary depends on the concentration of these two compounds.[57]

Ursolic acid is not an antioxidant; however, it strongly inhibits 12-O-tetradecanoylphorbol-13-acetate–induced inflammation and tumor promotion in the skin of mice.[58] Rosemary inhibits skin tumor initiation by benzo[a]pyrene in CD-1 mice.[59] Rosemary also inhibits 7,12-dimethylbenz[α]anthracene.[60]

Fresh rosemary may be added to food; however, therapeutic doses of rosemary can be obtained by getting freeze-dried or powdered rosemary and taking the capsules. I recommend 3 capsules twice daily as a starting dose. Rosemary tincture or botanical extract is also available. I begin with 60 drops three times daily. The tincture does contain the active constituents that exhibit tumor inhibition.

Languas galanga

COMMON NAME ■ Galangal

The rhizome is used to make medicine. Galangal is a member of the ginger family, *Zingiberaceae.* Dr. Bastyr did not teach about this remedy. I have been interested in this plant for the past 15 years. Galangal is one of the nonchewy, hard, woody spices found in soups in Thai restaurants, especially in the tom yum soups. It has a wonderful hot, gingerlike flavor. Galangal contains

(1′S)-1′-acetoxychavicol acetate (ACA), which inhibits tumor-promoter–induced Epstein-Barr virus activation.[61] ACA is known to be an inhibitor of xanthine oxidase, which generates superoxide anions from the substrates xanthine or hypoxanthine.[62] Research on mice shows that the inhibition of this anion by ACA inhibits tumor promotion.[63]

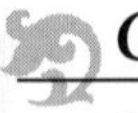

Glycyrrhiza glabra typica

COMMON NAME ■ Licorice root

The roots and rhizome are used to make medicine. Licorice contains many active constituents. Two of these constituents are glycyrrhizic acid, also known as glycyrrhizin, and glycyrrhetinic acid, which is the aglycone of glycyrrhizin. Both of these constituents inhibit 7,12-dimethylbenz[alpha]-anthracene–induced skin tumor initiation.[64]

When using licorice root, I initially monitor the blood pressure of the patient weekly. Some patients are subject to blood pressure elevation when taking this remedy. Other patients do not seem to have any problem. For an anticancer remedy, I begin with a dose of 30 drops of the botanical extract daily. I increase this dose if the patient responds well to this medicine.

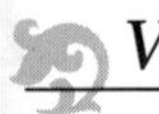

Viscum album

COMMON NAME ■ European mistletoe

The whole plant is used to make medicine. *Viscum* contains a large number of compounds, including flavonoids, triterpenes, vasoactive amino acids, polysaccharides, and alkaloids. It also contains caffeic acid and stigmasterol. The plant even takes on some of the constituents of the trees on which it grows. I have used *Viscum* predominantly as an anticancer agent. The effect of *Viscum* is to enhance macrophage phagocytic and cytotoxic cell-mediated abilities. It also enhances natural killer cell activity[65] and stimulates the thymus gland. The active principle may be the viscotoxins, which are polypeptides made from 26 amino acids. *Viscum* may be used to treat any cancer, although some literature suggests using it to treat breast cancer specifically. For the treatment of cancer, I recommend starting with a dose of 30 drops of tincture twice daily. More may then be prescribed depending on the patient's ability to tolerate the medicine.

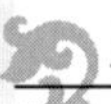

Hypericum perforatum

COMMON NAME ■ St. John's wort

The aerial parts are used to make medicine. There is some evidence that St. John's wort may be of some help in fighting brain cancer. Hypericin, one of the active constituents of *Hypericum*, inhibits the growth of neuroblastoma cells by stimulating apoptosis. Keep in mind this was an in vitro study.[66] Think of *Hypericum* when treating pituitary adenoma hypertrophy. Research has shown that hypericin inhibits protein kinase C and induces apoptosis in pituitary adenoma cell lines.[67] I have only treated two cases of pituitary adenoma and have lost track of both patients, so I cannot speak here from very much personal experience. However, *Hypericum* standardized to 80% hypericin might be worth a try. For starters, I would use 600 mg of standardized *Hypericum* capsules three times daily, which is double the normal dose used for depression.

Trifolium pratense

COMMON NAME ■ Red clover

The aerial parts of the plant are used to make medicine. *Trifolium* is an ingredient in anticancer formulas, such as Hoxey's formula. I use *Trifolium* as an anticancer agent. I recommend taking 60 drops of *Trifolium* twice daily or adding it to anticancer formulas. I have an elderly patient with suppurative and metastasized breast cancer who put herself on red clover and chaparral tea. Her dose was 3 tablespoons of each herb brewed into a quart of water. She drank the whole quart each day. For her this proved miraculously curative.

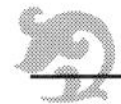

Tabebuia impetiginosa

COMMON NAMES ■ Taheebo, Pau'Darco, Bowstick

This plant may also be found as *Tecoma curialis*. The medicine is made from the inner bark of the LaPacho tree. I use taheebo to treat breast cancer together with 100 milligrams of coenzyme Q_{10} three times daily. It may also be used for blood and bone marrow cancers. I think of taheebo in the treatment of blood and lymph cancers. It seems to be specific here. The dose that I recommend for helping to fight cancer in an adult is 2 teaspoons of the botanical extract twice daily in hot water. It makes a reasonable tasting tea that patients do not seem to mind. What arouses my interest is the concept that some cancers are initiated by what appear to be oncoviruses. Could taheebo possibly block cancer initiation and development by blocking the virus-cancer link?

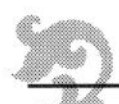

Ceanothus americanus

COMMON NAME ■ New Jersey tea

The dried bark of the root is used to make medicine. Dr. Bastyr mentioned that in lymphatic leukemia, *Ceanothus* can sometimes prolong the length and quality of life. Dr. Bastyr used the phrase "holds them" to describe this action. I have confirmed the use of *Ceanothus* for treating leukemia in two cases thus far. One of my cases was an 80-year-old man. He died 10 years later of leukemia, which had been the original diagnosis. During those 10 years, he remained mobile and pain free. It was not until the last 3 months of his life that he weakened noticeably. I was impressed that he remained healthy and active for all of those years. The dose that I recommend is 60 drops of tincture twice daily.

CHAPTER

7

ANTICOAGULANTS

CHAPTER • OUTLINE

Anticoagulants are agents that prevent clotting in a fluid, especially blood.

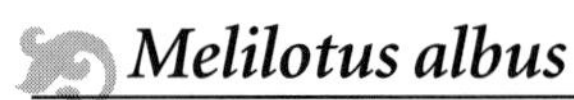

Melilotus albus

COMMON NAME ■ Sweet clover

Use the whole plant to make medicine. Sweet clover contains coumarin, which is the lactone of *o*-hydroxy-cinnamic acid. Coumarin itself is not an anticoagulant but contains dicumarol, which inhibits hepatic synthesis of the vitamin K-dependent coagulation factors. Drugs based on coumadin are used as anticoagulants. A decoction or a tincture of this plant may be used to prevent unwanted clotting. I prescribe 30 drops twice daily. This plant should not be considered for anticoagulant therapy directly after stroke or coronary events of a serious nature. For these more serious conditions, dicumarol-derived drugs are prescribed by medical professionals.

Dicumarol was originally isolated from spoiled sweet clover but is now produced synthetically. Once a coronary crisis has passed and the patient is stabilized, a less toxic plant medicine such as poplar or willow may be given.

Melilotus officinalis

COMMON NAME ■ Sweet clover—another variety

Melilotus is a member of the pea family, *Leguminosae.* The whole plant is used. This plant also contains substantial amounts of coumarin. Coumarin stimulates the reticuloendothelial system and the proteolytic power of macrophages.[26] Dr. Bastyr recommended a dose of 10 to 20 drops of tincture three times daily or 1 cup of the standard tea twice daily. He used *Melilotus* to help resolve venous stasis, which is a combination of venous and lymphatic insufficiency. He also used *Phytolacca* to help resolve this condition. He used 20 drops of *Melilotus* tincture and 10 drops of *Phytolacca* tincture three times daily.

Dipteryx odorata

COMMON NAME ■ Dutch tonka beans

The beans are used to make medicine. One may also use *Dipteryx oppositifolia.* The seeds of *Dipteryx* contain 1% to 3% coumarin. The coumarin compounds suppress the formation of prothrombin and factors VII, IX, and X by the liver. The advantage of using plant medicines is that they avoid toxicity reactions such as hypoprothrombinemia, which can occur with prolonged use of the more powerful dicumarols. Dr. Bastyr recommended a dose of 7 to 20 grains of the powdered tonka beans twice daily. He mentioned that tonka beans were once used as flavoring agents. They are now banned from such use because of their anticoagulant effect.

Anthoxanthum odoratum

COMMON NAME ■ Sweet vernal grass

The dried flowers are the medicinal part of this plant. Sweet vernal grass contains coumarin. A fluid extract was given by the eclectics in doses of 5 to 10 drops daily as an anticoagulant.

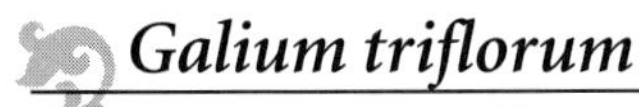

Galium triflorum

COMMON NAME ■ Sweet scented bedstraw

The whole dried flowering plant is used to make medicine. This plant contains coumarin and has been used by herbalists as a mild anticoagulant to supplement other natural therapies in dealing with circulatory disorders, strokes, and coronary occlusion disorders. Dr. Bastyr recommended that the powder be given in doses of 20 to 30 grains twice daily. As an alternative, he said that the fluid extract could be given in doses of 10 to 20 drops twice daily.

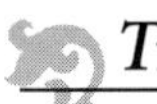

Trifolium pratense

COMMON NAME ■ Red clover

Medicine is made from the aerial parts of the plant. This plant contains coumarin. Eclectics and herbalists have given 3 to 4 cups of standard tea three times daily as a mild tonic and anticoagulant. *Trifolium* has been prescribed classically for convalescence from influenza or dysentery. I prescribe *Trifolium* to help prevent blood clots and strokes.

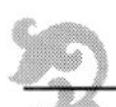

Trilisa odoratissima

COMMON NAME ■ Vanilla leaf

This plant contains coumarin. The leaves are used to make medicine. As an anticoagulant, Dr. Bastyr gave 20 drops of the tincture twice daily. This plant is very useful in convalescence from stroke. Elderly people may have small strokes that affect them in more minor ways. A stroke is not always a major event. Nevertheless, anticoagulant medicines should be considered for elderly patients who complain of strange, unexplained symptoms such as visual disturbances and dizziness that come on suddenly. These symptoms can coincide with sudden loss of cognition or memory, weakness in the arms, or loss of vocal crispness and sharpness. For an anticoagulant dose, I recommend 20 drops twice daily. Dr. Ed Madison taught me about the use of *Trilisa* for cerebral edema. Forty drops of the tincture is given twice daily for this.

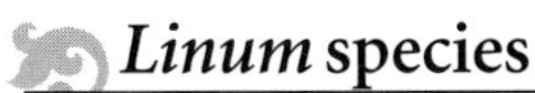

Linum species

COMMON NAME ■ Flaxseeds

Look for this under the name *Linum lewisii* or *Linum usitatissimum. Linum* is in the flax family, *Linacaea.* The oil of the seed is used for medicine. The oil of the flaxseed is about 40% omega-3 oil, which has a platelet anticoagulating effect by preventing platelets from becoming sticky.

Blood-clotting time increases when flax is consistently consumed. Our culture is beset by coronary arterial occlusion problems, and I prescribe flax seed oil for elderly and middle aged patients at a dose of 2 teaspoons daily. I have my patients store their flax oil in a dark bottle in the refrigerator because it is sensitive to light and heat. In addition, I tell them not to cook with it. Flax oil also helps to decrease symptoms of allergy in patients who are hypersensitive to foods.

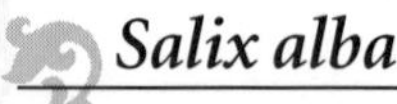

Salix alba

COMMON NAME ■ White willow tree

The bark is used to make medicine. Both the willows and the poplars belong to the *Salicaceae* family. Like aspirin, which contains acetylsalicylic acid, white willow is an anticoagulant. White willow contains salicin and other salicylic acid analogues. These salicylates act by blocking the formation of platelet-aggregating prostaglandins and thromboxanes. Wintergreen leaves and the bark of sweet birch also contain salicylic acid. The dose I give as an anticoagulant to prevent heart disease is 800 mg of white willow bark daily. The same dose of poplar bark may be used.

Zingiber officinale

COMMON NAME ■ Ginger

The root is used to make medicine. *Zingiber* inhibits platelet aggregation and so can be used to prevent blood-clotting tendencies. I have had dozens of cases where patients have been taking coumadins for blood thinning. Frequently, by using flax oil and *Zingiber*, patients can carefully wean themselves off coumadin drugs. This should be done with the help of their doctor. I give 2 capsules of *Zingiber* twice daily and 1 tablespoon of flax oil once daily. Eliminating greasy, sticky foods such as peanut butter is helpful in this process. Peanut flour enhances blood clotting, and all peanut products should be avoided when trying to prevent platelet aggregation.

CHAPTER

8

ANTIDEPRESSANTS

CHAPTER • OUTLINE

Antidepressants are medicinal materials that decrease depression or a feeling of isolated, fearful sadness. Dr. Bastyr did not present a section called antidepressants. I have added this section to the book because these remedies are important in treating this disorder. The eclectic physicians in the 19th and early 20th centuries sometimes referred to antidepressants as nervines and nerve tonics. It is important to remember that herbalists and eclectic physicians did not study antidepressants based on knowledge of neurotransmitters as do modern naturopathic physicians and herbalists. The scientific investigation of the active constituents of plant materials is creating new and expanded uses for plant medicines in the field of mental disorders.

Hypericum perforatum

COMMON NAME ■ St. John's wort

The leaves and flowers are used to make medicine. *Hypericum* is a little shrubby plant that likes to be around people. It probably finds us interesting. It probably wonders why it took us so long to find it interesting.

Hypericum contains an array of carotenes, flavonoids, xanthones, acids, essential oils, alcohols, and other phenolics. The antidepressant effects of *Hypericum* are likely caused by a variety of constituents, including hyperforin, xanthones, and hypericin, which is a naphthodianthrone. Although hypericin is a famous constituent, do not make the mistake of attributing all of *Hypericum*'s antidepressant activity to this constituent.

For thousands of years, physicians and herbalists have used *Hypericum*. Even the Greeks used *Hypericum* medicinally. Pliny and Hippocrates also used St. John's wort. You can bet that they didn't call it St. John's wort, however. St. John did not come along for another 600 years or so. The ancient Greek medical texts referred to *Hypericum* as a plant to drive away demons.

Hypericum's antidepressant effect seems to stem from a number of factors. The flavonoid content may have a moderating effect on monoamine oxidase. Catechol-o-methyl-transferase, an enzyme functionally similar to monoamine oxidase, may also be moderated by flavonoids and xanthones.[68] Inhibition of the reuptake of serotonin has also been shown, at least in a test tube, to be brought about by *Hypericum*.[69]

Curiously, gamma-aminobutyric acid receptors are also affected by *Hypericum*, which seems to inhibit the uptake of gamma-aminobutyric acid in the synapses and retard receptor binding. How this may deflect depression is as yet unknown.[70] *Hypericum* inhibits cytokines, which may partly explain its antidepressant action. Hypericin strongly inhibits protein kinase C. This inhibition affects the brain, as was shown in a study by Hamilton et al. in which hypericin inhibited cell growth and induced apoptosis in pituitary adenoma cell lines.[67] I think that the antidepressant ability of *Hypericum* is due to a combination of things, both known and unknown. One thing is certain—the relationship between *Hypericum* and humans is evolving.

The dose of *Hypericum* as an antidepressant is 300 mg three times daily. It is suggested that this dose be standardized to 3% hypericin. Frankly, I'm not so sure. Hypericin is a photodynamic sensitizer,[26] which is why sun exposure may be dangerous to patients taking this preparation. Sun exposure induces the formation of singlet oxygen in patients taking hypericin-enriched *Hypericum*. It may be worth looking into larger doses of *Hypericum* with lower hypericin levels, such as 1%.

Hypericum is a good example of a plant that may be better used as a whole plant entity rather than an extracted and enhanced medicine. *Hypericum* contains a rich supply of carotenoids and flavonoids, which are useful antioxidants. These antioxidants protect the patient from the photosensitization problems that come with the territory when taking *Hypericum*. Perhaps it would be wise to recommend that our patients enhance their diets with carotenoid- and flavonoid-rich foods when taking *Hypericum*. I'm sure that if Dr. Bastyr were alive today, he'd probably say, as you were leaving his office with your bottle of *Hypericum*, "Be sure to eat your carrots and kale."

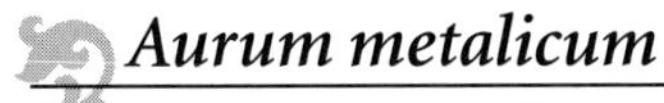

Aurum metalicum

COMMON NAME ■ Elemental gold

A homeopathic remedy is made from gold. I can't resist putting this remedy in at this time. For patients with depression, where there is a suicidal tendency, a 200X or a 200C potency of *Aurum* can make them feel like the light has been turned on. It is a fairly predictable remedy for depressed patients who are suicidal. This was a favorite remedy of the late Dr. Elder for this purpose. Dr. Elder was a contemporary of Dr. Bastyr. I recommend giving *Aurum* once daily until the symptoms abate. This may seem contrary to homeopathic prescribing. However, in practice I have found this to be efffective.

The happy formula

I combine the tinctures of *Armoracia, Cimicifuga, Glycyrrhiza glabra typica,* and *Dioscorea* in equal parts for what I call my "happy formula." This formula is a good antidepressant. The dose is 30 drops three times daily.

CHAPTER

9

ANTIDIARRHEALS

CHAPTER • OUTLINE

Potentilla tormentilla
Brown rice water
Croton tiglium
Kao-pectate
Tomato and sauerkraut

Antidiarrheals help stop diarrhea. Dr. Bastyr did not cover these remedies as a separate category. However, he did talk about these four remedies in other sections and mentioned their usefulness in treating diarrhea. They are grouped here for the convenience of the practitioner. The World Health Organization formula for electrolyte replacement for depletion from excessive diarrhea is 1 quart (liter) of water, 3.5 g sodium chloride, 2.5 g sodium bicarbonate, and 1.5 g potassium chloride. Clearly, persistent diarrhea calls for a definitive diagnosis to rule out serious disease. In naturopathic medicine, we don't automatically try to stop diarrhea. Acute diarrhea may be therapeutically purgative and the body's way of eliminating an intestinal toxin. The antidiarrheals are used for chronic, persistent, or life-threatening cases of diarrhea in which the patient is being dangerously depleted.

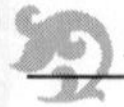

Potentilla tormentilla

COMMON NAME ■ Tormentil

One can also use *Potentilla erecta.* This plant is a member of the rose family, *Rosaceae.* The rhizome is used to make medicine. Tormentil contains more than 15% tannic acid, which makes this plant astringent. Dr. Bastyr used *Potentilla* for all types of diarrhea. He prescribed 60 drops of tincture twice daily. The powdered herb works better and is used in doses of $\frac{1}{4}$ teaspoon twice daily.

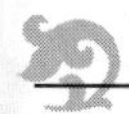

Brown rice water

This is an old folk remedy for curbing diarrhea. Boil brown rice in water for half an hour. Strain the rice and sip the liquid.

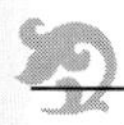

Croton tiglium

COMMON NAME ■ Croton seed

The medicine is obtained from the oil of the seed. *CAUTION: Even 1 drop of the oil of* Croton tiglium *will cause violent purgation.* This remedy is used homeopathically. I have often sent travelers on their way with a bottle of *Croton tiglium* 6X homeopathic potency with the instructions to melt 3 tablets under their tongues every half-hour until their diarrhea subsides. Dr. Bastyr thought highly of *Croton tiglium* 6X potency for the treatment of diarrhea. It is wise to give a vial of *Croton tiglium* to patients who are traveling. It can be life-saving in the case of violent, unstoppable diarrhea.

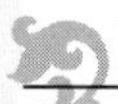

Kao-pectate

Kao-pectate is a product manufactured by Pharmacia and Upjohn. It's a good old-fashioned remedy that is worth mentioning because it is readily available from any drugstore. One of the ingredients is pectin, which is found plentifully in apples. I tell patients who are experiencing frequent bouts of diarrhea to eat several apples daily. The dose of Kao-pectate is given on the label and should be followed.

Tomato and sauerkraut

Dr. Bastyr used to prescribe 1 tablespoon of tomato juice and 1 tablespoon of sauerkraut every 15 minutes until the diarrhea stops.

CHAPTER

10

ANTIEMETICS

CHAPTER • OUTLINE

Amygdalus persica
Cerous oxalate
Cetraria islandica
Ballota nigra
Cephaelis ipecacuanha
Mentha veridis
Caryophyllus aromaticus
Nicotiana tobacum
Zingiber officinale

Antiemetics are remedies that are used to decrease the urge to vomit. Often, vomiting is a result of the body's need to expel something toxic. Because of this, the practitioner must consider the apparent cause of emesis before thinking about using an antiemetic. Overeating or overdrinking can also result in nausea leading to vomiting. Antiemetics are used to allay excessive vomiting or nausea in patients who are weak and debilitated. They are also used for nausea and vomiting of pregnancy and for general nausea of unknown origin as a palliative. Dr. Bastyr was careful in his teaching to encourage us to think before prescribing. We were reminded that one of the principles of naturopathic medicine is to do no harm.

Amygdalus persica

COMMON NAME ■ Peach tree

The leaves and twigs are used for medicine. *Amygdalus* leaf tea is helpful for stomach problems in which there is persistent nausea and vomiting. For nausea, Dr. Bastyr said that the dose of the tincture should be 5 to 30 drops as needed. The eclectics mention its use in nausea secondary to otitis media or otitis interna. I wonder if it might be useful in the nausea that often accompanies Meniere's disease. I haven't tried it for this yet.

Amygdalus was used in Hull's formula, which was sold as a tincture combination by Boericke and Tafel. The formula is equal parts of the tinctures of *Amygdalus, Chelone glabra,* and *Hydrastis.* The dose of this mixture is 5 to 10 drops in water before meals. The indications for Hull's formula include nervous or atonic dyspepsia, vomiting of pregnancy, and persistent vomiting from any cause other than organic disease. It was also given at the climacteric of disease as an intercurrent, which breaks into and modifies an existing disease.

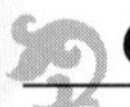

Cerous oxalate

COMMON NAME ■ Oxalate of cesium

For decades naturopaths have used the oxalate of cesium as an antiemetic. It is a white or slightly pink tasteless powder that is mostly insoluble in water. Dr. Bastyr used *Cerous* for nausea of pregnancy or nausea associated with gastric irritation and vomiting. He recommended that the patient take 3 grains three times daily, not to exceed 9 grains. Unfortunately, I have no practical experience with this remedy. I include it for historical reference.

Cetraria islandica

COMMON NAME ■ Iceland moss

The entire plant is used to make medicine. Herbalists use *Cetraria* for gastritis, dyspepsia, vomiting, cachexia, respiratory catarrh, and bronchitis. As an antiemetic, Dr. Bastyr suggested 1 to 2 mL daily.

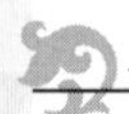

Ballota nigra

COMMON NAME ■ Black horehound

The dried aerial parts are used for medicine. Naturopaths and herbalists use *Ballota* to treat nausea, vomiting, and nervous dyspepsia. Dr. Bastyr suggested a dose of 1 to 2 mL twice daily. *Ballota* is useful in calming spastic coughing spells that could potentially cause vomiting. It contains marrubin, which is a lactone also found in white horehound, and is used medicinally in the same way that black horehound is used. *Ballota* also contains caffeic and ferulic acid derivatives, including chlorogenic acid.[25] For nervous dyspepsia, I mix $\frac{1}{2}$ teaspoon of glycine with *Ballota*. *Ballota* has a pleasant taste in and of itself; however, glycine can be used to sweeten this medicine further. Glycine also calms the mind.

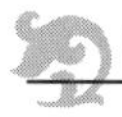

Cephaelis ipecacuanha

COMMON NAME ■ Ipecac

The root is used to make medicine. Ipecac contains a number of alkaloids, including emetine, a particularly active emetic, and psychotrine.

Ipecac causes nausea and vomiting and, per the law of opposites, is used homeopathically to prevent nausea. A 6X homeopathic potency was most often prescribed for the patients we saw as student clinicians when I attended National College of Naturopathic Medicine in the early 1970s. Dr. Bastyr was confident in this remedy. Two pellets are melted under the tongue as often as needed. A 6X potency dose of ipecac can be given every 15 minutes if necessary.

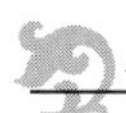

Mentha veridis

COMMON NAME ■ Spearmint

One may also use *Mentha spicata* and *Mentha cardiaca*. The leaves are used for medicine. There are a number of active constituents in the oil of spearmint such as carvone, alpha-pinene, and limonene. Dr. Bastyr said that this medicine will often stop vomiting when other remedies fail. Spearmint is most frequently given as a standard tea. Dr. Bastyr said to have the patient take 10 to 50 drops of tincture in water three or more times daily.

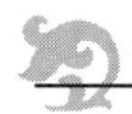

Caryophyllus aromaticus

COMMON NAME ■ Clove

There are several scientific names for clove, including *Eugenia caryophyllus* and *Eugenia caryophyllata*. The flower buds are used for medicine. Clove contains gallotannic acid, oleanolic acid, vanillin, and the chromone eugenin.

Dr. Bastyr said to add 2 drops of clove oil to 1 cup of water to relieve vomiting and nausea. Clove oil is also a famous remedy for relieving toothache pain. Clove oil is applied topically against the sore tooth and gum. Dr. Bastyr said that a pledget of cotton could be used to hold the oil nicely for this application.

Nicotiana tobacum

COMMON NAME ■ Tobacco

The medicine is made from the leaves. Of all of the antiemetic remedies, Dr. Bastyr spoke most often of ipecac and tobacco, both of which he used homeopathically. For nausea and vomiting, he typically gave a 6X homeopathic preparation of *Nicotiana* to be taken sublingually several times daily, or as needed. Dr. Bastyr said that this dose could be repeated frequently, even every 15 minutes if necessary.

Tobacco contains the alkaloid nicotine. Nicotine is very poisonous and is used in veterinary medicine to treat external parasites. Inhaling this material into the lungs is a dangerous practice.

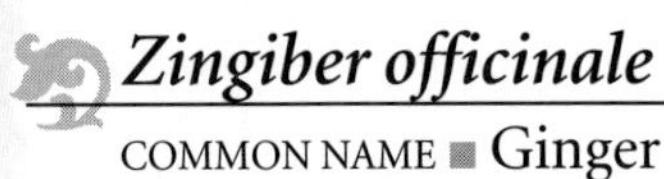

Zingiber officinale

COMMON NAME ■ Ginger

The root is used to make medicine. The active constituents in ginger are gingerol, shogaol, and zingerone. Ginger is used for motion sickness and has been shown to be more effective than Dramamine.[71] I prescribe two 200-mg capsules three times daily.

CHAPTER

11

ANTIHYPERTENSIVES

CHAPTER • OUTLINE

Veratrum viride
Rauwolfia serpentina
Tilia platyphyllos
Viburnum opulus
Allium tricoccum
Fumaria officinalis
Menyanthes trifoliata
Viscum album
Gelsemium sempervirens
Crataegus oxycantha
Cichorium intybus
Coleus forskolii

Antihypertensives are medicinal agents that decrease blood pressure. These natural remedies are especially important in light of the side effects of pharmaceutical antihypertensives, which include erectile dysfunction in men. The use of herbal antihypertensives, together with a program of nutritional management, is usually effective or at least helpful. Naturopaths use antihypertensive medicines temporarily until diet and lifestyle changes become effective. As blood pressure drops, the dose of the medicine can usually be lowered. When prescription drugs are needed, the dose is often minimized by adjunctive use of natural therapies.

Veratrum viride

COMMON NAME ■ American hellebore, Green hellebore

The roots and leaves are used for medicine. *Veratrum* contains a number of alkaloids, including veratramine and pseudojervine. *Veratrum* has been used to treat hypertension. It works on the afferent side of the nervous system, which it sensitizes to interpretation of blood pressure and consequently decreases the blood pressure reactivity. It lowers blood pressure and pulse rate.

Dr. Bastyr used 1 to 10 drops of tincture twice daily. He cautioned that this plant is toxic in large doses and told us to be careful when using it. I have used this tincture together with *Tilia europaea* and/or *Rauwolfia serpentina.* I prepare this remedy by mixing one part *Veratrum viride* tincture with four parts *Rauwolfia serpentina* tincture and four parts *Tilia europaea* tincture. The dose that I prescribe for hypertension is 20 drops of the formula twice daily.

Veratrum may be used for puerperal eclampsia. Dr. Bastyr suggested 30 drops of the tincture every 3 hours until the blood pressure drops. I would not suggest using *Veratrum* for eclampsia. Instead, I have found that eclampsia responds well to vitamin B_6 and magnesium in fairly high doses. These can be given in an intravenous push. According to Jonathan Wright, MD, the daily dose for preeclampsia is 500 mg of magnesium oxide three times daily and as much as 200 mg of vitamin B_6 four times daily.[72] In Dr. Bastyr's time, eclampsia was, and still is, life threatening. The use of high doses of botanicals was sometimes necessary to save the patient's life.

Rauwolfia serpentina

COMMON NAME ■ Rauwolfia

The root is used to make medicine. *CAUTION: Rauwolfia crosses the placental barrier and also enters breast milk.* Rauwolfia must be used respectfully. Overuse can result in severe depression in sensitive individuals. It is important that the patient be informed about Rauwolfia's potential side effects. It may cause depression and electrolyte depletion. The patient should be given a well-balanced mineral supplement at dinnertime when using Rauwolfia. This helps maintain electrolyte balance. In all my years of using Rauwolfia, I have never run into any problems with it.

Rauwolfia is a hypotensive. The main hypotensive agents in this herb are the tertiary indole alkaloids, reserpine, rescinnamine, and deserpidine. As an antihypertensive, Dr. Bastyr told us to use 150 to 200 mg daily for 1 to 3 weeks. He then suggested reducing the dose to 50 to 100 mg. The tincture dose as an antihypertensive is 10 drops twice daily. I combine *Rauwolfia* with equal parts of either *Viburnum opulus* or *Tilia europaea.* My formula for blood pressure control is equal parts of the tinctures of *Rauwolfia* and *Tilia* given in a dose of 30 drops twice daily. This dosage can be increased to 60 drops twice daily if the lower dose is ineffective.

I have frequently used *Rauwolfia* while I explore the cause of the patient's hypertension. Sometimes nutrition and lifestyle changes will lower blood pressure, at which point the patient can discontinue *Rauwolfia.* However, there are times when long-term treatment of persistent hypertension may require a continued dose of *Rauwolfia.*

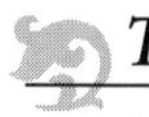

Tilia platyphyllos

COMMON NAME ■ Lime flowers

The flowers are used to make medicine. Dr. Bastyr used *Tilia* for hypertension associated with arteriosclerosis. The dose of the tincture is 30 drops two to three times daily or 15 to 30 grains of the powder three times daily. I use *Tilia,* together with other remedies, in almost every case of hypertension that I treat. *Tilia* is one of my favorite remedies for this purpose. To me, it is reassuring to know that *Tilia* is very safe, as so many other hypertensive remedies may have negative side effects.

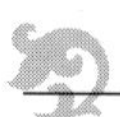

Viburnum opulus

COMMON NAME ■ Black haw

Also look for this plant under the name *Viburnum prunifolium.* The berries and seeds are used to make medicine. *Viburnum* contains isovaleric acid and tannins. Isovaleric acid is related to the butyrates, which gives *Viburnum* its peculiarly pleasant odor.

This herb is a mild hypotensive. I use 90 drops of tincture twice daily. For a stronger antihypertensive action, I use equal parts of *Viburnum* and *Rauwolfia* and give 20 drops of the mixture twice daily. In addition, Dr. Bastyr used *Viburnum* as an antispasmodic for any tubular organs such as the stomach, intestines, or bladder. This is a time-honored and tested remedy.

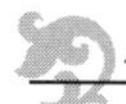

Allium tricoccum

COMMON NAMES ■ Galix, Wild leek

The root is used to make medicine. *Allium* is an antihypertensive. Dr. Bastyr said to boil the root in water and drink the resulting fluid. He also mentioned steeping *Allium* in vinegar and water. The resulting mixture is taken in doses of 1 cup twice daily. All of the plants in the *Allium* genus, especially garlic, prolong the action of insulin by means of disulfide inhibition of insulinase. Thus, in hypertension associated with diabetes, garlic is a good remedy.

Fumaria officinalis

COMMON NAMES ■ Fumitory, Earth smoke

The whole herb is used to make medicine. *Fumaria* is antihypertensive. The dose is 1 cup of the standard tea two to three times daily. I give 60 to 120 drops of the tincture three times daily. Its antihypertensive action may be the result of its diuretic action. I have found that a combination of equal parts of *Fumaria, Usnea,* and *Petroselinum,* taken in doses of 60 drops several times daily, is an excellent diuretic that can lower blood pressure and eliminate fluid accumulated in the extremities. The eclectics used *Fumaria* for plethora, a condition of redness and fullness of the face caused by excess body fluids.

I had a conversation with Dr. Bastyr at one of the naturopathic conventions in which he mentioned to me that *Fumaria* could be used in cases of increased blood viscosity.

Menyanthes trifoliata

COMMON NAME ■ Buckbean

Use the leaves for medicine. Dr. Bastyr used *Menyanthes* as an ingredient in antihypertension remedies. He, as well as many other herbalists, suggested making a standard tea and drinking a cup in mouthful doses. The tincture can be taken in doses of 15 drops three times daily. The bitter taste of buckbean is caused by a number of iridoids, including loganin, menthiafolin, and dihydromenthiafolin.

Viscum album

COMMON NAME ■ Mistletoe

The leaves and berries are used to make medicine. *Viscum* contains a large variety of pharmacologically active compounds, including lectins, viscotoxins, alkaloids, polysaccharides, and phenylpropanes. *Viscum* has several actions. It is a hypotensive, a cardiac depressant, and a sedative. Historically European herbalists have used *Viscum* to control postpartum hemorrhage because it has oxytocic effects.

Dr. Bastyr said to use 20 drops of tincture three times daily. He cautioned that this medicine is somewhat difficult to use because of its toxicity. He told us to be careful when prescribing it. He did not, however, discourage us from using this remedy. There were very few remedies that he discouraged us from using.

The key to using *Viscum* as a hypotensive is to use it in combination with several other botanicals. Try it with *Tilia* and either *Rauwolfia* or *Crataegus.* Use equal parts of *Viscum, Tilia,* and *Rauwolfia* and give 30 drops twice daily. It works well; however, I like to see a patient progress to the point where these medications are not needed.

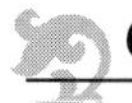

Gelsemium sempervirens

COMMON NAME ■ Yellow jasmine

Medicine should be made from the green root rather than from the dried plant if possible. *Gelsemium* contains several extremely toxic alkaloids, including gelsemine and gelsemicine.

Gelsemium is an antihypertensive. As such, Dr. Bastyr recommended a dose of 5 drops of tincture twice daily. In severe hypertension, he suggested a full dose of 30 drops.

In addition to discussing *Gelsemium*'s antihypertensive effects, Dr. Bastyr had several other curious things to say about this plant. He said that it was useful in cases where the eye is deviated to the side or upward or downward. He also talked about using *Gelsemium* to offset high doses of quinine. The antidote for *Gelsemium* is atropine.

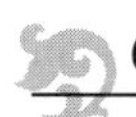

Crataegus oxycantha

COMMON NAME ■ Hawthorn

The berry is used to make medicine. Hawthorn is a mild antihypertensive, but it does not necessarily work immediately. I remember Dr. Bastyr telling us to be very persistent in its use. It may take a month to see any hypotensive effect. It is, however, a remedy worth considering in cases of hypertension. Hawthorn is nourishing to the heart. Even though its hypotensive effect is very mild, the cardioprotective effects of hawthorn make it especially appealing in light of the adverse side effects of the beta-blockers used by allopathic physicians. A study of rabbit aortas found that the size of extant arteriosclerotic plaques was reduced with dietary hawthorn.[73]

Hawthorn provides a number of procyanadin molecules that serve as antioxidants to the tissue of the arteries. Dr. Madison, a brilliant naturopath who taught at Bastyr University in the 1980s, told us that the dimeric proanthocyanidins found in hawthorn berry stabilized and strengthened the connective tissue in arteries and veins. Hawthorn mildly dilates the arteries. It is useful in hypertension and angina. The solid extract may be given in a dose of $\frac{1}{2}$ teaspoon daily.

Cichorium intybus

COMMON NAME ■ Chicory

Chicory is in the sunflower family, *Compositae*. The medicinal parts are the dried leaves and roots. Naturopaths have used chicory as a mild hypotensive agent. Herbalists recommend 90 drops of tincture twice daily for this purpose. We also use chicory as a cholagogue. The most famous use of chicory is as a coffee substitute. The roots are dried and ground up into a powder. This drink is good for the stomach and has been used to treat stomachaches. Infuse $\frac{1}{2}$ teaspoon of chicory in a cup of water.

Coleus forskolii

COMMON NAME ■ Coleus, Forskolin

The root of this plant is used to make medicine. *Coleus* is a hypotensive and an antispasmodic. Its main active principle is a diterpenoid called forskolin. The modus operandi of forskolin is its ability to activate the enzyme adenylate cyclase, which in turn activates adenosine monophosphate (cAMP) in cells. The physiological effects of increasing cellular cAMP are profound. These effects include inhibiting inflammation that is caused by mast cell degranulation and histamine release, relaxing arterial smooth muscles and thus lowering blood pressure, and relaxing bronchial smooth muscles. In addition, increasing cellular cAMP increases the force of the heart's pumping action, increases thyroid function, decreases platelet aggregation, and stimulates fat cells to burn fat more effectively and readily.

The best use of *Coleus* is in the treatment of hypertension and psoriasis and in the energizing of the aged. This plant is an excellent addition to geriatric tonics. I prescribe 30 drops of the tincture twice daily for elderly patients who are low in energy. In the case of hypertension, I use *Coleus* in combination with other hypotensives. I have found that combining equal parts of *Coleus, Rauwolfia, Tilia,* and *Viburnum* makes a useful hypotensive formula. I prescribe 30 drops of the tincture formula three times daily, or more if necessary.

CHAPTER

12

ANTIINFLAMMATORIES

CHAPTER · OUTLINE

Curcuma longa
Ananas comosus
Glycyrrhiza glabra typica
Chrysanthemum parthenium
Urtica dioica
Silybum marianum
Phytonadione
Salix alba
Colchicum autumnale

Antiinflammatories are remedies that decrease swelling and inflammation. Dr. Bastyr did not discuss a separate section called antiinflammatories. I have added this section in response to the current level of interest expressed by practitioners about antiinflamatory remedies. Keep in mind that inflammation is a normal body process, and that naturopathic physicians mostly use antiinflammatory remedies to check inflammation that threatens to become out of control or is causing great pain.

Curcuma longa

COMMON NAME ■ Turmeric

The root of this plant is used to make medicine. Turmeric is a member of the ginger family. Curcumin, the main active constituent, is extracted from turmeric. Naturopaths use curcumin in the treatment of inflammatory conditions. Use curcumin for joint inflammation, autoimmune inflammations, myalgia, and neuralgia and in cases where nonsteroidal antiinflammatory drugs would be used. In experimental studies, curcumin requires endogenous cortisol to work as an antiinflammatory agent. Thus, I often use licorice with curcumin to maximize its antiinflammatory effect. Licorice spares endogenous cortisol by increasing its half-life.

In a recent talk given by my good friend David Winston, a Cherokee medicine man and skilled herbalist, I was reminded that turmeric contains many active compounds, including alpha-curcumene. He cautions us to use whole turmeric rather than the extracted curcumin.

Although a huge amount of turmeric powder would be needed in order to receive an effective dose of curcumin for certain inflammatory conditions, there are many antioxidants in turmeric besides curcumin. I believe that it is beneficial to use both curcumin capsules and whole turmeric capsules. I encourage my patients to take $\frac{1}{2}$ teaspoonful of turmeric powder in the mouth directly and swallow it with water.

Curcumin depletes substance P, which is a neurotransmitter of pain.[74] Capsaicin, derived from cayenne pepper, is more widely known as a substance P depletor.

Turmeric has a long history of use in India for treating hepatic disorders and jaundice. I recommend 500 mg of curcumin three times daily for these conditions.

Ananas comosus

COMMON NAME ■ Pineapple

Bromelain, which is the active constituent, is extracted principally from the core and stem of the pineapple fruit. Bromelain increases fibrinolysis by enzyme activation. It also activates plasminogen to form plasmin. The plasmin then depolymerizes fibrin, thereby helping to prevent fibrin-clogged veins.[33] This helps to disperse localized edema and encourages adequate tissue drainage.[33] Inflammation is reduced as the edema decreases. I prescribe 1000 mg of bromelain twice daily. I have frequently prescribed bromelain for sports injuries and for aches and pains from muscle strain caused by overwork.

Bromelain may be used in the treatment of thrombophlebitis.[75] I give at least 200 mg of 1200-μU bromelain twice daily. I also have the patient eat blueberries. The anthocyanins in the berries protect the vascular system.

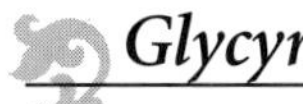

Glycyrrhiza glabra typica

COMMON NAME ■ Licorice root

The root is used to make medicine. *Glycyrrhiza* contains two interesting antioxidants, glabrin and glabrene, and a number of chalcones that inhibit leukotriene formation.[76] Specifically, chalcones block leukotriene B_2 and B_4, which decreases inflammation. *Glycyrrhiza* is a useful antiinflammatory in part because of these compounds. *Glycyrrhiza* blocks 5-beta reductase and thereby inhibits the breakdown of adrenal cortical hormone. Adrenal cortical hormone is the body's innate antiinflammatory substance. I give 30 drops of the fluid extract daily to reduce inflammation. I usually prescribe this dose at lunchtime to bolster flagging adrenal levels. *Glycyrrhiza* should not be forgotten in the fight to decrease allergy symptoms. I use 60 drops of the fluid extract together with 500 mg of quercetin twice daily for adults in the early stages of treatment for inhaled or ingested antigens.

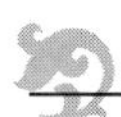

Chrysanthemum parthenium

COMMON NAME ■ Feverfew

CAUTION: Do not use this plant during pregnancy because it causes uterine contractions. The dried aerial parts of the plant are used to make medicine. An important active component in *Chrysanthemum* is the sesquiterpene lactone, parthenolide. *Chrysanthemum* blocks the eicosanoid cascade, preventing allergic reactions. One of the enzymes blocked is phospholipase-A_2. *Chrysanthemum* may be used to treat most inflammatory diseases including asthma and arthritis. I give 30 drops of tincture twice daily as an antiinflammatory. For allergic reactions, I use *Chrysanthemum* together with 500 mg of quercetin twice daily and 200 μg of selenium to decrease inflammation.

Urtica dioica

COMMON NAME ■ Nettles

The leaf of the nettle plant is used for preparing medicine. *Urtica* is a source of chlorophyll, which is considered by herbalists to be a general body tonic. *Urtica*'s ability to tonify and support mucous membranes is important for treating intestinal inflammation caused by diarrhea. It holds a special place in the herbal materia medica for its effectiveness in treating childhood diarrhea. For children I prescribe one 200-mg capsule two to three times daily.

Urtica decreases the symptoms of hay fever. I have often used it for this purpose with satisfying results. The dose I use is two 200-mg capsules three times daily. Some of my patients swear by it. By the way, an excellent remedy for hay fever that is sometimes almost miraculous is *Euphrasia officinalis* 6X potency. Melt 2 pellets under the tongue hourly at first, and then the dose can be taken several times daily. It has worked quickly for some patients.

Urtica contains both free and glycosylated sitosterol. Sitosterol decreases the synthesis of prostaglandins in the prostate and may be useful to treat benign prostatic hypertrophy.[77]

I have also found *Urtica* to be invaluable for treating migraine headaches. Some patients have reported feeling relief from their migraines within 15 minutes of taking the *Urtica*. The dose I use is 2 capsules every 2 hours at the first sign of migraine. I prescribe this for up to five doses.

Silybum marianum

COMMON NAME ■ Milk thistle

The seeds are used to make medicine. I cannot resist the temptation to add *Silybum* to the list of antiinflammatory remedies. I use it to treat inflammation of the joints, especially if the wrists are involved. Patients using *Silybum* tell me that their joints feel better. I've been using it together with other joint antiinflammatories. Don't overlook this plant when treating myalgia or fibromyalgia. The dose is 300 mg three times daily. *Silybum* can also be used effectively together with vitamin B_6 for the treatment of carpal tunnel syndrome. Of course, *Silybum* is used in cases of hepatic inflammation because it contains a mixture of three flavonolignans, chiefly silybin, silydianin, and silychristine, which are hepatoprotective.

Phytonadione

COMMON NAME ■ Vitamin K

Vitamin K is a fat-soluble vitamin, as are vitamins A, E, and D. All of the fat-soluble vitamins are polymers of isoprene units, so they are structurally similar. Vitamin K, which is contained in dark leafy greens, is an antiinflammatory in several ways. It is needed to mature the calcium-managing proteins in the bloodstream, including osteocalcin, kidney protein, protein C, and protein S. Inflammation is calcium-mediated. Therefore the proper management of calcium decreases runaway inflammation. Remember that the basic function of vitamin K is to add a carboxy group to the end-chain glutamic acid in calcium-managing proteins.

Vitamin K also decreases runaway inflammation in the management of hypercomplementemia in which vitamin K, by maturing a protein called complement-binding protein B4, facilitates the localization of complement to the wound or infection site and prevents excessive systemic activated complement, or fluid complement. Patients with inflammatory diseases and/or autoimmune diseases must be cautioned against the indiscriminate use of calcium.

I have used vitamin K for the management of cancer-related pain. The dose for pain management is 10 mg twice daily.

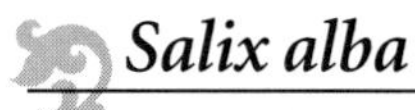

Salix alba

COMMON NAME ■ White willow bark

The bark is used to make medicine. This plant contains salicylates and acts as an antiinflammatory by blocking potentially inflammatory prostaglandins. It works like aspirin, which also contains salicylic acid. I recommend two 200-mg willow bark capsules three times daily. Dr. Bastyr talked about *Salix alba* as being the original source of aspirin.

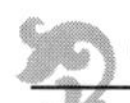

Colchicum autumnale

COMMON NAMES ■ Autumn crocus, Meadow saffron

The whole plant is used to make medicine. A major active ingredient in *Colchicum* is the alkaloid colchicine. Colchicine decreases the release of lactic acid and retards the movement of granulocytes into areas of inflammation. These actions mute the cycle that leads to an inflammatory response. Because of its action, colchicine has been used to treat gout. Another interesting use of *Colchicum* is in the treatment of Peyronie's disease.[78] The dose that I prescribe is 10 drops of tincture twice daily. I also give these patients 1600 IU of vitamin E daily.

CHAPTER

13

ANTIOXIDANTS

CHAPTER • OUTLINE

Hordeum vulgare
Carotenoids
Zingiber officinale
Sesamum indicum

Antioxidants prevent oxidation. The prevention of oxidation helps to inhibit premature aging, cancer, and rheumatic problems and, to some extent, limits autoimmune damage to tissues. In vivo, lipid peroxidation disrupts the normal precise arrangement of proteins and enzymes in membrane systems. As a result, there is damage to, impairment of, or loss of the activities in these biological systems.[79]

There are hundreds of antioxidants. Throughout this text I have written about dozens of plants and medicinal compounds that exhibit antioxidant activity. In this section, I will cover a number of these materials. In addition, I have discussed the antioxidant effects of many other plants where they are listed under other categories.

Dr. Bastyr did not lecture specifically on antioxidants as a group. I added this section because it is especially relevant for the prevention of tissue-damaging diseases.

Hordeum vulgare

COMMON NAME ■ Green barley leaves

Barley leaves contain a flavonoid, 2″-O-glycosylisovitexin that exhibits antioxidant activity by inhibiting malonaldehyde by 99%.[80] This flavonoid exists in the tincture of the dried barley leaves. Barley leaves also contain minerals and carotenoids that are good for the body. Carotenoids themselves are antioxidants and especially help to quench singlet oxygen.

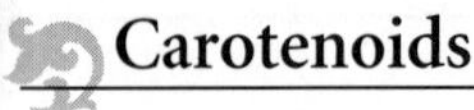

Carotenoids

COMMON NAMES ■ Carotene, Xanthophylls

So much has been written about the antioxidative effect of carotenoids that little needs to be added here. The longer the polyene chain of a carotenoid, the more effective it is as an antioxidant. It has been suggested by some researchers that carotenoids be consumed in the diet. Dietary carotenoids are usually of the cis structure rather than the trans structure. Some of the carotenoids in capsule form consist of rather large quantities of trans-carotenoids. Trans-carotenoids should be avoided.

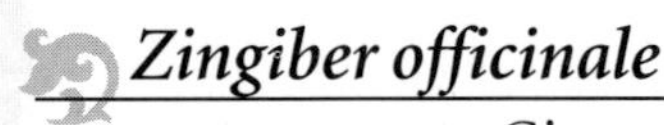

Zingiber officinale

COMMON NAME ■ Ginger

The root of this plant is used to make medicine. Many antioxidant constituents have been isolated from ginger rhizomes, including fourteen gingerol-related compounds and seven diarylheptanoids.[81]

For antioxidant use, 2 capsules of ginger root should be taken daily with meals. The flavonoids are better absorbed if taken with food. In addition, ginger is an appetite stimulant and a stomach-warming herb. It is also good for arthritis and rheumatism. This is probably because of the rich source of antioxidant and antiinflammatory constituents in the root.

Also noteworthy is that the diterpene dialdehydes in ginger inhibit 5-lipoxygenase as strongly as the alpha-sulfinyl disulfides found in onion.[82] These dialdehydes also inhibit platelet aggregation. It is postulated that adenosine diphosphate binding sites on platelets may be masked by labdane dialdehydes. As a result, the activation of platelets is suppressed, inhibiting platelet aggregation.[83]

Sesamum indicum

COMMON NAME ■ Sesame

The seeds are used to make medicine. Sesame seeds contain a number of lignan antioxidants.[84] Several of these lignan-phenol compounds include sesamol, sesaminol, and sesamolinol. Sesamol appears to be of major importance as an antioxidant among the constituents in sesame seeds.[85] Sesaminol is unaffected by heating and, when added to corn oil, depresses the degradation of tocopherol in the corn oil. I recommend putting ground sesame seeds on oatmeal or on any breakfast cereal as an antioxidant. I like the little seed grinders available in hardware stores and food co-ops.

CHAPTER

14

ANTIRHEUMATICS

CHAPTER • OUTLINE

Bryonia alba
Senecio jacobaea
Chimaphila umbellata
Harpagophytum procumbens
Apium graveolens
Lonicera periclymenum
Rhus toxicodendrum
Apis mellifera
Betula alba

Antirheumatics are remedies that relieve or prevent rheumatism. Rheumatism is defined by *Dorland's Illustrated Medical Dictionary* as "any of a variety of disorders marked by inflammation, degeneration, or metabolic derangement of the connective tissue structures of the body, especially the joints and related structures, including muscles, bursae, tendons, and fibrous tissue. It is attended by pain, stiffness, or limitation of motion of these parts. Rheumatism confined to the joints is classified as arthritis."[86]

Bryonia alba

COMMON NAME ■ White bryony

The root of this plant is used for medicine. *CAUTION: Bryonia is a toxic plant.* Even five or six berries of this plant will cause abdominal distress in children. The stomach should be pumped and activated charcoal given. Dr. Bastyr often gave *Bryonia* as an antirheumatic in the form of a homeopathic remedy. A 3X or 6X potency was frequently used by the early naturopaths. Dr. Bastyr pointed out that the classic indication for *Bryonia* is rheumatic pains made worse by motion. A plant that he talked about in the same breath was *Rhus toxicodendrum*, a rheumatic remedy for pain that is decreased by motion—just the opposite of *Bryonia*. *Bryonia* can be used for connective tissue pain almost anywhere in the body.

Senecio jacobaea

COMMON NAMES ■ European ragwort, St. James' wort

Do not confuse this with St. John's wort. The dried aerial parts are used for medicine. *CAUTION:* Senecio *contains a number of pyrrolizidine alkaloids,*[87,88] *including retronecine, seneciphylline, and senecionine. Large doses of these alkaloids, used over prolonged periods, are hepatotoxic.* This plant is an antirheumatic and is also used for myalgia and sciatica. Dr. Bastyr said that a dose of 20 drops of tincture four times daily should be given. *Senecio* may be used as a lotion. I have found that vitamin B_{12} shots also help sciatica. The dose of the shot is 2 mL per week.

Chimaphila umbellata

COMMON NAME ■ Pipsissewa

The root of this plant is used for medicine. This antirheumatic works by improving kidney function. Improved kidney function increases the body's elimination of water-soluble waste products. Those waste products are eliminated from connective tissue and other water-soluble compartments, decreasing their ability to inflame tissues. Pipsissewa contains arbutin, which is classified as a diuretic and a urinary antiinfective. I use 90 drops of tincture three times daily as a diuretic and give 120 drops of *Chimaphila* four times daily as a urinary antiseptic for cystitis. Pipsissewa is frequently combined with *Berberis aquifolium* for the treatment of cystitis.

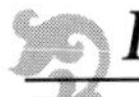

Harpagophytum procumbens

COMMON NAME ■ Devil's claw

The tuber is used to make medicine. *Harpagophytum* is native to southern and eastern Africa and is collected in regions bordering the Kalahari Desert. This medicine is specifically used by herbalists for arthritis and arthralgia. The dose I use is $\frac{1}{2}$ teaspoon of powder or 90 drops of tincture three times daily.

Dr. Bastyr included *Harpagophytum* in an antirheumatic and antiarthritic formula that consisted of equal parts of *Harpagophytum, Cimicifuga*, yucca, and *Larrea*. He also occasionally used *Achillea* in this formula. He probably gave these herbs in tincture form. Currently they are available in capsule form. The dose is 2 capsules twice daily.

This plant has an intriguing chemical structure. It contains free and glycosylated phytosterols and flavonoids, both of which may account for some of the antirheumatic activity. In addition, it has a number of iridoids, chief among which is harpagoside.[89] Harpagoside is an analgesic.[90]

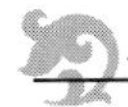

Apium graveolens

COMMON NAME ■ Celery

Use the seeds of this plant to make medicine. *Apium* contains a bicyclic sesquiterpenoid called beta-selinene, which may have an antiinflammatory effect on the tissues of the body. *Apium* is an antirheumatic and can also be used in urinary tract infections as an antiseptic. Dr. Bastyr mentioned that this remedy is useful in rheumatoid arthritis. When I say that Dr. Bastyr "mentioned" a remedy, I say that because that is frequently what happened. Dr. Bastyr would mention a remedy as an aside, without giving a specific dose or providing very much information about it.

Herbalists have used *Apium* for gout and arthritis of all kinds. When questioned, Dr. Bastyr's said to use 20 to 60 drops of the tincture three times daily. Patients with rheumatism and arthritis should drink ample fluids. In fact, I give these tinctures with a large glass of water specifically to encourage the consumption of adequate amounts of fluid.

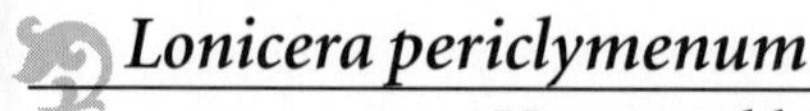

Lonicera periclymenum

COMMON NAME ■ Honeysuckle

This antirheumatic is made from the flowers of the plant. The antirheumatic effect is most likely caused by the salicylic acid present in this herb. Herbalists recommend 2 cups of the standard tea per day.

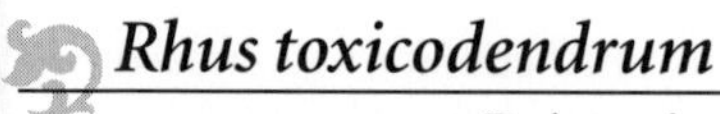

Rhus toxicodendrum

COMMON NAME ■ Poison ivy

Naturopaths have always used the homeopathic preparation of the leaves. Dr. Bastyr commonly used either a 6X or 12X potency for rheumatic and connective tissue pain, especially in cases where the pain is decreased by motion. Motion improves the blood supply of nutrients to the connective tissue. The physiological picture of *Rhus toxicodendrum* is one of edema and itching. The itching is caused by the phenolic antigen, urushiol. Edema can occur in the system when the capillary exchange network is inadequate to pick up excess tissue fluid or when it deposits excess fluid as the result of inflammation-induced osmolality imbalances. *Rhus toxicodendrum* is helpful in these cases. I also remember one instance in which Dr. Bastyr prescribed a 200X potency of *Rhus toxicodendrum* for a severe case of herpes zoster. It was helpful in this case.

Apis mellifera

COMMON NAME ■ Bee sting

Dr. Bastyr spoke extensively about the homeopathic use of *Apis* for inflammation in connective or dermal tissues. In addition, I have used *Apis* as an antirheumatic in cases of stubborn edema secondary to bruise-type trauma in which the edema persists for a prolonged time. Dr. Bastyr said to use a 3X to 6X potency several times daily. I have found that *Apis* is slow acting but persistent. I have used *Apis* homeopathically for cysts and for general edema or swelling. Sometimes cysts will respond to a 6X potency of *Apis* used three times daily for up to 3 months.

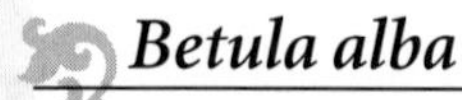

Betula alba

COMMON NAME ■ White birch

Use the young leaves and the bark to make medicine. *Betula* contains flavonoids such as hyperoside, as well as quercetin and luteolin flavonoids combined with sugar groups. The probable antirheumatic effect derives from the methyl salicylate content in the oil of the plant.

Betula is a diuretic, which may account for its use in treating edematous swellings and the pain of rheumatism. One can think of using *Betula* much as one would use aspirin. I prescribe 60 drops of tincture three times daily. I also use quaking aspen and poplar for rheumatic symptoms. Both contain salicylates.

The advantage of using salicylate-containing herbs rather than aspirin is that the herbs contain a variety of flavonoids, minerals, and other secondary plant constituents that are generally good for the body. For example, the quercetin glycosides in *Betula* stop inflammation caused by the production of hydroperoxy fatty acids and leukotrienes by the mast cells. Given the salicylate and quercetin content of this plant, one can see that *Betula* decreases inflammation by at least two pathways.

CHAPTER

15

ANTISEPTICS

CHAPTER • OUTLINE

Calendula officinalis
Oxyquinoline sulfate
Creosote
Hypericum perforatum
Guaiacum officinale
Potassium permanganate
Hydrogen peroxide
Sulfur flowers
Gnaphalium uliginosum
Hydrastis canadensis
Valeriana officinalis
Nasturtium officinale
Glycyrrhiza glabra typica
Iodine
Rum

Antiseptics inhibit the action of microorganisms, thereby preventing infection. This category principally focuses on remedies that are applied to the surface of the skin or mucous membranes. This section includes a number of materials that are not botanicals. These materials were discussed by Dr. Bastyr in class and were commonly used by naturopaths in the 1960s and 1970s when Dr. Bastyr was practicing.

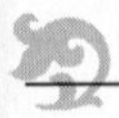

Calendula officinalis

COMMON NAME ■ Marigold

The flowers are used to make medicine. *Calendula* contains calendulin, carotenoids, which are saponins that yield oleanolic acid after hydrolysis, and a bitter principle called caledin. It also contains the flavonoids isorhamnetin and quercetin. *Calendula* is useful against most of the common pathogenic bacteria that frequent the throat, including *Staphylococcal* and *Streptococcal* organisms. Dr. Bastyr taught us that *Calendula* tincture is excellent as a throat swab. He suggested swabbing the throat three to four times daily. This tincture may also be applied to skin infections with good benefit. Dr. Bastyr also taught us that *Calendula* tincture, added to water, could be used as an antiseptic vaginal douche for bacterial vaginitis.

Oxyquinoline sulfate

COMMON NAMES ■ Kollesol, Collesol, Sulfax

This material is a sulfate of the coal tar derivative, quinoline. Oxyquinoline sulfate was very popular among the naturopaths of Dr. Bastyr's time, especially mixed in water to make an antiseptic vaginal douche for bacterial vaginitis. The dose he recommended was 1 to 4 grains mixed in a cup of water. He said to have the patient douche once daily for 3 days. I have treated several intractable cases of vaginitis using oxyquinoline sulfate douches with good results.

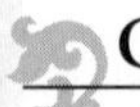

Creosote

A main component of creosote is creosol, which occurs in beechwood tar. External applications are used for their antibacterial and antifungal effects. Coal tar derivatives have been used to treat psoriasis, although I prefer other less smelly applications.

Dr. Boucher from Canada once told me about the use of coal oil on severe frostbite. He spoke of a man whose hands were black from frostbite. What saved his hands from certain amputation was the application of coal oil or stove oil to the hands. The same was done for his feet. Dr. Boucher was one of the founders of the National College of Naturopathic Medicine. He traveled from Vancouver, British Columbia, to Seattle to teach when I was a first- and second-year student at NCNM in 1972-1973. He taught willingly, enthusiastically, and without pay, as did the other naturopaths of his day. His lectures were incredibly inspiring.

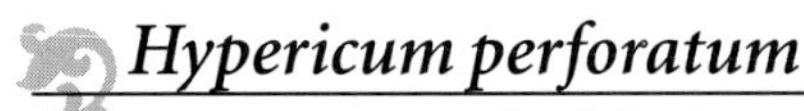

Hypericum perforatum

COMMON NAME ■ St. John's wort

Use the flowering tops and leaves to make medicine. The antibacterial property of *Hypericum* is attributed to the acylphloroglucinol, hyperforin.[42] Apply *Hypericum* tincture externally three times daily as an antiseptic to treat bacterial skin infections. *Hypericum* is also a useful diuretic. The diuretic dose is 20 to 30 drops of tincture three times daily.

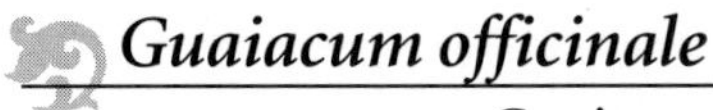

Guaiacum officinale

COMMON NAME ■ Guaiacum

One of the active constituents of *Guaiacum* is guaiacol, which is part of the resin from this plant. This antiseptic is useful in otitis externa and otitis media. Dr. Bastyr said that the dose is low, 1 to 2 drops of tincture in the ear twice daily. The tincture can also be used on skin conditions. I use a drop or two in the mouth for sore throat. Curiously, it tastes rather good.

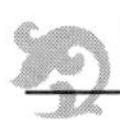

Potassium permanganate

The chemical formula for potassium permanganate is $KMnO_4$. Potassium permanganate is the potassium salt of permanganic acid. It is bactericidal, fungicidal, astringent, and oxidizing. Dr. Bastyr said that it is useful as an antiseptic douche and is also applied locally to wounds to treat infection. In addition, he used it as a gastric lavage for bacterial sepsis in the colon.

Hydrogen peroxide

The chemical formula for hydrogen peroxide is H_2O_2. Hydrogen peroxide is applied to wounds to "boil them out." Repeat this application as long as the boiling action persists. Dr. Bastyr taught us that this remedy could be used in otitis media to clear the ear canal and as an antibiotic. It may be put in a spray bottle and used as a household spray on moldy or dirty areas to kill organisms. It also loosens dirt to help clean surfaces or areas between tiles, which may be helpful for mold-sensitive individuals. The body makes hydrogen peroxide from superoxide by an enzymatic process involving superoxide dismutase.

Sulfur flowers

Sulfur flowers are antiseptic. Dr. Bastyr taught that sulfur flowers could be used in an ointment base for scabies. A 3X homeopathic potency is used for intense itching. This is our great sporicide. For scabies I recommend using Kwell, a product manufactured by Reedco, Inc. Although this remedy is allopathic, scabies is so miserable, causes so much inconvenience, and is so contagious that I like to choose a remedy that I know will be effective.

Gnaphalium uliginosum

COMMON NAME ■ Marsh cudweed

The whole plant is used to make medicine. *Gnaphalium* is used as an antiseptic for catarrhal pharyngitis. Herbalists have recommended a dose of 1 to 3 mL of the tincture, gargled and swallowed. Dr. Bastyr said that *Gnaphalium* is a good antitussive. I can't remember his dosage recommendations or any other specifics.

Hydrastis canadensis

COMMON NAME ■ Goldenseal

The root is used to make medicine. This wonderful plant is useful for skin infections including *Staphylococcus* infection. I recommend applying it four times daily for this purpose. For thrush, apply a pinch of powder in the mouth. It works very well. Internally, *Hydrastis* is a great antimicrobial. I use 30 drops of the tincture four times daily. More may be used depending on the case.

Valeriana officinalis

COMMON NAME ■ Valerian

Use the root to make medicine. The alkaloids chatine and valerine have been shown to possess antibacterial activity against gram-positive bacteria. The Thompson Indians of British Columbia pulverized roots between stones and applied the mash to injuries. I've used the same technique in the mountains. Dry roots were used as an antiseptic and the leaves were applied to cuts and wounds as poultices.

Nasturtium officinale

COMMON NAME ■ Watercress

The flowering aerial parts are used to make medicine. *Nasturtium* contains a glucosinolate called glucotropaeolin. This material, when hydrolyzed, releases benzyl isothiocyanate, which is a known antibacterial and antifungal.[26] This is an antiseptic herb. *Nasturtium* seeds are used in preparations to fight worms. The seeds contain high levels of erucic acid, which makes them somewhat toxic.

Nasturtium also functions as a heart tonic. Dr. Bastyr said that the general dose is $\frac{1}{2}$ teaspoon of fresh juice three times daily. *Nasturtium* flowers are great in salads. In conversations with herbalists, I have learned that *Nasturtium* tea mixed with honey and lemon is a terrific cough medicine.

I have little experience with this plant and include it for historical reference. Unfortunately, while talking about *Nasturtium*, we were sidetracked into a conversation with Dr. Bastyr about his Nubian goats and the wonderful milk he got from them. Frankly, I can't remember what else he said about *Nasturtium* after that.

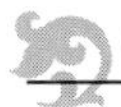

Glycyrrhiza glabra typica

COMMON NAME ■ Licorice root

The roots and rhizome are used to make medicine. Topically, isoflavanoid compounds of licorice are useful against *Candida* and *Staphylococcus aureus*. Licorice decreases sepsis caused by severe burns. This can be lifesaving in severe cases. I use licorice internally for coughs as a moisturizing expectorant and antiseptic. It is excellent for this. The dose I prescribe is 30 drops of the fluid extract twice daily. Licorice is a plant that has so many uses that it could appear in probably a third of the medicinal categories in this book.

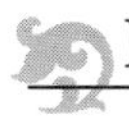

Iodine

Used topically, povidone iodine is a great antiseptic against almost all microbes. It is available in ointment form. I often mix iodine ointment with zinc cream, vitamin A cream, and tea tree ointment as a general antimicrobial vulnerary treatment.

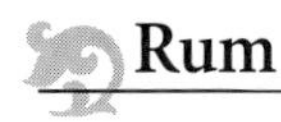

Rum

Dr. Bastyr mentioned the use of good old, 151-proof rum as a topical antiseptic for wounds when nothing else was available. One ounce can be put in a little juice and given for internal use for undue pain.

CHAPTER

16

ANTISPASMODICS

CHAPTER • OUTLINE

Conium maculatum
Solanum carolinense
Datura stramonium
Urba delpasmo
Strychnos castelnaei
Oenanthe crocata
Atropa belladonna
Gelsemium sempervirens
Passiflora incarnata
Ammi visnaga
Dioscorea villosa
Lobelia inflata
Hyoscyamus niger
Matricaria chamomilla
Piscidia erythrina
Petasites hybridus

Antispasmodics are remedies that relieve contractions and cramps in both smooth and skeletal muscles.

Conium maculatum

COMMON NAME ■ Poison hemlock

The whole plant is used to make medicine. *CAUTION: This plant is tremendously poisonous.* It was used to execute criminals in ancient Greece. Socrates is thought to have been executed this way. Evidently, he was convicted of thinking. The plant contains several nicotine-like alkaloids such as coniine and conhydrine, as well as an alkaloid called gamma-coniceine. *Conium* was used to treat painful spasms by eclectic physicians during the late 19th and early 20th centuries. This antispasmodic has been prescribed when there are nervous and jerky muscular movements. Dr. Bastyr said that a tincture dose of 1 drop is used; however, a 3X potency may be safer. He recommended *Conium* homeopathically for Landry's paralysis. In addition, Dr. Sarkar suggests *Conium* 200X potency for bicycle rider's prostatitis.[91]

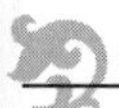

Solanum carolinense

COMMON NAMES ■ Horse nettle, Bull nettle

Use the whole plant and root to make medicine. *Solanum* contains the steroid alkaloid, solanidine, which may have an effect on the smooth and/or skeletal muscles. It also contains the alkaloid solanine, which has been categorized as a sedative and an anticonvulsant. Use this remedy for treating coughs, epilepsy, pertussis, eclampsia, and convulsions. It is antispasmodic and antitussive. Dr. Bastyr used 15 to 30 drops of tincture three times daily. I mix *Solanum* with other appropriate plants such as licorice or gumweed for the treatment of coughs. Dr. Bastyr recommended higher doses for Parkinson's palsy.

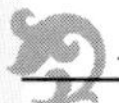

Datura stramonium

COMMON NAME ■ Jimsonweed

The leaves and seeds are used to make medicine. This plant is similar biochemically to belladonna in that it contains atropine and scopolamine. *Datura* also contains a significant amount of the anticholinergic alkaloid hyoscyamine. *Datura* is an anticholinergic, a sedative, an antispasmodic, an anodyne, a narcotic, and a hallucinogenic. It quiets peristaltic intestinal contractions. Eclectic physicians used *Datura* for asthma, paralysis agitans, and Sydenham's chorea. The dose of *Datura* as an antispasmodic is 2 drops of tincture two times daily. Dr. Bastyr taught us that *Datura* could be used for the chronic alcoholic who talks to himself/herself. While it won't stop the behavior, it will allow the person to enjoy the conversation a lot more.

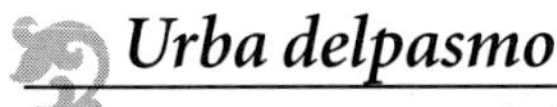

Urba delpasmo

COMMON NAME ■ Aplopappus

Dr. Bastyr said that this antispasmodic is used to treat hysteria, convulsions, and epilepsy. A standard infusion is used. I don't know how to find this plant or whether its name has been changed; it is included for historical purposes.

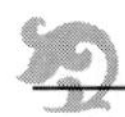

Strychnos castelnaei

COMMON NAME ■ Curare

The bark of this plant is used to make medicine. *CAUTION: Large doses will paralyze the patient.* The constituent tubocurarine chloride is responsible for the paralyzing effect on voluntary muscles. This plant decreases the activity of motor nerves and decreases peristalsis by sedating smooth muscles. I advise using the homeopathic preparation of curare. Dr. Bastyr used a 3X to 30X potency. If using the tincture, he recommended $\frac{1}{4}$ drop daily.

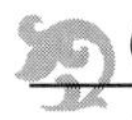

Oenanthe crocata

COMMON NAME ■ Hemlock

The root is used to make medicine. *Oenanthe* contains toxic nicotine-like alkaloids such as coniine, gamma-coniceine, and conhydrine. In addition, it contains a long-chain acetylenic alcohol, oenanthotoxin, and a less toxic long-chain acetylenic ketone, oenanthetone.

Dr. Bastyr taught us to use this remedy in a 3X to 6X homeopathic preparation for seizures associated with petit mal epilepsy. It is given four times daily. Many patients who have seizures will be taking phenobarbitol or dilantin. If so, supplementing magnesium and vitamin B_6 will help offset the toxic effects of these drugs.

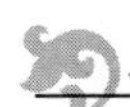

Atropa belladonna

COMMON NAME ■ Deadly nightshade

The root and leaves are used to make medicine. This plant is a smooth muscle antispasmodic. I give the tincture in doses of 10 drops several times daily for chronic intestinal cramping. I have used this plant primarily for spastic colon disease. In emergency medicine, atropine, an alkaloid from belladonna, is given subcutaneously at a dose of 1 mg for intestinal obstruction deemed life threatening.

Gelsemium sempervirens

COMMON NAME ■ Yellow jasmine

The root is used to make medicine. *CAUTION: Gelsemium should be avoided for patients with congestive heart failure and for elderly patients whose hearts are simply too weak. Gelsemium* is an energetic antispasmodic. Dr. Bastyr used 30 drops of *Gelsemium* tincture for women in labor in whom the cervical os would not dilate. At first it stimulates, then depresses, much like *Conium* or tobacco. As a general antispasmodic, Dr. Bastyr used 1 to 5 drops of the tincture twice daily. I add *Gelsemium* to antispasmodic formulas rather than using it alone. A good smooth muscle antispasmodic formula that I've developed and use is two parts belladonna, one part *Gelsemium*, five parts *Dioscorea*, and six parts *Hydrangea*. I give this tincture mixture in doses of 20 drops four times daily. The formula may look a little strange, but it works well.

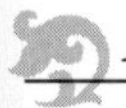

Passiflora incarnata

COMMON NAME ■ Passionflower

The whole plant is used to make medicine. The harman compounds in *Passiflora* act as monoamine oxidase inhibitors. The plant also contains oxy-coumarins. Coumarins have been noted for their potential antispasmodic properties. Dr. Bastyr recommended the use of *Passiflora* for childhood convulsions, tetanus-type convulsions, and repeated seizure activity. All of these are serious problems, and accurate diagnosis is required. For these conditions, *Passiflora* is used as an adjunctive therapy. *Passiflora* can be sweetened with $\frac{1}{2}$ teaspoon of glycine to increase its calming effect.

Ammi visnaga

COMMON NAME ■ Khella

The seeds are used for medicine. The most active constituent in khella is khellin. In addition, khella contains two other crystalline compounds, visnagin and khellol glucoside. Khella is extremely bitter and yet has a curious flowery taste. It is antispasmodic and relaxes the smooth muscle of tubular structures such as the bronchi, stomach, intestines, ureter, bladder, and uterus. Dr. Bastyr mentioned its use for bronchial asthma or bronchitis. For the above conditions, I give 30 to 60 drops of khella three times daily.

For relaxation of the ureter, I mix equal parts of the tinctures of khella and *Hydrangea*. The dose is 120 drops of the mixture three times daily. This combination is useful for passing kidney stones that are smaller than 7 mm.

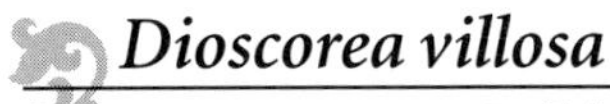

Dioscorea villosa

COMMON NAME ■ Wild yam

The root is used for medicine. *Dioscorea* is antispasmodic and relaxes the muscles of the gastrointestinal tract. Dr. Bastyr suggested 30 drops of tincture two to three times daily. For a stronger antispasmodic effect on the intestines, I combine *Dioscorea* with a little belladonna. I mix 30 drops of *Dioscorea* with 10 drops of belladonna. Give this mixture twice daily.

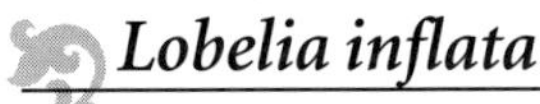

Lobelia inflata

COMMON NAMES ■ Lobelia, Indian tobacco

The whole plant is used to make medicine. *Lobelia* contains many alkaloids, three of which are lobeline, lobelanidine, and lobelanine. Lobeline is the most important antispasmodic constituent. Dr. Bastyr used *Lobelia* as an antispasmodic in asthma and bronchospasm. The dose of the tincture is 5 to 10 drops twice daily. In severe asthma, he recommended a dose of 30 drops of *Lobelia* to stop status asthmaticus. He also recommended mixing *Capsicum* with *Lobelia* to improve its antispasmodic effects.

Dr. Bastyr mentioned the use of *Lobelia* in natural childbirth to lessen the strength of uterine contractions. For infantile colic, he taught us to mix 5 drops of *Lobelia* in $\frac{1}{3}$ cup of water and give this a teaspoon at a time throughout the day. The old Thompsonian herbalists used excessive doses of *Lobelia* as a purgative. It was given basically in toxic doses to induce vomiting.

Hyoscyamus niger

COMMON NAME ■ Henbane

Dr. Bastyr suggested that we obtain the medicine from the second-year growth of the flowering tops and roots of *Hyoscyamus*. This plant contains hyoscyamine. The alkaloids in henbane are synthesized in the roots, and although the alkaloids are transported throughout the plant, the highest concentration is in the roots. The foul odor of henbane is caused by tetramethylputrescine. In addition to alkaloids, a number of pyrrolidines such as hygrine are found in the roots. Henbane is antispasmodic to the smooth muscles of the gastrointestinal tract. Dr. Bastyr taught us that it is also a useful remedy for uterine cramps. His suggested dose was 5 to 10 drops twice daily. I have found that in most cases the dose of the tincture is quite variable, depending on the individual patient, and can often be increased.

Matricaria chamomilla

COMMON NAME ■ German chamomile

The dried flowers are used to make medicine. Several of the active constituents in *Matricaria* are bisabolol sesquiterpenes. These constituents may account for the antispasmodic action of this plant. *Matricaria* is sedative and antispasmodic to the gastrointestinal tract. I have found it to be useful in spastic colitis. I prescribe 90 drops of tincture three times daily for this condition.

Dr. Ed Madison, who was one of my classmates, has pointed out that German research has demonstrated this plant's ability to reduce blood urea nitrogen levels. The dose is 120 drops three times daily.

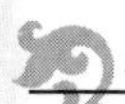

Piscidia erythrina

COMMON NAME ■ Jamaican dogwood

The bark is used to make medicine. One of the active constituents of *Piscidia* is piscidic acid. *Piscidia* is an excellent uterine antispasmodic for dysmenorrhea. I use this remedy frequently and with confidence for painful cramping during menstrual periods. In my opinion, its best use is for relief of uterine cramping. Here it is positively curative. I give 2 capsules every 2 hours until full relief is attained. This is frequently accomplished with the first dose. *Piscidia* may also be used for myalgia caused by muscle spasms in low back syndromes. I have found it useful in cases of viral myalgia, such as one would find in flu. The dose for this purpose is 1 capsule four times daily. Dr. Ed Madison introduced me to this plant.

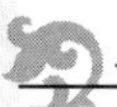

Petasites hybridus

COMMON NAME ■ Butterbur

Also look for this plant under the name *Petasites officinalis.* Butterbur is a member of the daisy family, *Compositae.* The whole plant is used to make medicine. Butterbur is a spasmolytic, effective for both gastrointestinal cramps and ureter spasms. I would suggest giving high doses of this plant. An excellent way to use butterbur is 30 drops of the tincture hourly until relief is attained. Thankfully, it has a pleasant taste.

CHAPTER

17

ANTIVIRALS

CHAPTER • OUTLINE

Allium sativum
Glycyrrhiza glabra typica
Zinc
Tabebuia impetiginosa
Bioflavonoids
Heat
Melissa officinalis
Camellia sinensis

Antiviral remedies fight viral infections. The list of antiviral remedies has grown over the last decade as a result of an immense amount of research directed at viral infections, especially immune-compromising viruses such as human immunodeficiency virus (HIV). This research has spilled over into the plant medicine realm as well. I do not remember Dr. Bastyr talking about antiviral remedies as a separate category. Instead he discussed remedies that were effective against colds and flu, childhood viral disorders, herpes zoster, and polio. All of these conditions are recognized as disorders caused by viruses. The antiviral remedies discussed by Dr. Bastyr, as well as other antiviral remedies, are presented here as a separate category for the practitioner's convenience.

Allium sativum

COMMON NAME ■ Garlic

One may also use *Allium campanulatum*. Garlic is from the lily family, *Liliaceae*. The bulb is used for medicine. Garlic oil contains sulfur compounds such as allicin, which is the material responsible for the plant's odor. Garlic is a good source of organic sulfur.

Garlic oil is useful in otitis media caused by bacterial or viral infection. Macerated garlic can be applied topically to wounds to prevent infection. I prescribe both fresh garlic and garlic oil in capsule form for the treatment of viral disorders. I give 5 cloves four times daily, or 2 capsules three times daily, for colds and flu. When confronted with an infection, whether viral, rickettsial, bacterial, or fungal, I usually find garlic to be useful. I give garlic together with a handful of other antimicrobial medicines that I have chosen for the specific case. I think along these same lines with *Echinacea*. Both of these medicines are good general antimicrobials and, as far as I have experienced, go well with other prescribed botanicals.

Murray and Pizzorno have done a nice job of summarizing the effects of garlic in *The Encyclopedia of Natural Medicine*.[92] They include hypotensive effects, antitumor effects, antiviral effects, and anthelmintic effects, a use for garlic that goes back to the Egyptian medical papyrus dating to about 1550 BC.[19]

Glycyrrhiza glabra typica

COMMON NAME ■ Licorice root

The roots and rhizome are used to make medicine. Licorice demonstrated antiviral effects against herpes I, polio, DNA and RNA viruses, and Newcastle disease.[43] Glycyrrhetic acid is one of the main constituents in licorice root. Ed Madison, ND, said to apply glycyrrhetic acid compounds to the mouth four times daily for relief from canker sores. I use licorice as a main ingredient in my upper respiratory formula for viral bronchitis. My formula is two parts licorice fluid extract, mixed with two parts *Grindelia* tincture, one part *Sanguinaria* tincture, one part *Tussilago* tincture, and 50 drops lomatium isolate. I mix the above in a 2-ounce dropper bottle and prescribe 90 drops four times daily.

I use licorice root almost daily in my practice. It has a wide range of benefits, most notably its ability to increase one's energy and sense of well-being while fighting disease. This uplifting effect should not be missed and is probably caused by the ability of licorice root to prolong the half-life of adrenal hormones. Licorice root is also excellent for allergies.

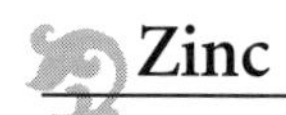

Zinc

One study I read long ago, for which I cannot recall the source, mentioned the virostatic activity of zinc by inhibition of viral replication by means of polypeptide cleavage inhibition. The study reported 85% to 90% inhibition of viral replication in vitro with 3 mg zinc chloride. Zinc is often forgotten in the management of colds and flu. It should be included in the daily multiple vitamin and supplemented further at the very first sign of upper respiratory distress. Make sure that the multiple vitamin/mineral that the patient takes contains at least 25 mg of zinc. Daily use of zinc helps to prevent colds and flu. At the first sign of upper respiratory distress, I prescribe 100 to 200 mg of zinc daily for the duration of the cold and flu. In addition to zinc, Dr. Bastyr recommended cod liver oil daily as a viral disease preventive.

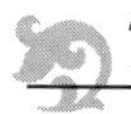

Tabebuia impetiginosa

COMMON NAMES ■ Taheebo, Pau'Darco, Bowstick

Look for this plant also under the name *Tecoma curialis*. The medicine is made from the inner bark of the LaPacho tree. The active constituents in taheebo are a host of quinones divided into two general types, the anthrequinones and the naphthoquinones. The anthrequinones and naphthoquinones in taheebo are as follows[93]:

Naphthoquinones: Lapachol, alpha-lapachone, beta-lapachone, menaquinone-1, and deoxylapachol.

Anthraquinones: 2-acetoxymethylanthroquinone, anthraquinone-2-aldehyde, 2-hydroxymethylanthraquinone, 1-hydroxyanthraquinone, and 1-methoxyanthraquinone.

Of some interest to me is the use of taheebo in fighting viruses. It has been shown that this plant, especially its beta-lapachone and lapachol, is active against a number of viruses, particularly herpes type I and II, influenza virus, vesicular stomatitis, and polio virus.[94,95] It is no wonder that taheebo has gained favor with native peoples in South America as a medicinal plant. Taheebo has been used by the natives of South America to help cure acute and chronic illness. According to the writers who have spoken to native peoples, the tea of the bark seems to have antiviral and antineoplastic activity. Taheebo can be used against *Candida*, although I prefer oregano oil at a dose of 1 capsule twice daily.

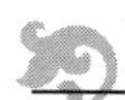

Bioflavonoids

The berry and vegetable bioflavonoids are particularly useful in the general prevention of illness. In viral diseases I have found that it is useful to give the bioflavonoids together with vitamin C and cod liver oil. In my opinion, one probable modus operandi of bioflavonoids is to strengthen the interstitial tissue and prevent rampant spread of viral particles. I use berry anthocyanins, rutin, hesperidan, and pycnogenol either alone or in combination as a daily supplement. I have found that the incidence of disease decreases when using these materials. Patients frequently tell me that their colds resolved faster and were far less severe than when not taking the bioflavonoids.

Heat

I cannot resist the obvious. Patients will sometimes run low-grade fevers during viral flu. I encourage this temperature elevation by giving hot fluids and keeping the patient bundled up. This philosophy opposes that of well-meaning doctors who encourage the use of aspirin or acetaminophen at the first sign of fever. Viruses do not like heat. Saunas can be useful in treating viral disease if plenty of replacement water and electrolytes are given adjunctively.

A study by Steve McDougal at the Centers for Disease Control and Prevention in Atlanta showed that exposing the acquired immunodeficiency syndrome to heat at 140°F to 155°F kills it.[96] The amount of time needed to kill the virus at 150°F is just a couple of minutes.[96] The obvious problem with simply running the blood through a temperature circuit is that this virus resides in many tissues in addition to the bloodstream. Whereas the viral load may be temporarily decreased, the virus is likely to return, seeded by particles residing in the tissues.

I have found that most common cold and flu viruses respond well to the following regimen. I have the patient drink 3 cups of hot yarrow tea and bundle up in a sleeping bag or extra covers to increase the body temperature. I have the patient smear Vicks VapoRub, a product manufactured by Procter & Gamble, liberally on the head, chest, and neck. The patient then spends the night sweating. The patient generally wakes up much improved. I have been practicing medicine for 25 years and have only missed half a day of work partly because every time I am coming down with something I follow the above procedure exactly.

Once when I was at Dr. Bastyr's clinic, I remember seeing an elderly woman wrapped in a mummy bag, lying down on a table with hot water bottles surrounding her. Dr. Bastyr was using hyperthermia to treat her. She had cancer. Application of heat was very important in Dr. Bastyr's practice. He used infrared lamps, hot-pack applications, diathermy, and ultrasound. I have followed in that tradition by realizing the importance of heat application as a therapeutic modality in the treatment of disease.

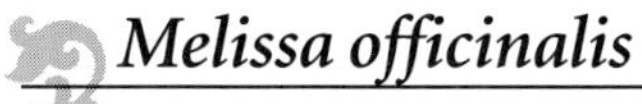

Melissa officinalis

COMMON NAME ■ Lemon balm

The dried aerial parts are used to make medicine. A preparation of this lovely plant is helpful in treating mouth herpes. A lemon balm salve is applied four times daily. I have found that patients do quite well on this preparation. Lemon balm tea can be consumed internally for colds and flu. I mix 30 drops of lemon balm tincture with equal parts of yarrow tincture in a cup of hot water. This is taken twice daily. The oil contains citral a, citral b, and citronellal, which give lemon balm its lemon odor.

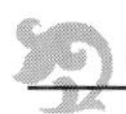

Camellia sinensis

COMMON NAMES ■ Green tea, Black tea

The leaves contain the active principles. The theaflavins occur in black tea and are oxidation products of green tea catechins. Green tea polyphenols and black tea theaflavins are strong inhibitors of HIV-reverse transcriptase.[54] For the polyphenols to be effective HIV-reverse transcriptase inhibitors, it is essential for a galloyl moiety to be present in the catechin or theaflavin structure. Especially effective are (-)-epicatechin gallate and (-)-epigallocatechin gallate, both of which have a galloyl moiety in their structure.[54] Because HIV-reverse transcriptase is an enzyme unique to retroviruses and is requisite for retroviral infection, the inhibition of this enzyme is an appropriate target in the fight against acquired immunodeficiency syndrome.

I have the patient take 2 capsules of decaffeinated green tea polyphenols three times daily. The dose may be increased if the patient tolerates the capsules well. It is also helpful to drink a high-quality green and black tea combination. I have the patient take a green tea bag and a black tea bag and infuse them in 2 cups of boiling hot water. Let the teabags sit in the water for 15 minutes while the water is cooling. This tea solution can then be consumed. Do not add milk to this tea as it binds to the polyphenols and may affect the potency of the medicine.

CHAPTER

18

ASTRINGENTS

CHAPTER • OUTLINE

Argentum nitrate
Alum
Quercus robur
Uncaria gambir
Krameria triandra
Pterocarpus marsupium
Hamamelis virginiana
Coffea arabica
Rubus species
Commiphora abyssinica
Camellia sinensis

Astringents are agents that cause contraction of tissue. Tannins in these plants, which precipitate the proteins with which they come into contact, may accomplish this. Astringents often reduce mucous membrane secretions. Because astringents are contracting, they are often antihemorrhagic. There are many astringents. I have listed some of them in the section entitled Gastrointestinal Tonics, Astringents, Stimulants. Following are a group of the more active astringents.

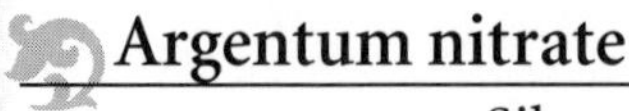

Argentum nitrate

COMMON NAME ■ Silver nitrate

This remedy is an astringent and an antigonorrheic. A 1% to 2% solution is dropped in the newborn's eye to prevent infection at childbirth. This practice is being revised. The solution is used as an antiseptic and an astringent when applied to lesions of the skin.

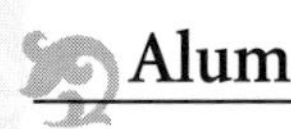

Alum

Alum is prepared from bauxite and sulfuric acid, with the addition of ammonium or potassium. Alum is a local styptic and astringent. It is used principally as an astringent to contract mucous membranes. Dr. Bastyr said that alum is used in cases where there is atony of the mucous membranes. He said that a gargle of 1% to 5% solution is used. This solution may also be used as a douche. Because there are many good plant astringents, I consider this an unnecessary, and a somewhat toxic, astringent. It is mentioned here only for its historical interest as an extremely powerful astringent. I generally discourage using any preparation containing aluminum. Although Dr. Bastyr taught about alum in class, I am not sure that he used it for his own patients.

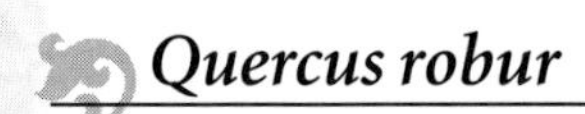

Quercus robur

COMMON NAME ■ Oak tree

The bark is used to make medicine. Most of the oaks have a very astringent gall. *Quercus* contains a number of tannins as well as gallic acid, which occurs when tannins are hydrolyzed by alkaline or acid reactions. Dr. Bastyr said that *Quercus* is used as an astringent for douches, for gargles, and in the treatment of wounds. It must be diluted to form a gargle. In addition, he said that it has been used in gastrointestinal bleeding when the bleeding is not too severe. *CAUTION: Rule out severe gastrointestinal disease in patients with persistent bleeding or black stools.* I primarily use *Quercus* in annoying and persistent diarrhea. I recommend 20 drops of the tincture three times daily. The old eclectics like Ellingwood used *Quercus* for dysentery and cholera infantum. When Dr. Bastyr taught botanical medicine at the National College of Naturopathic Medicine, he frequently referred to Ellingwood's work.

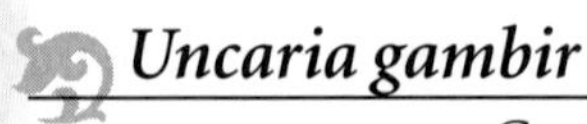

Uncaria gambir

COMMON NAME ■ Gambir

The leaves and twigs are used to make medicine. This is a powerful astringent. Dr. Bastyr taught that this plant is used to contract tissues and check secretions.

He said that it is used as a gargle in pharyngitis or as a mouthwash in stomatitis. Use it three times daily for these conditions. This plant contains tannic acid, as do *Quercus* and many other astringent botanicals. It also contains catechin, which is a bioflavonoid.[97]

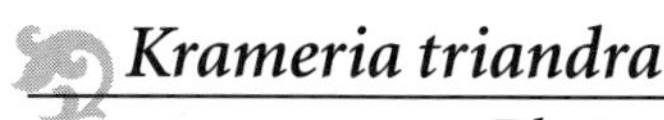

Krameria triandra

COMMON NAME ■ Rhatany

The roots are used to make medicine. The active astringent ingredient in *Krameria* is a *Krameria*–tannic acid. Dr. Bastyr taught the use of this plant topically as an astringent. It is also a good hemostatic. Herbalists have used it in regional ileitis, gastritis, and proctitis. The dose is 20 to 40 drops three times daily. It may be diluted to form an enema for proctitis.

Two benzofuran derivatives from rhatany, ratanhiaphenol I and II, are effective ultraviolet light filters, making this plant potentially useful in sunscreen preparations, perhaps in combination with A*esculus hippocastanum*, or horse chestnut, which also has sunscreen potential. Ed Madison, ND, has done extensive work with *Aesculus* as a sunscreen.

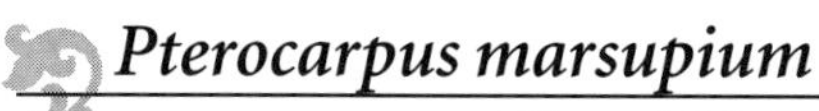

Pterocarpus marsupium

COMMON NAMES ■ Kino, Malabar kino

The bark of the tree is used to make medicine. *Pterocarpus* contains phlobatannins. Dr. Bastyr taught the use of *Pterocarpus* as an astringent for catarrhal inflammations of the mucous membranes. He said to use doses of 10 drops three times daily. I have little experience with this plant, other than having tasted it.

Hamamelis virginiana

COMMON NAME ■ Witch hazel

The leaves, bark, and twigs are used to make medicine. Witch hazel contains a variety of tannins, including gallotannins, ellagitannins, hamamelitannin, and gallic acid. It also contains proanthocyanidins.

Witch hazel may be used internally as an astringent to check bleeding and decrease inflammation. For painful, protruding hemorrhoids, a cloth soaked in a strong witch hazel solution may be applied and left on for an hour or so. Dr. Bastyr also suggested soaking towels in witch hazel and applying them to varicose veins on the legs. He said that an extract of witch hazel could be taken in teaspoon doses three times daily for varicose veins as well. I use large doses of the berry anthocyanins and other bioflavonoids internally for the health of the veins. I have found that hawthorn berry, blueberry, elderberry, and blackberry anthocyanins work well.

A number of authors, such as Kuts-Cheraux,[28] have mentioned a poultice application for postpartum vulval bruising. (Do not forget *Arnica* here as a 6X homeopathic potency taken sublingually.) I mix witch hazel with goldenseal and a little salt and add it to the water of the neti pot to do a sinus rinse in cases of nasopharyngeal catarrh and hyperemic membranes with or without bleeding. A neti pot is a small pot used to irrigate the sinuses.

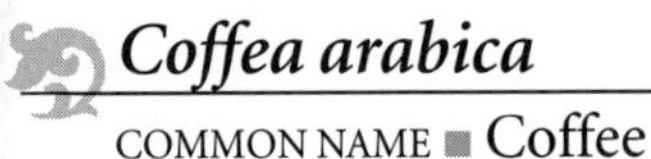

Coffea arabica

COMMON NAME ■ Coffee

The seeds are used to make medicine. The active alkaloid in coffee is caffeine. Coffee can be used as an antidote in many alkaloidal poisonings. It is astringent and may be taken as a strong decoction. Coffee is a tonic to the intestinal tract and colon and may be helpful to stimulate a bowel movement.

If you want to remove coffee from the patient's diet, you should first question the patient about his or her bowel movements. Many patients rely on coffee to help produce a stool and removing it from the diet may result in constipation. I recommend that my patients take fairly high doses of vitamin C and magnesium to offset the constipation caused by removing coffee from their diets.

Rubus species

COMMON NAME ■ Blackberry

Blackberry roots are used to make an astringent medicine. Kuts-Cheraux[28] mentions the curious use of blackberry in gastrointestinal disorders caused by anorexia. Using blackberry root tea for this purpose sounds interesting; however, I have not tried this myself with patients. I have primarily used blackberry leaf tea as a tonic for women, blackberry anthocyanins to relieve venous congestion, and blackberry extract to help stop stubborn cases of diarrhea. For diarrhea, I use a teaspoon of blackberry extract twice daily. Charlie Black, ND, a naturopathic physician in the state of Washington and a 1975 graduate of NCNM, told me about the use of the blackberry preparations for diarrhea.

Commiphora abyssinica

COMMON NAME ■ Myrrh

The resin of this plant is used to make medicine. *Commiphora* is astringent. It contains alpha-, beta-, and gamma-commiphoric resin acids. Dr. Bastyr said that it is useful as a mouthwash in periodontal disease or as an antiseptic mouthwash. He said to use about $\frac{1}{2}$ dram of the tincture in a mouthful of water as a gargle. The remarkable characteristic odor of myrrh comes from furanosesquiterpenes.[98]

Camellia sinensis

COMMON NAME ■ Tea leaves

The leaves are used to make medicine. Most of the black teas are astringents. A strong cup of black tea contains a large number of tannins and is one of the safest astringents. Dr. Bastyr said to apply tea bags to bleeding gums after tooth extractions. Tea contains about one third of the amount of caffeine contained in coffee. It also contains theobromine, which is an alkaloid that has been used to treat asthma. I recommend green tea to my asthmatic patients. I have them steep the dried leaves in hot water for about 5 minutes. The dose is 2 cups of the standard infusion per day.

Green tea polyphenols inhibit the growth of *Streptococcus mutans*, and they also inhibit the extracellular glucosyl-transferase activity of *S. mutans*.[99] These actions may inhibit the formation of dental caries and plaque.

CHAPTER

19

BITTERS

CHAPTER • OUTLINE

Achillea millefolium
Gentiana lutea
Chelone glabra
Centaurium erythraea
Tanacetum vulgare
Marrubium vulgare
Chelidonium majus
Humulus lupulus

Bitters are medicinal agents that have a bitter taste. They are used as digestive tonics, especially for the stomach. They exert tonic effects by a number of mechanisms. For example, they may increase the excitability of the sympathetic nervous system, or they may act by stimulating the appetite. I do not recall Dr. Bastyr talking about bitters as a separate group of remedies.

I have listed bitters below, many of which Dr. Bastyr talked about during the course he taught us in botanical medicine. Recall that during the 19th century, digestive enzyme tablets were not available. The closest thing to a digestive aid was the introduction of ox bile in the early 20th century. Instead of digestive enzyme capsules, herbalists used bitters to stimulate digestion. The use of bitters was especially popular for elderly patients to support failing digestive systems.

Achillea millefolium

COMMON NAME ■ Yarrow

The aerial parts are used to make medicine. *Achillea* contains sesquiterpene lactones, including achillin, achillicin, achillifolin, millefin, dihydroparthenolide, balchanolide, and leucodin.[20,26] *Achillea* was considered a panacea by the Native Americans of the Southwest. It is a plant that has a wide range of actions and uses. I suggest using 20 drops of tincture as a bitter digestive stimulant before main meals.

I use *Achillea* in one way that may be less common. I use it as a bitter for people with elevated blood pressure. I prescribe 30 drops three times daily for this purpose. It is a mild hypotensive and a good bitter to help the gastric phase of digestion. For this I suggest 10 drops of the tincture per meal.

Gentiana lutea

COMMON NAMES ■ Gentian root, Yellow gentian

The underground plant organs and aerial parts are used to make medicine. Dr. Bastyr used to say that *Gentiana* was the best plant to increase the production of hydrochloric acid. One bitter principle in *Gentiana* is gentiopicrin. Gentiopicrin is also an antimalarial. Another bitter principle in *Gentiana* is amarogentin, which is one of the most bitter glucosides known.

Dr. Bastyr advised 10 drops of the tincture at mealtime to promote the production of saliva and gastric juices and to promote duodenal and pancreatic output. It generally tones the digestive system. I like to mix it with *Zingiber* to excite the digestion and warm the stomach. Certainly, hydrochloric acid itself may be given to hypochlorhydric patients, but the naturopathic idea is to try to improve the patient's own ability to produce hydrochloric acid in response to a protein-containing meal.

Chelone glabra

COMMON NAME ■ Balmony

The fresh, flowering herb is used to make medicine. Herbalists teach that this bitter is useful for stimulating digestion and aiding in liver function. Strong liver function is essential for a healthy appetite and for processing absorbed nutrients. This is why the appetite is lacking in patients who have liver cancer. The body simply cannot handle the nutrients that are absorbed. *Chelone* can be taken in doses of 60 drops of tincture at mealtimes. A good tincture of *Chelone* will have a peppery taste when held on the tongue. I suggest that a combination of equal parts of bromelain and curcumin be taken at mealtimes as well.

Bromelain is an excellent proteolytic enzyme, whereas *Curcuma longa* is one of the best liver antioxidants.

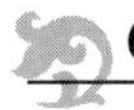

Centaurium erythraea

COMMON NAME ■ Centaury

Also look for this plant under the name *Centaurium umbellatum.* It was formerly called *Erythaea centaurium.* The aerial parts of the flowering plant are used to make medicine. The bitter principles in centaury are the secoiridoids. These include sweroside, centapicrin, swertiamarin, and others. Centaury is a classic bitter that can be counted on to enhance gastric motility and stimulate gastric secretions. It is used for sluggish digestion. I use 30 to 60 drops of the tincture per meal to aid digestion.

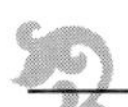

Tanacetum vulgare

COMMON NAME ■ Tansy

The dried leaves and flowering top are used to make medicine. *CAUTION: Avoid during pregnancy. Tanacetum* oil contains thujone, which is also found in the cedar tree. I use this bitter in small doses, for example, 5 drops of tincture per meal, to aid digestion. In addition, *Tanacetum* can be used in large doses to kill worms.

Marrubium vulgare

COMMON NAME ■ White horehound

The whole plant is used to make medicine. *Marrubium* contains a bitter diterpene lactone called marrubiin. *Marrubium* numbs the tongue. As a bitter and tonic to most of the digestive tract, 15 drops of the tincture are taken per meal. Herbalists teach that doses of 30 drops in a cup of hot water promote diuresis and diaphoresis. *Marrubium* can also be used as a respiratory remedy.

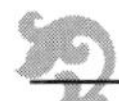

Chelidonium majus

COMMON NAMES ■ Greater celandine, Tetterwort

The whole plant is used to make medicine. I use *Chelidonium* frequently. This bitter remedy is famous in the arena of hepatic disorders. Many practitioners miss the opportunity to use it as a bitter and digestive stimulant. This plant helps in sluggish liver conditions such as Gilbert's syndrome or in conditions in which the liver is overtaxed. Remember that when the liver is functioning poorly, digestive function will be depressed. The body will react to liver congestion either by diarrhea or by decreasing appetite. Nausea may also be present. I recommend 15 drops of *Chelidonium* per meal as a digestive bitter and stimulant. *Chelidonium* is a five-star remedy. Dr. Bastyr suggested that we use *Chelidonium* and *Chionanthus* together to improve liver function.

Chelidonium has a wonderfully complex bittersweet characteristic. It contains chelerythrine, chelidonic acid, and chelidonine. Chelidonine has been looked at for its reverse transcriptase activity.

Humulus lupulus

COMMON NAME ■ Hops

Known as a flavoring agent in beer, hops can be used as a bitter or, in larger doses, as a calmative and a hypnotic. Beta-myrcene, humulene, and a number of other constituents account for the characteristic bitter taste of hops. When using hops as a bitter, I suggest 15 drops per meal.

I could discuss many other bitters; however, the above list will give the practitioner various herb choices that can be used to improve digestion and the management of food.

CHAPTER

20

CALMATIVES

CHAPTER • OUTLINE

I have chosen to include several remedies under the category of calmatives because this category suggests something other than sedatives. A calmative quiets the restless energy of the body in a gentle way, without the drugged aftereffect that is frequently felt after taking a sedative. Dr. Bastyr did not cover a group of remedies called calmatives; however, he did lecture about most of these remedies at other times.

Glycine

Glycine is an amino acid. It is the shortest and simplest amino acid in nature, occurring in all protein-containing foods. The reader may find it interesting that some scientists who study the origins of living matter think that glycine may be one of the first molecules formed 4 billion years ago.

There are glycine receptor sites in the brain and in the spinal cord that respond to glycine by decreasing the activity of the central nervous system. For example, glycine binds to the locus ceruleus in the midbrain, decreasing the release of norepinephrine. The effect is to calm the mind and spirit. Excess activity of the locus ceruleus can lead to feelings of anxiety and panic. The dose of glycine that I recommend is $\frac{1}{2}$ to 2 teaspoons per day. I often prescribe glycine as a calmative before bedtime.

Glycine has a sweet taste and can be used to sweeten other plant medicines. These plant medicines can have a calming effect in and of themselves. They include *Matricaria matricarioides, Matricaria recutita, Passiflora, Scutellaria,* and *Humulus.*

Matricaria matricarioides

COMMON NAMES ■ Pineapple weed, Pineapple mayweed

Also look for this plant under the names *Matricaria discoidea* and *Matricaria suaveolens.* This plant grows in the cracks of sidewalks and driveways and all over the city where other plants cannot grow. It is small and looks like little green pineapples on the end of short stalks. The little pineapple-like tops are used to make medicine. This plant is underused. It is a gentle calmative and strengthens the vital force of the body. I make tea from this plant. I use 3 or 4 tops for 1 cup of tea and recommend drinking 2 cups daily.

Matricaria recutita

COMMON NAME ■ Chamomile

The *Anthemis nobilis* variety, or Roman chamomile, works as well. For hundreds of years this plant has been used as an antispasmodic and a calmative for anxiety. Tea bags are available in most grocery stores. When I prescribe *Matricaria* as a calmative, I recommend 60 drops of the tincture three times daily.

Passiflora incarnata

COMMON NAME ■ Passionflower

The whole plant is used to make medicine. The active ingredients in *Passiflora* include a number of alkaloids, including harmine, harman, harmaline, and harmalol. *Passiflora* also contains a large number of bioflavonoids such as apigenin, kaempferol, and quercetin. Dr. Bastyr talked about *Passiflora* as a calmative. I suggest 90 drops of the tincture three times daily as a calmative. This plant may be combined with other calmatives. For example, I sweeten *Passiflora* with glycine. Dr. Bastyr said that *Passiflora* is useful to help people sleep better. In my own experience with *Passiflora*, I have found that very large doses are required as a sleep aid. I prescribe 1 teaspoon of tincture in a small amount of water at bedtime.

Dr. Ellingwood, an eclectic physician, suggests its use for restless sleep and wakefulness at night. The use of *Passiflora* has not always met my expectations, and patients often come back asking for something stronger. I usually suggest reading oneself back to sleepiness.

Piper methysticum

COMMON NAME ■ Kavakava

The root of this plant is used to make medicine. The active constituents are pyrone derivatives, or kavalactones. It is pretty clear when one takes this plant that it is a calmative. Forty drops of the tincture has a nice calming, almost sedating effect on the body. I have patients use it sparingly and only when really necessary because it is a powerful herb. I give 50 to 60 mg of the standardized kavalactones twice daily as a calmative. I have found that using a 200-mg capsule of the powdered plant twice daily is also sometimes effective.

Ironically, I have found that taking large doses of kava can produce a stimulating effect on the body. This is a personal experience on my part. In one case, when I took very large doses of kava, my muscles became agitated and I wanted to exercise to use up this energy. Having found that kava can act as either a sedative or a stimulant, I would suggest that when prescribing kava for your patients, you follow their progress closely to determine what effect kava has on them.

CHAPTER

21

Cardiac Remedies

CHAPTER • OUTLINE

Cactus grandiflorus
Digitalis purpurea
Strophanthus kombe
Convallaria majalis
Lycopus virginicus
Adonis vernalis
Cytisus scoparius
Apocynum cannabinum
Crataegus oxyacantha
Iberis amara
Nerium oleander
Ammi visnaga
Anemone pulsatilla
Erythroxylum coca
Amyl nitrite
Viola tricolor
Glonoin
Urginea maritima
Helleborus niger

Cardiac remedies affect the heart. Some of these remedies slow the heart rate as they strengthen the heartbeat. Others correct tachycardia, correct arrhythmias, or treat the pain of angina. We were taught to try to improve the strength and function of the heart muscle itself. For this purpose, Dr. Bastyr had some favorite remedies, including *Crateagus oxycantha* and *Cactus grandiflorus.* He used these alone and in combination with other remedies.

In Dr. Bastyr's day, and indeed in the days of the early herbalists both in Europe and in the United States, heart surgery was unknown. Reliance on herbal remedies was critical because there were no choices to fall back on.

I would suggest that the administration of cardiotonics to elderly patients be combined with treatment to improve the strength and integrity of the vascular system. This can be accomplished by giving the patient $\frac{1}{2}$ cup of blueberries daily for 1 month. This provides anthocyanins that improve the strength and resilience of the vascular system.

Cactus grandiflorus

COMMON NAME ■ Night blooming cereus

The flowers are used to make medicine. *Cactus* was one of Dr. Bastyr's favorite remedies. He frequently used it in his own practice and lectured on it extensively. The constituents of this plant include cactoid and cactine. Dr. Bastyr said that *Cactus* could substitute for *Digitalis* as a cardiac remedy; however, the patient must be weaned off *Digitalis* slowly and with careful monitoring. A small amount of *Cactus* may be introduced as the patient is being weaned off *Digitalis.* Dr. Bastyr told us that *Cactus* did not cause the gastrointestinal symptoms found with *Digitalis.*

Cactus can correct an irregular pulse. I use magnesium and potassium together with any cardiac remedy to correct an irregular pulse. I prescribe 100 mg of each three times daily.

Dr. Bastyr said that *Cactus* could be used even with mild valvular lesions. He said that for angina, 10 drops of the tincture of *Cactus* could be given in a little warm water every 10 minutes until the symptoms subsided. When *Cactus* is used as a cardiac tonic, he recommended 10 to 20 drops of the tincture twice daily.

Dr. Bastyr said that *Cactus* could be used in bradycardia because it is an active sympathetic stimulant. He taught us that *Cactus* helps in heart diseases resulting from disordered innervation. It can also be used to help with aortic regurgitation. He said that if the patient feels constriction in the chest, as though iron bands were around it, *Cactus* could help. If these symptoms come on suddenly or for the first time, suspect a medical emergency. It is essential that all cardiac patients be properly diagnosed. This helps the cardiologist and the naturopathic physician make the right choices in the patient's care.

Digitalis purpurea

COMMON NAME ■ Foxglove

The leaves are used to make medicine. *CAUTION: Potassium deficiency increases the toxicity of* Digitalis. Furthermore, it is dangerous to give calcium with *Digitalis* because calcium potentiates the effect of *Digitalis* on the heart. Its main active ingredient is a cardiotonic glycoside called digitoxin.

We should probably pause here to give credit to William Withering, who introduced foxglove as a medicinal agent in 1785.[100] His famous monograph details the physiological activity of this plant. Foxglove is a stimulant to the contractile strength of the heart. It decreases the heart rate and so is used in patients with tachycardia or irregular heart rate.

Dr. Bastyr told us to notice the jugular veins of our patient. He said that if they are distended, this is an indication for *Digitalis.* In addition, he said that for a fluttering, fast, and feeble pulse, *Digitalis* is well indicated. The daily maintenance dose is 0.1 to 0.2 mg per day. Dr. Bastyr used *Digitalis* for congestive heart failure and atrial fibrillation.

A patient is initially given a higher dose of *Digitalis* for acute cardiac dysfunction, followed by a maintenance dose. This is termed digitalization of the patient. *Digitalis* leaf itself is strongly nauseating if overused. The resulting emesis is protective because it rids the body of what would otherwise be a toxic dose. When digoxin is extracted from the *Digitalis* leaf, as is done in making the drug digitalis, the nauseating principles are left behind. The refined digoxin does not have the intestinal symptoms and is therefore more dangerous. Typically, nature has some built-in safeguards. The dose of the tincture of *Digitalis* is 10 drops twice daily. In addition to being a cardiant, *Digitalis* is also a diuretic.

Strophanthus kombe

COMMON NAME ■ Strophanthus

The dried ripe seeds are used for medicine. *Strophanthus hispidus* or *Strophanthus gratus* may be used. *Strophanthus* normalizes respiration. It is a cardiac stimulant and a strong diuretic. It contains a glycoside called ouabain. This polyhydroxylated aglycone is responsible for the diuretic and cardiotonic actions of *Strophanthus.*

Dr. Bastyr told us that we should not use this plant in an aqueous menstruum because it precipitates. He suggested that we have the patient take the tincture straight. Therapeutically, *Strophanthus* is long lasting. Dr. Bastyr said to use it for patients with weak, rapid heartbeats, where there is muscular weakness or fatty deterioration of the heart. He said that it is used for atony of the heart after prolonged disease and inactivity.

Dr. Bastyr used *Strophanthus* in place of *Digitalis*. I remember him saying that the two remedies are similar in action. The dose of *Strophanthus* tincture is 3 to 8 drops up to four times daily. In my own practice, I use *Strophanthus* with hawthorn berry to strengthen the heart. I have more confidence in hawthorn to strengthen both the heart and the blood vessels. I prescribe $\frac{1}{2}$ teaspoon of the soft extract of hawthorn berry daily. You can also use 2 teaspoons of fluid extract daily.

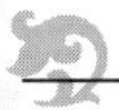

Convallaria majalis

COMMON NAME ■ Lily of the valley

The root is used to make medicine. This plant contains more than 30 glycosides. One of the glycosides is convallatoxin, which is cardioactive. Dr. Bastyr said that *Convallaria* is another substitute for *Digitalis*. It is used in organic heart weakness and valvular insufficiency. It strengthens the heart action and slows a rapid, feeble pulse. I use *Convallaria* with magnesium to correct arrhythmia.

Dr. Bastyr told us to use 5 to 20 drops of tincture per day. In cases of rheumatic carditis and pericarditis, he suggested that we combine one part *Convallaria* with five parts *Echinacea* and one part *Phytolacca* to retard involvement of the valves. In both American and European herbal traditions, *Convallaria* is used to improve coronary circulation. When Dr. Bastyr taught about this remedy, he specifically used the term "mitral insufficiency." Because *Convallaria* is also a diuretic, patients may notice increased urination during its use. Another interesting comment that Dr. Bastyr made was that this remedy helps correct dyspnea caused by heart disease.

I give patients with pericarditis 5 drops of *Convallaria* tincture twice a day. I use 60 drops of *Hydrastis* tincture four times a day. If I use capsules, I have the patient take 2 capsules four times a day. I use 2 cloves of garlic four times daily as an internal bacteriocide. In addition, I use 2 teaspoons of *Crataegus* fluid extract twice daily and 1000 mg of bilberry bioflavonoids three times daily. You can also use other anthocyanins, particularly those from elderberry or blueberry.

Lycopus virginicus

COMMON NAME ■ Bugleweed

The whole plant is used to make medicine. *Lycopus* is an astringent tonic and a weak diuretic. It decreases the heart rate as it increases the contractile force of the heart. When I used it as a heart tonic, I prescribe 60 drops of tincture twice daily. *Lycopus* has been used to treat peripheral vasoconstriction and is somewhat antihemorrhagic as well. Dr. Bastyr said that it is used to treat paroxysmal tachycardia. The old eclectics used *Lycopus* to treat Graves' disease with cardiac involvement.

Adonis vernalis

COMMON NAME ■ Pheasant's eye

The whole plant is used for medicine. Its primary cardioactive glycosides include adonitoxin, cymarin, and K-strophanthin. This plant decreases heart rate and increases cardiac tone. In addition, it helps slow the respiratory rate. Dr. Bastyr used 1 to 3 drops of the tincture twice daily, or the homeopathic remedy. He said that *Adonis* is indicated for the patient who has cardiac incompetence, a shallow electrocardiogram, poor ambulation, dyspnea, and fluid retention. He mentioned that *Adonis* 30X homeopathic potency is excellent for dyspnea. *Adonis* is a diuretic and has been used for cardiorenal affectations in which albuminuria is present. It has been used for asthma with cardiac feebleness and for neurocirculatory asthenias. It can be used in hydrothorax as a diuretic.

Cystisus scoparius

COMMON NAME ■ Scotch broom

Another genus name for scotch broom is *Sarothamnus scoparius*. The dried aerial parts of this plant are used to make medicine. *CAUTION: Avoid in patients with hypertension and pregnancy.* This is a bush with magnificent yellow flowers that blooms in the early summer. It contains a number of flavonoids including the C-glycosylflavone scoparin. It also contains quinolizidine alkaloids, mainly (-)-sparteine.

Scotch broom is a cardiac stimulant, a peripheral vasoconstrictor, an antihemorrhagic, an oxytocic, and a diuretic. It is also used in cases of hypothyroidism. I recommend a dose of 10 to 20 drops of tincture twice daily.

I use broom flowers to increase my awareness of the environment. Scotch broom is a mild psychotropic drug. It is not nearly as strong as the commonly misused drugs, but it has the effect of allowing one to be more aware of the world. It is as though one can see with the third eye, as odd as that may sound. I think that this is an important thing to do at this time, as humans attempt to rediscover a benevolent interaction with nature. Plants do affect us. Understanding the deeper messages coming to us through interactions with plants is important for our survival.

Apocynum cannabinum

COMMON NAME ■ Canadian hemp

The root is used to make medicine. *Apocynum* is a cardiac tonic, a diuretic, and a kidney tonic. As with many of the cardiac remedies, *Apocynum* increases the force of the heart's contraction as it decreases the heart rate. Use it in small doses of 5 drops of tincture repeated as often as four to five times daily. The dose of the powder is 5 to 10 grains twice daily.

Curiously, Dr. Bastyr mentioned that *Apocynum* might be helpful for intractable cases of sciatica. He cautioned us not to use this plant to treat structural damage to the kidneys.

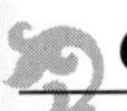

Crataegus oxyacantha

COMMON NAME ■ Hawthorn

The berries are used to make medicine; however, the flowers and leaves are also rich in procyanadins. The main active ingredient in *Crataegus* is procyanadin B_2. This plant does not contain cardiac glycosides such as we see in *Digitalis.* In my practice I have found that *Crataegus* is a gentle and effective heart medicine. It is perhaps the most reliable heart medicine in the *Materia Medica. Crataegus* is a consistent and gentle strengthener of the heart, a protector of the arteries and veins, and an all-around great botanical citizen. Dr. Bastyr recommended prolonged use of *Crataegus* as a cardiotonic. It increases coronary circulation. The dose that I suggest is $\frac{1}{2}$ teaspoon of the solid extract daily. The fluid extract may be used at the 2-teaspoon level, and the powdered extract may be used in doses of $\frac{1}{2}$ teaspoon or more. I have seen hundreds of patients who have been able to function better, even with seriously compromised hearts, after just 1 week of treatment with *Crataegus.* I encourage the use of the bioflavonoids in treating arterial disease as well. Dr. Dirk Powell recalls Dr. Bastyr cautioning us not to withdraw the dose of *Crataegus* abruptly.

Iberis amara

COMMON NAME ■ Bitter candytuft

The whole plant is used to make medicine. *Iberis* is indicated for conditions that include heart-related vertigo, weakness, and rheumatism. In addition, Dr. Bastyr mentioned that sea legs, or wobbly legs, respond to *Iberis.* The dose that he recommended for any of these conditions was 5 drops of tincture twice daily. I list *Iberis amara* for historical purposes; however, I have no personal experience with this particular plant. My efforts to obtain it have been fruitless. In the case of difficult-to-obtain plants, I often plan trips to wildcraft these medicines. It makes for vacations to interesting places. I definitely encourage practitioners to obtain plants this way.

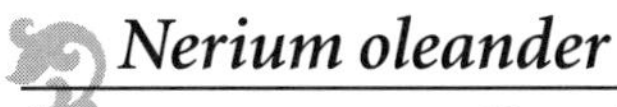

Nerium oleander

COMMON NAME ■ Rose laurel

This plant may also be found under the name *Nerium odoratum.* The leaves are used to make medicine. Dr. Bastyr used this plant in exactly the same way that he used *Strophanthus* for heart problems. Rose laurel contains a number of cardenolides; chief among them is oleandrin.

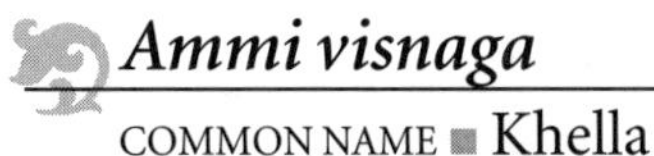

Ammi visnaga

COMMON NAME ■ Khella

The medicine is made from the seeds. Khella is a member of the carrot family, *Umbelliferae.* It is an antispasmodic, a relaxant, and a cardiant. It dilates the coronary arteries. Dr. Bastyr used this plant to treat angina pectoris. The results in angina are mixed. Higher doses are needed for nonresponsive patients. The active constituent, visnadine, is one of the ingredients responsible for the dilation of coronary arteries. Another major constituent is khellin, which is a furanochromone that has a spasmolytic action on both the coronary arteries and the bronchi. Dr. Bastyr said to use 10 to 60 drops of the tincture twice daily.

Anemone pulsatilla

COMMON NAMES ■ Wind flower, Pasque flower

The dried aerial parts of the plant are used to make medicine. *Pulsatilla* contains ranunculin, protoanemonin, and anemonin. Dr. Bastyr said that *Pulsatilla* is a heart tonic. He said that it is useful for heart consciousness where there is no particular functional disease but where there may be problems associated with tension, stress, and insomnia. The patient may complain of tachycardia, bradycardia, dyspnea, or syncope in an otherwise normal heart. The tincture dose is 3 drops three times daily in a small amount of water. Dr. Bastyr said that one might also use a 3X potency twice daily.

Erythroxylum coca

COMMON NAME ■ Cocaine

The leaves of this plant are used to make medicine. *Coca* is a cardiac stimulant. It acts as an adrenergic stimulant by blocking noradrenaline reuptake.[26] Alkaloids constitute the active ingredients, three of which are cocaine, cinnamoylcocaine, and hygrine. Chewing the leaves stimulates respiration.

It also stimulates the brain. Because of its addictive nature, or perhaps more correctly, the patient's addictive nature, *coca* should be avoided. Dirk Powell reminded me that Dr. Bastyr mentioned the use of *coca* for altitude sickness. Cocainc is illegal and therefore must not be used. However, historically it has been used for its medicinal properties.

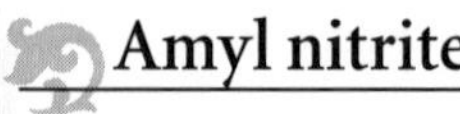

Amyl nitrite

COMMON NAME ■ Smelling salts

This material dilates the coronary arteries and has been used medically to counteract cyanide poisoning. It forms a complex with the cyanide, forming cyan-methemoglobin, which is nontoxic.

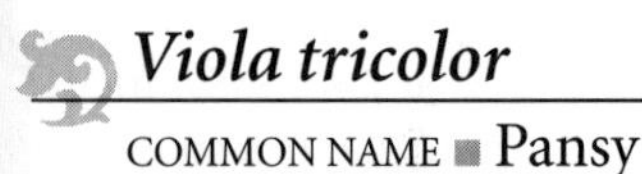

Viola tricolor

COMMON NAME ■ Pansy

The whole herb is used to make medicine. Herbalists have used *Viola* as a mild heart tonic and a hypotensive. A cup of the standard tea is taken daily in mouthful doses. The tincture dose is 5 to 10 drops three times daily. It has also been used traditionally as a cough medicine. *Viola* contains caffeic acid, which is a phenolic acid present in many plants. Caffeic acid is somewhat hepatoprotective, but its exact mechanism of action is still being explored.

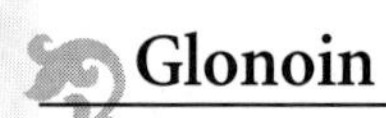

Glonoin

COMMON NAME ■ Nitroglycerin

This is for emergency dilation of the coronary arteries. Dr. Bastyr considered this a good remedy to keep in your doctor's bag for emergencies only. A pill form is used sublingually. The dose is $\frac{1}{150}$ of a grain. Dr. Powell said that Dr. Bastyr used higher potencies of *Belladonna* for headaches caused by glonoin.

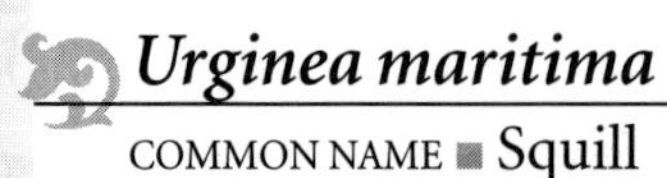

Urginea maritima

COMMON NAME ■ Squill

This plant is a member of the lily family, *Liliaceae.* The bulbs are used to make medicine. Squill contains more than a dozen cardioactive glycosides, chief of which is scillaren A. A steroidal skeleton forms the bulk of the molecule. Herbalists often start with 10 drops of tincture twice daily as a cardiotonic. This dose can be slowly and carefully increased to the patient's tolerance. One may use up to 20 drops twice daily.

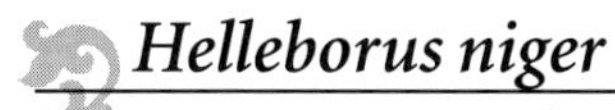

Helleborus niger

COMMON NAME ■ Christmas rose

The rhizome has been used to make medicine. However, in ancient Greek medicine, Paracelsus suggested using the leaves to make medicine. The leaves make a gentler and better tolerated medicine to use as a heart tonic for the elderly. This plant is contained in Paracelsus' "Elixir for Long Life." When using *Helleborus* as a cardiotonic, I prescribe 5 drops of the tincture twice daily.

CHAPTER

22

CARMINATIVES

CHAPTER • OUTLINE

Carminatives are agents that dispel stomach or intestinal gas and relieve pain associated with the accumulation of gas in the gastrointestinal tract.

Mentha piperita

COMMON NAME ■ Peppermint

The leaves are used to make medicine. Peppermint contains many compounds, including flavonoids, triterpenes, and carotenoids. Menthol and menthone are especially prevalent active compounds. The oil of peppermint inhibits contractions of the smooth muscles of the intestine by reducing calcium influx into muscle tissue. It may be used to relax the sphincters of the stomach and thus allow gas to pass out of the stomach and into the duodenum. In addition, peppermint slightly increases circulation and secretions in the stomach. I use it for flatulent dyspepsia and stomach bloat as well as for spastic colitis. In fact, peppermint is specific for spastic colitis. The dose of the oil of peppermint is 1 capsule prior to meals.

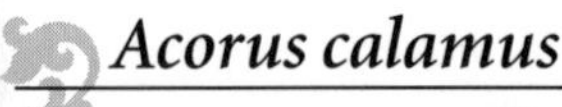

Acorus calamus

COMMON NAMES ■ Sweet flag, Calamus

The rhizome is used to make medicine. The oil of sweet flag contains a variety of monoterpenes and sesquiterpenoid derivatives, including camphene, beta-gurjunene, linalol, alpha- and beta-asarone, and others. This remedy is a gentle gastric stimulant and a carminative. The beta-asarone is probably the strongest spasmolytic and may account for the main carminative effect. I say "may" because the exact mechanism of action of a plant with so many active constituents is hard to pin down relative to the exact activity of each component. The dose of the tincture is 120 drops three times daily.

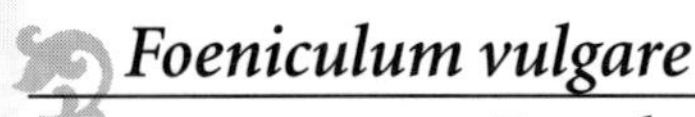

Foeniculum vulgare

COMMON NAME ■ Fennel

The seeds of this plant are used to make medicine. Fennel belongs to the carrot family, *Umbelliferae.* This plant is a carminative and a stomachic and is useful in flatulence. Dr. Bastyr considered fennel to be one of the best remedies for dispelling stomach and intestinal gas. Fennel contains anethole and estragole, which is also called methylchavicol. The constituent most related to fennel's action as a carminative is anethole.

The dose of the fluid extract of fennel is 30 to 60 drops several times daily. The standard dose recommended by herbalists is $\frac{1}{2}$ teaspoon of the powdered seeds brewed as a tea and taken in doses of 1 ounce throughout the day.

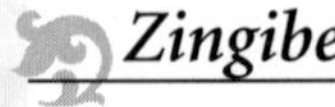

Zingiber officinale

COMMON NAME ■ Ginger

The root of the ginger plant is used to make medicine. The pungent taste comes from the gingerols. This plant is a warming carminative and a gastrointestinal stimulant. Capsules or tincture may be used. The dose as a carminative is 2 capsules, or 30 drops of tincture, three times daily.

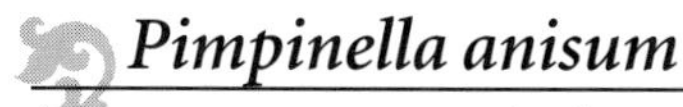

Pimpinella anisum

COMMON NAME ■ Anise

The seeds are used to make medicine. This plant has a number of primary actions. It is an antispasmodic, a carminative, and a respiratory expectorant. As a carminative, herbalists say to crush 1 teaspoon of the seeds just before use and make an infusion. I recommend drinking several cups daily. Anise is relaxing to the gastrointestinal tract and helps relieve flatulence. Dr. Felter, an eclectic physician, considered anise good for infant colic. In infant colic, the diet of the mother should also be considered if she is breast-feeding. Chocolate, colas, and foods that the mother may be allergic to can produce colic in nursing babies.

Anise seeds contain E-anethole, linalool, estragole, alpha-terpineol, and anisaldehyde. Of these, E-anethole is present in the highest concentrations in this plant. Historically, anise has been known as a galactagogue, probably because it contains several estrogenic-type molecules such as E-anethole. In addition, it has been added to other medicinal preparations to improve the flavor of bad-tasting combinations.

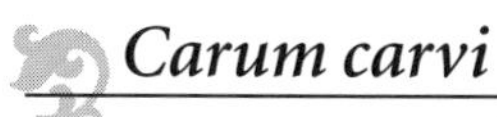

Carum carvi

COMMON NAME ■ Caraway

This plant is from the carrot family, *Umbelliferae.* The seeds are used to make medicine. The principal active ingredients are carvone and d-limonene. As a carminative, herbalists say to crush a heaping teaspoon of seeds and make an infusion. Strain and drink the tea to help relieve intestinal and stomach gas. This treats both meteorism and dyspepsia.

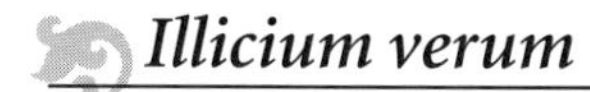

Illicium verum

COMMON NAME ■ Staranise

The fruit and seeds are used to make medicine. Staranise contains chavachol methyl ester, limonene, and fenchone. This plant can be used as a carminative. A good way to take staranise is to put the whole star in soup. I remember having lunch with Dr. Madison one afternoon at his house and he had made soup with the whole herbs in it. It was excellent. As a tea, herbalists say to take four or five stars and crush them up. Make an infusion, strain, and drink.

CHAPTER

23

CHOLAGOGUES

CHAPTER • OUTLINE

Chelidonium majus
Chionanthus virginicus
Taraxacum officinale
Euonymus atropurpurea
Peumus boldus
Iris versicolor
Leptandra virginica
Juglans cinerea

Cholagogues are medicines that increase the flow of bile from the gallbladder into the duodenum. I have chosen eight plants that I have used extensively as cholagogues. This section is included for the convenience of the practitioner. In class, Dr. Bastyr included these remedies with what he called the greater and lesser liver remedies.

There are many cholagogues available. Frankly, to choose the right plant for a patient, the health care professional will have to spend many years tasting, using, and experimenting with various plants. Eventually, the practitioner achieves a feeling for the plants and the ability to choose the exact combination of plants needed to improve the patient's condition.

I encourage a more thorough study of these plants. David Hoffmann has a nice treatment of the cholagogues in his book *Therapeutic Herbalism.*[46]

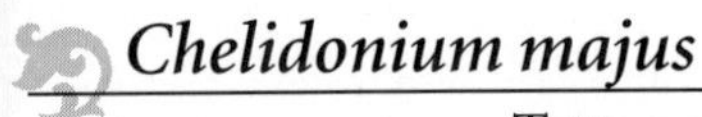

Chelidonium majus

COMMON NAMES ■ Tetterwort, Greater celandine

The medicine is obtained from the dried aerial parts of the plant. *Chelidonium* increases bile flow, stimulates hepatic action, and slightly dilates the bile passages. I use *Chelidonium* for liver congestion when there is mild jaundice. I have found it to be an excellent remedy for Gilbert's syndrome. Of all the cholagogues, *Chelidonium* is the one I use most frequently. Dr. Bastyr said to use 20 drops of tincture three times daily. He almost always mixed *Chelidonium* with equal parts of *Chionanthus* tincture.

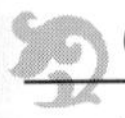

Chionanthus virginicus

COMMON NAME ■ Fringe tree

The bark is used to make medicine. It contains saponins and lignane glycosides. *Chionanthus* is an excellent cholagogue. It is specific for gallbladder disease in which either stones or sludge is present. I usually mix it with equal parts of *Chelidonium*, as recommended by Dr. Bastyr. Dr. Bastyr said that the dose of *Chionanthus* is 30 drops twice daily. I use this remedy for all forms of hepatitis. Dr. Bastyr said that *Chionanthus* should not be overlooked in the treatment of cancerous or noncancerous pancreatitis. In my experience, I have found that foot reflexology is one of the most effective treatments for pancreatitis.

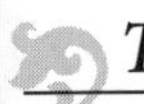

Taraxacum officinale

COMMON NAME ■ Dandelion

Taraxacum is a member of the sunflower family, *Compositae*. The root is used to make medicine. *Taraxacum* contains a monohydroxy triterpene called taraxasterol and a bitter sesquiterpene lactone called taraxinic acid glucoside.[20] These bitter compounds stimulate bile flow. Dr. Bastyr recommended giving 60 drops of tincture three times daily as a liver medicine.

Taraxacum also contains large quantities of fructose and inulin. The inulin content in the root of the dandelion reaches 40% in the fall. Inulin stimulates complement, and therefore using dandelion root has an immunostimulatory effect. In the spring, the root has the greatest fructose content, which accounts for the sweeter taste of the spring roots. The bitterness of all parts of the plant is caused by sesquiterpenoid lactones such as germacradienolides and eudesmanolides. The leaf is more specific as a diuretic.

This is one of the plants that I always include as a spring tonic to get the patient going after the long winter's nap. The spring tonic that I recommend is equal parts of the tinctures of *Taraxacum* root and leaf, *Eleutherococcus*,

Euonymus atropurpurea, Glycyrrhiza, and *Zingiber.* I prescribe 30 drops of this combination at mealtimes.

Dr. Dirk Powell reminded me that Dr. Bastyr suggested that the patient hold strong *Taraxacum* tea in the mouth for canker sores.

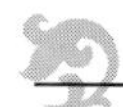

Euonymus atropurpurea

COMMON NAME ■ Wahoo

The medicine is made from the bark of the root. *Euonymus* contains cardenolide glycosides, which are mild cardiotonics. Among these are euatroside, euatromonoside, and digitoxigenin.[20] This is a great liver remedy to decongest the liver and encourage the flow of bile. I have found that this remedy is especially effective for the patient who eats too much, doesn't get any physical exercise, is overstressed, and is generally toxic. Many Americans fit into this category. *Euonymus* is useful in these cases to stimulate hepatic function. The taste of the herb is bitter and rather active tasting. I dose *Euonymus* at 30 drops of tincture three times daily.

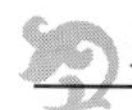

Peumus boldus

COMMON NAME ■ Boldo

The leaves are used to make medicine. Boldo is a cholagogue and a mild diuretic. It is a joy to taste because of its complex flavor. Boldo contains monoterpenoids, flavolol glycosides, and aporphinoid alkaloids. Among these alkaloids is boldine, which is the primary active cholagogue, and isocorydine, isoboldine, laurolitsine, and norisocorydine. Boldo is another gallbladder remedy that helps with gallstone dissolution and removal. Use 30 drops of the tincture three times daily for this purpose. I have noticed that, after taking boldo, the patient will appreciate a warming effect in the gallbladder region. This is one of my favorite liver remedies. It is often overlooked, unfortunately.

Iris versicolor

COMMON NAMES ■ Iris, Blue flag

Blueflag is in the iris family, *Iridaceae.* The dried rhizome is used to make medicine. The active constituent in *Iris* is the triterpenoid iriversical. This cholagogue is a remedy that I count on frequently for cases of psoriasis in which the liver seems to be involved. Believe me, the liver is frequently involved. I mix equal parts of *Iris,* boldo, and *Chionanthus* and give 30 drops three times daily.

Leptandra virginica

COMMON NAME ■ Culver's root

The medicinal part is the dried rhizome with the root. Dr. Bastyr told us that *Leptandra* stimulates the flow of bile. The dose he recommended was 10 drops of tincture at meal times. It is a bitter-tasting herb that is useful in cholecystitis. The active constituents are cinnamic acid derivatives such as 4-methoxycinnamic acid and 3,4-dimethoxycinnamic acid. It also contains tannins. I have used it for general fatigue as a liver and intestinal tonic.

Juglans cinerea

COMMON NAMES ■ White walnut, Butternut

This plant is a member of the *Juglandaceae* family. The inner bark is used for medicine. This bark contains juglone, which is a naphthoquinone. It also contains tannins and a number of volatile oils. *Juglans* is most frequently used as a cholagogue.

This plant is a liver stimulant and cholagogue that mildly increases the secretion of bile. Large doses are cathartic. Eclectics used this in medium doses to treat clay-colored stools. The general dose is 5 to 30 drops per meal. The tincture has a dark color and a whiskey-pepper flavor that comes at you slowly.

CHAPTER

24

CHOLESTEROL-LOWERING MEDICINES

CHAPTER • OUTLINE

Commiphora mukul
Panthethine
Cynara scolymus
Allium sativum

These plants lower cholesterol. Other lipids, such as triglycerides, are also often affected. Dr. Bastyr did not teach these remedies as a group. I have added this important section to help the practitioner select from among a list of natural remedies that show promise in dealing with the management of both familial and idiopathic hypercholesterolemia. I have used all of these remedies in my practice and am impressed with their effectiveness in most cases.

Clearly, a comprehensive program of dietary management is indicated for these patients. This program includes the management of fat and fiber intake, fluid intake, food quantity, and an eating schedule. Other cholesterol management tools include exercise programs, stress reduction techniques, and healthy time management tools. The following remedies, when combined with the application of the aforementioned therapeutic categories, are often very effective in improving the lipid profiles of patients.

Commiphora mukul

COMMON NAME ■ Mukul myrrh tree

The resin from the bark is used to make medicine. The active constituent of this plant is the lipid-soluble fraction of the resin of the tree. This resin is called gum guggul. The specific medicinal material responsible for lowering cholesterol is called E-guggulsterone and Z-guggulsterone.

This plant is promising because animal studies have shown that mukul lowers total cholesterol and levels of triglycerides, low-density lipoproteins, and very-low-density lipoproteins and elevates levels of high-density lipoproteins.[101,102] This plant does not have side effects. The LD-50, or 50% lethal dose, in mice is 1600 mg/kg.[103] That is quite a bit. To lower cholesterol, I give 3 capsules of gugulipid per day. Each capsule will generally contain between 400 and 500 mg of the powdered plant material. There have also been reports that *Commiphora mukul* stimulates the thyroid gland.[104] As a result, this plant has been used in weight loss programs.

Panthethine

Panthethine is a pantothenic acid derivative. Panthethine lowers total cholesterol and low-density lipoprotein and triglyceride levels and elevates high-density lipoprotein levels. The dose is 300 mg three times daily. I use this remedy for nearly all of my patients who have hypercholesterolemia, whether it is idiopathic or familial. It is very effective.

Cynara scolymus

COMMON NAME ■ Artichoke

The leaves of this plant are used to make medicine. An extract of artichoke leaves standardized to 0.06% cynarin has been shown effective for treating hypocholesterolemia.[105] In a study by Montini et al, patients given *Cynara* extract showed 20% lower cholesterol levels and 15% lower triglyceride levels as compared to their levels at the onset of the study.[105] The suggested dose is 500 mg of *Cynara* extract daily. What is impressive about this approach to lowering cholesterol is that the remedy is safe and effective. Follow-up studies of some of the stronger prescription drugs used to lower cholesterol have reported some very disconcerting side effects with prolonged use. Patients should consult their doctor if these prescription medications have been prescribed.

Dr. Ed Madison taught about the use of *Cynara* at Bastyr University in the mid-1980s, stressing the use of the leaves as a liver medicine.

Allium sativum

COMMON NAME ■ Garlic

The bulbs are used as medicine. Garlic is a safe remedy to use to lower both total and low-density lipoprotein cholesterol in the blood.[106] A number of active compounds in garlic, such as ajoene and diallylthiosulfinate allicin, inhibit 3-hydroxy-3-methylglutaryl-coenzyme A reductase, which is an enzyme needed to produce cholesterol in the human body. I have patients take several cloves of garlic twice daily to lower cholesterol. If taken before meals, the odor is decreased.

CHAPTER

25

Circulatory Tonics and Stimulants

CHAPTER • OUTLINE

Circulatory tonics and stimulants increase the flow of blood to body tissues in general. These remedies may act by a variety of methods, including dilation of blood vessels, improvement of coronary output, or general tonification of the vital force of the body.

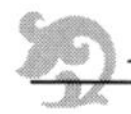

Ruscus aculeatus

COMMON NAME ■ Butcher's broom

This plant is a member of the lily family, *Liliaceae*. The herb and rhizome are used to make medicine. I have used butcher's broom as a circulatory tonic for years. Thirty drops of tincture three times daily has a healthy effect on the general circulation. It is a favorite of one of my elderly patients, Lucille Tennyson, who introduced me to this wonderful plant in 1991.

Ruscus contains a sapogenin called ruscogenin, which has been scientifically placed in the therapeutic category of hemorrhoid treatment. Ruscogenin is an antiinflammatory, which possibly accounts for its effectiveness as a constituent in hemorrhoid preparations.

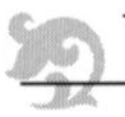

Vinca minor

COMMON NAME ■ Lesser periwinkle

This plant is a member of the *Apocynaceae* family. The whole flowering plant is used to make medicine. *Vinca* contains an indole alkaloid called vincamine. Vincamine increases cerebral circulation, increases oxygen availability, and tonifies cerebral function.[107] I recommend 10 drops of tincture twice daily as a circulatory stimulant.

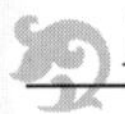

Rosmarinus officinalis

COMMON NAME ■ Rosemary

Rosemary is a member of the *Labiatae* family. The rosemary leaves are used for medicine. Rosemary is a general circulatory tonic. It can be used for hypotension or for any chronic circulatory inefficiency. The great German hydrotherapist Sebastian Kneipp prescribed rosemary wine as a tonic for the elderly. The patient should take 15 drops of the tincture two to three times daily.

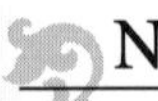

Niacinamide

COMMON NAMES ■ Niacin, Vitamin B_3

Niacin increases circulation to the skin. To cleanse and purify both the blood and skin, I sometimes use niacin in conjunction with a brief sauna. I have patients consume several glasses of water beforehand. The amount of niacin necessary to produce a flush varies greatly from patient to patient. I have found that taking 100 mg per day will often result in flushing, and a single 500-mg tablet usually produces the flush. Patients with Raynaud's disease should take niacin daily.

Ginkgo biloba

COMMON NAME ■ Ginkgo

The leaf of the *Ginkgo* plant is used to make medicine. *Ginkgo* is an ancient plant, unchanged since long before the Jurassic period. No wonder it is useful for improving memory. *Ginkgo* is native to all northern latitudes including Europe, China, and the United States. For example, there are petrified *Ginkgo* trees in eastern Washington State worth visiting.

Ginkgo contains a number of interesting constituents, such as the flavonoid quercetin, kaempferol, and isorhamnetin. It also contains a number of ginkgolide structures and a novel amentoflavone, which is a combination of two flavones linked together. *Ginkgo* also provides a unique terpene called bilobalide. The flavonols have sugar units called glycosides attached to them and are thus called flavonoid glycosides. The organic acids in *Ginkgo* make tea from the leaves particularly water soluble. Of interest historically, the flavone kaempferol was named after Engelbert Kaempfer, a German botanist who first catalogued the *Ginkgo* tree in Europe.

Ginkgo should be considered a true circulatory tonic and stimulant. It stimulates both prostacycline and endothelium-derived releasing factor, causing relaxation of the blood vessels.[108] This action improves blood perfusion to tissues. Platelet aggregation is inhibited as well. *Ginkgo* is particularly helpful in cerebral ischemia. The dose is 500 mg of powdered *Ginkgo* twice daily for an adult. A standardized *Ginkgo* extract has been used in doses of 40 mg three times daily.

I have seen a number of cases of tinnitus improved by using 40 mg of the standardized extract three times daily. I have found that it is especially effective when given in combination with 50 to 100 mg of niacin. Along the same lines, cochlear deafness is helped by *Ginkgo*.

Sikorsa, writing in the *Journal of Urology* in 1989, reported that erectile dysfunction caused by decreased blood flow might be helped by taking *Ginkgo*.[109] For further studies and applications of *Ginkgo*, I would suggest reading Michael Murray's book, *The Healing Power of Herbs*, ed 2,[110] which is well written and profusely documented.

CHAPTER

26

CONDIMENT MEDICINALS

CHAPTER • OUTLINE

Pimpinella anisum
Armoracia rusticana
Dentaria laciniata
Salvia officinalis
Myristica fragrans
Ocimum basilicum
Cinnamomum zeylanicum
Coriandrum sativum
Origanum majorana

This group of remedies consists of condiments or spices that are of medicinal value when used properly. Many plants that we consider to be foods are also medicines. These plants are easy for your patients to obtain, which makes them especially attractive as medicines. I have used them to treat a number of patients who have called me from remote areas to request medical assistance. For example, there have been several cases in which I have been telephoned from tribal reservations for assistance in treating elders of the tribe. The problem with calls for assistance from remote areas is the lack of availability of medicines that I would normally be able to supply. Having thorough knowledge of kitchen medicines comes in handy in these cases. For this reason, I consider this section to be especially important to naturopathic doctors and herbalists.

My grandmother saved my life with one of these remedies. I remember my family visiting my grandparents in Minonk, Illinois, when I was 5 or 6 years old. I had such bad asthma one night that I honestly couldn't breathe without great difficulty. My grandmother took a half of a teaspoon of Vicks VapoRub, a drugstore product manufactured by Procter & Gamble, and stuck it in my mouth and told me to keep it there. Within 15 minutes, I could breathe again. I was so happy. To this day I can still recall my feelings of mental and physical relief.

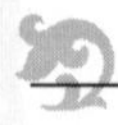

Pimpinella anisum

COMMON NAME ■ Anise

The fruit of this plant is used for medicine. Anise is a carminative, an antispasmodic, a tonic, and an anticolic medicine. The carminative activity of the plant is caused by its anethole content. Anise also contains chlorogenic acid and estragole. Chlorogenic acid is a good liver antioxidant. Estragole is responsible in part for the distinct flavor of anise. Herbalists have told me that anise makes a good cough medicine. The dose that I recommend is 1 teaspoon of tincture twice daily.

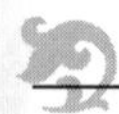

Armoracia rusticana

COMMON NAME ■ Horseradish

The root is used to make medicine. Horseradish is a winter source of vitamin C. It contains beta-glucopyranoside, sinigrin, gluconasturtin, and the flavonoid kaempferol. I tell my patients to add horseradish to food to help clear nasal passages. In addition, I use horseradish to treat sinusitis. It is a reasonable urinary antiseptic and a stimulating diuretic, which is not widely known. I prescribe $\frac{1}{2}$ teaspoon of tincture three times daily. More may be used if needed.

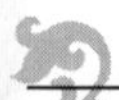

Dentaria laciniata

COMMON NAME ■ Cutleaf toothwort

I have included this plant for historical purposes. I have no direct experience with it. Dr. Bastyr said that *Dentaria* could be used in a manner similar to that of *Armoracia*, which I have described above.

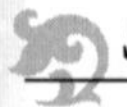

Salvia officinalis

COMMON NAME ■ Sage

The medicinal part of this plant is the dried leaves. *Salvia* contains resins, tannins, and bitter principles. *Salvia* is a good remedy for night sweats. Dr. Bastyr suggested that we prescribe a dose of 20 to 40 drops of tincture twice daily or make a standard tea from the leaves using 1 teaspoon of the herb per cup of water. Take 1 to 2 cups of this tea per day in tablespoon doses.

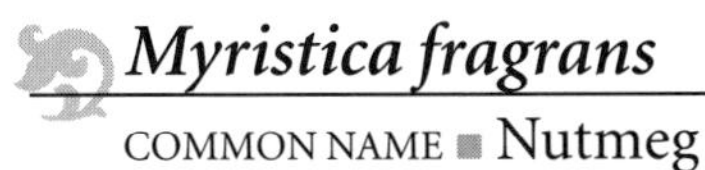

Myristica fragrans

COMMON NAME ■ Nutmeg

The medicine is the dried ripe seed. *CAUTION: Nutmeg is hallucinogenic in large doses and should be used carefully.* The psychotropic activity of nutmeg is probably caused by myristicin. Some authors believe that the phenyl-propanoids, such as myristicin, are transaminated within the body into 3-methoxy-4,5-methylenedioxyamphetamine.[26] The oil of nutmeg contains eugenol, myristicin, and safrole. It also contains terpenoid hydrocarbons such as sabinene, alpha- and beta-pinenes, and limonene.[26] There are also several neolignans, fragransol-C, and several myristicanols in nutmeg. Eugenol and isoeugenol prevent platelet aggregation by inhibiting cyclooxygenase.

Dr. Bastyr used the oil in doses of 1 to 5 drops for flatulence and gastrodynia. Tyler, Brady, and Robbers make the interesting statement that nutmeg may be of use in treating cancer-associated diarrhea.[33] I use 10 to 20 drops of tincture as a mild stimulant.

Ocimum basilicum

COMMON NAME ■ Sweet basil

Use the whole herb as medicine. The oil of basil contains estragol, cineole, fenchol, linalool, and methyleugenol. This medicine is tonifying and stimulating. It may be used in a similar fashion as peppermint in cases of spastic colon to relax the smooth muscles of the gastrointestinal tract. For this purpose, Dr. Bastyr recommended 60 drops of tincture twice daily. Peppermint oil is more predictable as a smooth muscle relaxant. It tends to elevate the spirit and is considered by many, including myself, to be a sacred food. I have my patients take 15 to 30 drops of the tincture twice daily to combat sadness.

Cinnamomum zeylanicum

COMMON NAME ■ Ceylon cinnamon

The bark of this plant is used to make medicine. Cinnamon can be found in herbal texts as far back as 2700 BC, where it is mentioned in the Chinese herbals. Cinnamon is a carminative, an antiseptic, and a pungent aromatic flavoring material. It contains an aldehyde oil called cinnamaldehyde, as well as polycyclic diterpenes and proanthocyanidinoid oligomers. The aldehyde oils are also contained in orange oil, lemon oil, witch hazel, and citronella. Dr. Bastyr said that the dose of the oil of cinnamon as a carminative should be 1 drop twice daily. The essential oil of cinnamon has been shown in vitro to be a potent antibacterial and antifungal medicine.[26]

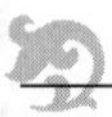

Coriandrum sativum

COMMON NAME ■ Coriander

The seeds are used to make medicine. Coriander is a carminative, a stimulant and a stomachic, and it can help with stomach gas and belching. Think of this plant when treating patients with mild digestive disorders. I recommend taking $\frac{1}{4}$ teaspoon of crushed seeds after meals.

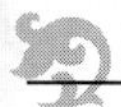

Origanum majorana

COMMON NAME ■ Marjoram

This plant is from the mint family, *Labiatae.* The whole flowering plant is used to make medicine. It contains several interesting polar antioxidants, including rosmarinic acid and an acylated arbutin called 6-O-p-hydroxybenzylarbutin.[54] In addition to tasting good, this plant is an excellent antioxidant.

CHAPTER

27

DEBRIDING AGENTS

CHAPTER • OUTLINE

Hydrogen peroxide
Urea
Proteolytic enzymes
Streptokinase

Debriding agents help to remove foreign materials and contaminated or damaged tissue. Although some of these agents are not plant medicines, they should be considered in the practice of natural medicine. Dr. Bastyr did not cover these remedies as a group.

Hydrogen peroxide

I use this liquid as an external application to debride wounds. I also use it to debride material in the ear canal. Hydrogen peroxide may be added to gargles to help clear the mouth of excess debilitated cells.

Urea

Urea, also called carbamide, is a debriding agent. Various preparations of urea have been used as ear drops in conditions involving otitis. Interestingly, in the paper industry, urea is used to soften cellulose.

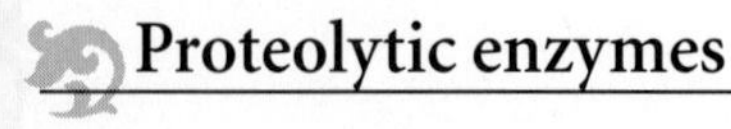

Proteolytic enzymes

Bromelain and papain are the most frequently used natural proteolytic enzymes. Dr. Bastyr suggested mixing bromelain with glycerin to form a debriding solution, which can be applied to warts and wounds.

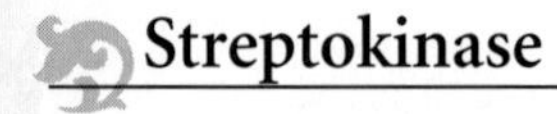

Streptokinase

This material is used allopathically as a debriding agent.

CHAPTER

28

DEMULCENTS AND EMOLLIENTS

CHAPTER • OUTLINE

Tussilago farfara
Malva rotundifolia
Coptis trifolia groenlandica
Ulmus fulva
Lithospermum tinctorium
Acacia senegal
Prunus amygdalus
Althaea officinalis
Anogeissus latifolia

Demulcents are medicines, ointments, or preparations that help allay inflamed mucous membranes or soothe irritated tissue. Emollients also soothe membranes, and have a tendency to soften skin.

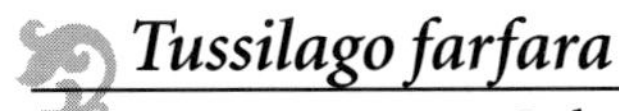

Tussilago farfara

COMMON NAME ■ Coltsfoot

The flowers and the leaves are used to make medicine. *Tussilago* is a mild astringent, an expectorant, and an emollient. It may be used to soothe and allay irritation of the bronchial and gastric membranes. Dr. Bastyr pointed out that *Tussilago* allays cough caused by irritation of the mucous membranes. Use it for dry cough, laryngitis, pharyngitis, bronchitis, and asthma. Dr. Bastyr said to use 30 drops of tincture four times daily.

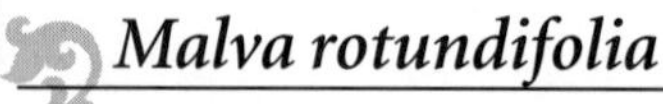

Malva rotundifolia

COMMON NAME ■ Round-leaved mallow

One may also use *Malva sylvestris.* The whole herb is used to make medicine. Dr. Bastyr said that this plant makes an excellent hand lotion, especially when mixed with alcohol, Irish moss, and glycerin. *Malva* is useful in all types of respiratory inflammations (the "itises" of the upper respiratory tract). I recommend a dose of 30 drops of tincture three times daily.

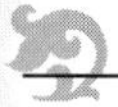

Coptis trifolia groenlandica

COMMON NAME ■ Goldthread

Medicine is made from the roots. I have no experience with this plant; it is included for historical purposes. Dr. Bastyr said that it is a good emollient mouthwash to use for thrush and mouth sores. He said to add 1 teaspoon of the tincture to $\frac{1}{4}$ cup of water for this purpose.

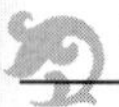

Ulmus fulva

COMMON NAME ■ Slippery elm

The inner bark is used to make medicine. *Ulmus* contains mucilage composed of galactose. I use this plant as a soothing medicine for irritated intestinal lining in most types of gastrointestinal diseases. The patient may steep the slippery elm bark in water until a mucilaginous substance is formed. This is then taken internally as a demulcent as needed. Dr. Bastyr said that this plant could be used externally on eczema and other skin disorders, including hemorrhoids. He said to use an infusion for vaginitis and proctitis. It also helps in cases of enteritis caused by irritative materials and foods. *Ulmus* is a valuable emollient for dysentery. I have found that capsules are the best way to administer *Ulmus.* Take 2 capsules three times daily.

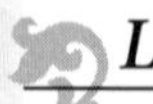

Lithospermum tinctorium

COMMON NAME ■ Common gromwell

The root is used to make medicine. Dr. Bastyr taught us that this plant is a good emollient when mixed with petroleum jelly or coconut oil. As an emollient, it had been used in acute and chronic cystitis. An infusion is prepared by mixing

2 tablespoons of the dried, chopped root in 1 cup of water. Two teaspoons of the infusion is taken every 2 hours as needed. It contains a phenolic acid derived from cinnamic acid called lithospermic acid. I have included this plant for historical purposes.

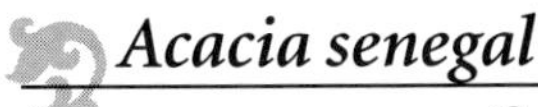

Acacia senegal

COMMON NAME ■ Gum arabic

Acacia belongs to the pea family, *Leguminosae.* The closely related plant, *Acacia laeta,* is also used for its gum contents.[111] The medicine is made from the stems and branches of the plant, which provide a dried gummy exudate. *Acacia* consists mostly of arabin, which is a mixture of calcium, potassium, and magnesium salts complexed with arabic acid. This plant is a useful demulcent and emollient. Dr. Bastyr said to take 1 to 4 drams of the syrup of *Acacia* twice daily.

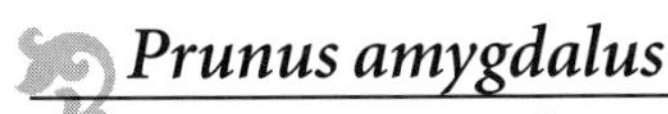

Prunus amygdalus

COMMON NAME ■ Almond

The kernels are used to make medicine. The oil of this plant is used as an emollient in cosmetics and skin lotions. Dr. Bastyr mentioned its use internally for intestinal irritation. Unfortunately, I do not know how he used it. I was too busy writing down whatever he had been saying previously to ask pertinent questions about almond.

Althaea officinalis

COMMON NAME ■ Marshmallow

This plant is a member of the mallow family, *Malvaceae.* The medicinal parts are the leaves, flowers, and roots. *Althaea* has 10% mucilage and 2% asparagine, making it demulcent. It contains polysaccharide chains that make up the mucilaginous characteristics. There are a number of these polysaccharides, one of which contains four sugars: L-rhamnose, D-galactose, D-galacturonic acid, and D-glucuronic acid. *Althaea* is an excellent demulcent. The most famous use of this plant is as a demulcent for intestinal disorders such as colitis. Dr. Bastyr was fond of *Althaea* as a soothing remedy for enteric inflammations. I recommend taking 2 capsules of the powdered herb three times daily to soothe the intestinal tract. The tincture may be taken in doses of 120 drops three times daily. I remember Dr. Bastyr suggesting that the medicine could be obtained by chopping up the plant and letting it soak in cold water for 3 or 4 hours. This tea makes an excellent demulcent in gastroenteritis.

I have used this medicine for peptic ulcers with good results. It is especially effective when used with deglycyrrhizinated licorice root powder. The dose of deglycyrrhizinated licorice powder that I recommend is $\frac{1}{2}$ teaspoon three or four times daily. I have found that this combination is nearly always curative as long as the patient maintains a reasonable diet. *Althaea* is also effective as a soothing ingredient in cough medicines.

Anogeissus latifolia

COMMON NAME ■ Ghatti gum

This tree is a native of Sri Lanka and India and belongs to the *Combretaceae* family. The gum of the tree is used to make medicine. It is used occasionally as a substitute for *Acacia* gum, although the dispersions are thicker than those made with *Acacia*. This gum can be used as an emollient and an emulsifying agent. I have no experience with this medicine.

CHAPTER

29

DIAPHORETICS

CHAPTER • OUTLINE

Achillea millefolium
Eupatorium perfoliatum
Asclepias tuberosa
Zingiber officinale
Polemonium reptans
Verbena hastata
Crocus sativus
Xanthoxylum americanum
Capsicum frutescens
Salvia officinalis

Diaphoretics are agents that promote or increase perspiration. The skin is a semipermeable membrane through which the body eliminates wastes. It is also a protective membrane and a vital part of the immune system. Sweating, fasting, emesis, and the use of colonics are methods of ridding the body of toxins.

The ancient Greeks noticed that disease often resolved after a fever. Hippocrates wrote extensively in his tracts on the "Epidemics" about the course of disease, noting the resolution of some problems after the febrile stage. Historically, these remedies were important to eclectics and herbalists, who used them as part of the detoxification program. Fever therapy has also been practiced by modern herbalists and naturopathic physicians. Natural healers have become familiar with the remedies that produce diaphoresis to aid the body in ridding itself of poisons during the febrile stage of disease. The patient must be given copious amounts of hot liquids and bundled up to induce and even prolong fevers.

In the current practice of naturopathic medicine, there remains a place for colonics, fasting, and diaphoresis, where indicated and where appropriate. As time goes on, fever therapy should be explored more thoroughly as a means of improving the immune response.

Achillea millefolium

COMMON NAME ■ Yarrow

This plant is a member of the sunflower family, *Compositae.* The whole plant is used to make medicine. Among other things, yarrow is a diaphoretic, an antiviral, a diuretic, an astringent, and a good bitter. Yarrow is useful in treating just about everything, which sounds zany, but anyone familiar with yarrow will know what I am talking about. Use 90 drops in a cup of warm water twice daily as a diaphoretic. Dr. Bastyr said to take the tea at night along with plenty of hot fluids. He said to apply extra covers at bedtimes to sweat the disease out. I use this tactic to treat my own colds and flu with great success.

As far as I know, *Achillea millefolium* is the oldest remedy in the *Materia Medica* that people have actually used as a medicine. *Achillea* was found in the graves of Neanderthals.

Eupatorium perfoliatum

COMMON NAMES ■ Boneset, Feverwort

The flowering tops and leaves are used to make medicine. *Eupatorium* contains a number of sesquiterpene lactones. Dr. Bastyr said that *Eupatorium* is an excellent diaphoretic. He said that a standard tea should be made and $\frac{1}{4}$ cup should be drunk every 30 minutes until results are obtained. He was fonder of *Eupatorium* as a flu remedy than he was of it as a remedy for broken bones, as the common name boneset would imply. In fact, this was one of his favorite flu remedies.

I frequently use *Eupatorium* in flu remedies. Hot tea made from the leaves induces sweating in flu and colds, which speeds resolution of the illness. The tea stimulates the immune system, which may account for its success treating flu epidemics in the 19th century. The dose is 30 drops four times daily in hot water. This is one of our finest flu remedies. I like to mix it with *Sambucus,* or elder flowers and buds, in the treatment of flu with accompanying muscular aches.

Tom Brown, the tracker who learned a great deal of herbal medicine from Stalking Wolf, an Apache Indian, mentions boneset tea being drunk by many elders to ward off arthritic complaints. As I write these words, I am taking boneset tincture to nurse my broken arm back to health. Boneset is pleasant to take on the tongue in tincture form. It has a powerful, penetrating feel to it.

This is a good plant to have on hand just to experience its uplifting quality. Tom Brown further mentions a badly broken hand that he suffered. The doctors expected that it would take 6 weeks to heal, but after taking boneset tea, he was able to have the cast removed after 2 weeks.[112]

Asclepias tuberosa

COMMON NAMES ■ Pleurisy root, Butterfly weed

The rhizome of this plant is used to make medicine. This plant is a powerful diaphoretic. The diaphoretic and diuretic effect may be caused by cardioactive steroids called cardenolids. These materials may strengthen the heart contraction and allow better fluid removal as an effect of improved circulatory force. Dr. Bastyr told us to have the patient put 20 drops of the tincture in a cup of hot water every hour until diaphoresis has been achieved.

Zingiber officinale

COMMON NAME ■ Ginger

The root is used to make medicine. This plant is a warming diaphoretic and a stimulant. The diaphoretic action of *Zingiber* makes it useful in viral colds. *Zingiber* tea will often stop a cold if taken at the first signs. I recommend 60 drops of the tincture in a cup of hot water. This dose may be repeated 1 hour later if diaphoresis is not produced. The patient must be kept warm, of course. One of the active constituents, zingerone, is antibacterial against *Salmonella typhi* and *Vibrio cholerae.*

Polemonium reptans

COMMON NAME ■ Abscess root

The root is used to make medicine. Abscess root is a diaphoretic. Dr. Bastyr said to take 1 to 2 fluid ounces of the infusion four times daily. He used abscess root for respiratory complaints, febrile diseases, acute inflammation, and flu. Remember to drink adequate amounts of water when using diaphoretics. During acute illness, never drink cold liquids because this can weaken the body by requiring it to expend excess energy to heat up the liquid.

Verbena hastata

COMMON NAME ■ Blue vervain

The whole plant is used to make medicine. *Verbena* is a diaphoretic. It is used to treat fevers and colds, and it helps clear congestion in bronchial conditions.

Dr. Bastyr said to use the tincture as a diaphoretic in doses of 20 drops three to four times as needed to produce sweating. I have found a curious use for *Verbena*: the tea helps to clear the voice.

Crocus sativus

COMMON NAMES ■ Autumn crocus, Saffron

The stigma and style are used to make medicine. This plant is one of my favorite medicinal plants. It is a diaphoretic, antioxidant, cerebral antiinflammatory, and brain tonic. I recommend taking 6 stigmas in water daily as a health drink. *Crocus* contains rare water-soluble carotenes. Most carotenes are fat soluble. One of the main pigments in saffron is crocin, which upon hydrolysis yields crocetin and glucose.[113,114]

Dr. Bastyr said to take 10 stigmas in a large cup of hot water as a diaphoretic. If the tincture is used for diaphoresis, I recommend a dose of 40 drops per cup of hot water. This plant, together with *Trilisa odoratissima,* may be used to decrease edema after brain surgery or spinal cord injury.

The interesting odor of saffron comes from safranal, which is contained in the essential oil of saffron. Several other interesting compounds found in saffron are picrocrocin and mangicrocin. Mangicrocin is a novel adaptogenic xanthone carotenoid glycosidic conjugate from saffron.[115]

Dr. Ed Madison, in his lectures at Bastyr University, mentioned the significance of saffron in providing adequate oxygen nourishment to the brain and in protecting and improving blood vessel competency. The gist of the analysis had to do with a number of factors, especially the role of crocetin as a water-soluble carotenoid. Of extreme interest is Gainer and Chisolm's study wherein intramuscular injections of crocetin into rabbits fed a cholesterol-containing diet resulted in greatly reduced severity of atherosclerosis. Serum cholesterol levels were reduced by 50%.[116]

In my opinion, saffron is an underused botanical medicine of extreme importance. It is curious that saffron is one of the most expensive botanicals on the market. It costs in excess of $4000 a pound, yet 2 cups of saffron tea daily is far less expensive than the price of a double tall latte.

Xanthoxylum americanum

COMMON NAME ■ Northern prickly ash

The bark or the berries are used to make medicine. This plant is a good diaphoretic and a tonic to the whole system. Dr. Bastyr said that 1 dram of the plant material should be decocted in 4 ounces of boiling water for about 5 minutes. Let it infuse for another 15 minutes and drink warm. He said that another option is to take 10 to 30 drops of the tincture three times daily in hot water.

I have found this plant effective in producing salivation. For dry mouth, I combine 20 parts *Xanthoxylum* with one part *Pilocarpus jaborandi* and give 30 drops of this preparation twice daily. Leg cramps and cold extremities respond to prickly ash as well. The guiding problem here is circulatory feebleness or deficiency. I have found that this plant may be given to the elderly with *Crocus* as a general tonic.

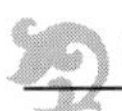

Capsicum frutescens

COMMON NAME ■ Cayenne

Look for this remedy also under the name *Capsicum fastigiatum. Capsicum* is a member of the nightshade family, *Solanaceae.* The fruit of the plant is used to make medicine. Capsaicin appears to be the chief constituent responsible for the pungent flavor of the pepper. When it is used as a diaphoretic, Dr. Bastyr said that $\frac{1}{4}$ teaspoon of dried powder of *Capsicum* should be taken and washed down with warm water.

In treating cancer patients, I frequently add *Capsicum* to the food because it is rich in vitamin C and carotenoids, including capsanthin, capsorubin, and capsaicin. Cayenne depletes substance P, which is a pain transmitter. Thus the pain of mouth sores frequently associated with chemotherapy may be avoided.

Quite a number of applications of *Capsicum* have been cropping up lately, especially topical applications of *Capsicum* salves. Because of *Capsicum*'s ability to deplete the neurotransmitter substance P, salves applied to inflammatory conditions are suggested. For example, a *Capsicum* salve may be applied to herpes zoster lesions to relieve pain, to psoriatic lesions to decrease inflammation,[117] to facial nerves to treat trigeminal neuralgia, and to the hands and feet to treat arthritis.

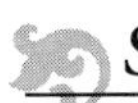

Salvia officinalis

COMMON NAME ■ Sage

The aerial parts are used to make medicine. I have used *Salvia* as a diaphoretic at the first sign of a cold. *Salvia* is a diaphoretic alterative in that hot sage tea induces diaphoresis and cold sage tea helps to restrain the sweating. I suggest giving 40 drops of tincture in a cup of hot water twice daily as a diaphoretic. This use of sage in eclectic medicine can be traced back to Dr. Harvey Wickes Felter.[118] Dr. Felter was an MD who practiced eclectic medicine around 1910.

CHAPTER

30

DIGESTANTS

CHAPTER • OUTLINE

Ananas cosmosus
Hydrochloric acid
Ingluvin
Pancreatin
Carica papaya
Pepsin
Aspergillus oryzae
Ficus carica or *Ficus glabrata*

Digestants are agents that improve the digestion of food, either directly because they contain digestive enzymes or indirectly because they stimulate the body to produce digestive enzymes. These remedies are especially important for our elderly patients who sometimes cannot digest their food adequately either because they do not produce enough hydrochloric acid or because their pancreas secretes insufficient enzymes in response to materials coming into the duodenum.

As a naturopathic physician, I encourage practitioners not to miss the simple diagnosis of maldigestion in elderly patients. The solution to gastric and intestinal upset is usually to aid the digestion, not to repress it with antacids and histamine blockers.

Digestants can often be used in harmony with bitters to improve the digestive health of our patients.

Ananas cosmosus

COMMON NAME ■ Pineapple

The core and fruit are used to make medicine. This plant contains bromelain, which is a proteolytic enzyme. The bromelain content is highest in the core. This plant is useful in treating arthritis, rheumatism, fibromyalgia, and polymyalgia rheumatica. It is also a good digestant. I use bromelain to help rid the body of internal fibrous tissue. The dose of bromelain for most problems is 1000 mg three times daily. I like to use curcumin with bromelain because, by preventing sulfhydral breakdown, curcumin spares bromelain and thus prolongs its effectiveness. Bromelain encourages healthy prostaglandin production. It encourages prostaglandin E_1 synthesis but has no effect on prostaglandin E_2.

Hydrochloric acid

Both betaine and glutamic acid are available as a source of hydrochloric acid (HCl). An acid environment is needed in the stomach to help convert pepsinogen to pepsin. Other acids may be used to create this acid environment, such as acetic acid from vinegar or citric acid from lemon juice. The dose for HCl as a digestant varies widely. Try 5 to 10 grains per meal initially; however, HCl may be dosed as high as 20 to 30 grains per meal. Dr. Bastyr said that *Gentiana lutea* was the best remedy for stimulating hydrochloric acid production in the stomach. He recommended 10 drops of *Gentiana* per meal. Sometimes the elderly experience a decrease in HCl production as they age, with a concomitant increase in gas production. *Gentiana* often helps these patients.

Dr. Bastyr taught that patients who require HCl have a thin or narrow tongue that often appears red. Sometimes patients have a dry brown coating on the tongue as well. I would add that the face might have a red flush or hyperemic skin on the upper cheek area. It could also have flaring of the nostrils out from the edge of the nose toward the lower ear. The lupus mask face is sometimes seen in people who need HCl.

Ingluvin

Dr. Bastyr said that ingluvin is extracted from chicken stomachs. He mentioned that it is one of the best remedies for indigestion when the patient has nausea with pains in the stomach. He said that vertigo might also be present. I would like to know more about ingluvin, but as yet I have little to offer. I have included this selection for historical purposes.

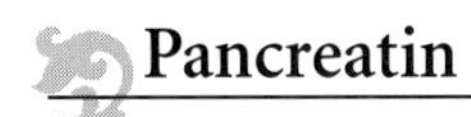

Pancreatin

This material is derived from animal sources, such as cows; however, there are also effective vegetable sources of this enzyme. Pancreatin is a digestive enzyme that digests protein, fat, and starch. It contains trypsin, chymotrypsin, amylase, and lipase. The dose of pancreatin is usually 3 or 4 capsules per meal.

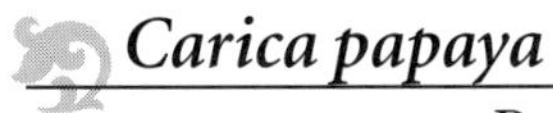

Carica papaya

COMMON NAME ■ Papaya

This plant contains papain, which is derived from the unripe fruit of the papaya. Papain is a proteolytic enzyme that aids in protein digestion in either an acid or an alkaline environment. Papaya can be used as a meat tenderizer. Evidently the meat is wrapped in papaya leaves. Naturopathic physicians prescribe 500-mg capsules at a dose of one or more per meal as a digestant.

Dr. Bastyr commented that the powdered papain could be used to clean wounds because it acts as a fibrinolytic. He said that it should be applied topically.

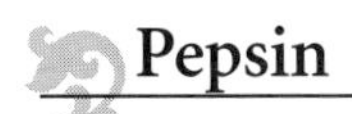

Pepsin

Pepsin is produced by the chief cells in the stomach. Medicinally, it is extracted from hog stomach. I prescribe 500 mg per meal to aid the digestion of protein.

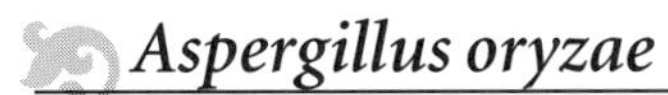

Aspergillus oryzae

COMMON NAME ■ Taka-diastase

Taka-diastase is a multienzyme from *Aspergillus*, which has many enzymatic functions. It is a microscopic fungus that converts starch into sugar and aids in the digestion of proteins and lipids. When it is used as a digestive aid, Dr. Bastyr said that the dose is 2 to 5 grains per meal. This is another material included for historical reference. I have no experience with this in my own private practice.

Ficus carica or *Ficus glabrata*

COMMON NAME ■ Fig

The fruit contains digestive enzymes. Ficin, which is the name of the proteolytic enzyme itself, is obtained by filtering and drying the latex of *Ficus glabrata*. Figs are also mild laxatives. A dose of 300 mg per meal may be used. According to Dr. John Lust, an early naturopathic physician, the stems and leaves contain an acrid milky juice that has been used to treat warts.

CHAPTER

31

DIURETICS

CHAPTER • OUTLINE

Arctostaphylos uva-ursi
Urtica urens
Coffea arabica
Petroselinum sativum
Triticum repens
Usnea species
Galium aparine
Levisticum officinale
Ononis spinosa
Orthosiphon stamineus

Diuretics increase urine excretion. The following list of remedies includes a handful of useful diuretics. I cover a number of diuretics in Chapter 40, Genitourinary Agents, and Chapter 41, Genitourinary Sedatives and Stimulants. For additional diuretic remedies, please consult these chapters. Give adequate hydration when using diuretics. Foods such as greens and liquids such as tomato juice and carrot juice help to maintain adequate electrolyte balance in patients who need diuretics either to flush the kidneys or for blood pressure management.

Arctostaphylos uva-ursi

COMMON NAMES ■ Upland cranberry, Bearberry

The medicine is obtained from the leaves of the *Arctostaphylos uva-ursi* plant. It is a fair diuretic and an excellent genitourinary antiseptic. The dose is 90 drops of tincture four times daily for either of these conditions. Dr. Bastyr recommended combining *Arctostaphylos* with *Chimaphila* for urinary tract infections. His dose was 60 drops of the formula three times daily in water.

The active ingredient in *Arctostaphylos* is arbutin, which is contained in the leaves. The leaves also contain tannin and quercetin, which is a flavone. Another constituent, ellagic acid, is present in some other berries, like raspberry. Ellagic acid is currently being looked at with interest as a neoplastic growth inhibitor in the treatment of cancer.

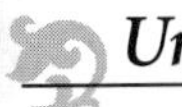

Urtica urens

COMMON NAME ■ Stinging nettle

The flowering plant is used to make medicine. The diuretic action of this plant helps to flush the renal pelvis, ureters, and urinary bladder. I have used *Urtica* to treat cystitis and nephritis. The dose I recommend is 90 drops of tincture four times daily. However, if preferred, 2 capsules may be taken four times daily. It may be of interest to the reader that there is a small amount of histamine in the stinging hairs of the leaves.

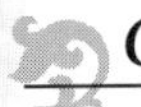

Coffea arabica

COMMON NAME ■ Coffee

The seeds are used to make medicine. Dr. Bastyr mentioned this plant as a diuretic, but he said that it must be diluted with water. He said to take a standard cup of coffee and dilute it with water—$\frac{1}{2}$ cup water to $\frac{1}{2}$ cup coffee. He said that the dose as a diuretic is 1 diluted cup twice daily. Excess use of this plant can cause heart palpitations and nervousness. Caffeine in excess of 200 mg per day becomes somewhat toxic to the nervous system.

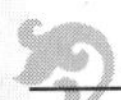

Petroselinum sativum

COMMON NAME ■ Parsley

Petroselinum sativum was the species name given when Dr. Bastyr taught about this plant. *Petroselinum crispum* is the scientific name of parsley as well. The whole plant, including the seed, can be used; however, the parsley fruit provides the best diuretic, followed by the root. This plant is a good diuretic. I recommend 90 drops of the tincture three times daily in a cup of water. *CAUTION: Large doses of parsley should not be used during pregnancy because parsley tends to stimulate the uterus.*

I have found that combining *Petroselinum* with *Usnea* makes one of the more effective diuretics. I mix equal parts of each plant tincture and prescribe a dose of 90 drops of the formula four times daily. I have found that this is a very good diuretic when other diuretics are not working for the patient. Among other things, parsley contains apiol, flavonoids, vitamin C, and myristicin.

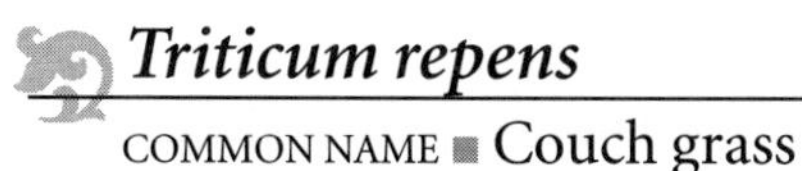

Triticum repens

COMMON NAME ■ Couch grass

Also look for this plant under the name *Elymus repens.* The rhizome is used to make medicine. This plant is a demulcent diuretic. The diuretic action is fairly mild. I use 150 drops of the tincture three times daily. This soothes the urinary tract. To soothe the urinary tract and relax the ureters, I often combine *Triticum* with *Hydrangea.* This combination is excellent. The plants are combined in equal parts, and the dose is 150 drops of the formula three to four times daily. This combination is so effective that I have used it a number of times for the passage of kidney stones less than 6 mm. I would suggest tasting the tincture for oneself. The soothing quality is apparent in the tasting experience.

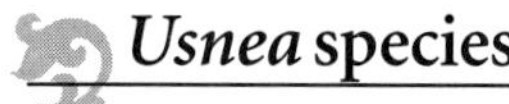

Usnea species

COMMON NAMES ■ Usnea, Beard moss

The whole lichen is used to make medicine. *Usnea* is an excellent diuretic. I prescribe 90 drops of the tincture three times daily. *Usnea* is mucilaginous and antimicrobial. It contains polyketides, which are lichen acids. Usnic acid, thamnolic acid, lobaric acid, stictinic acid, evernic acid, and barbatic acid are some of the lichen acids and give the *Usnea* tincture an acidic taste.[25]

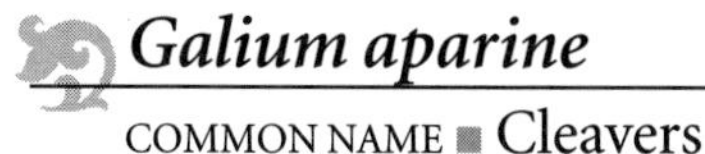

Galium aparine

COMMON NAME ■ Cleavers

Use the dried aerial parts for medicine. *Galium* contains the iridoid monoterpene asperuloside; several alkaloids, including the benzyl isoquinoline alkaloid; protopine; flavonoids; and a plethora of minerals. This plant is an important and excellent diuretic. It may be given in high doses—90 drops of the tincture four to five times daily. Even higher doses may be considered. This plant should also be remembered when treating the lymphatic system for conditions such as lymphostasis and lymphadenopathy. I combine three parts *Galium* with one part *Phytolacca* and five parts *Echinacea* to create an effective formula for this purpose.

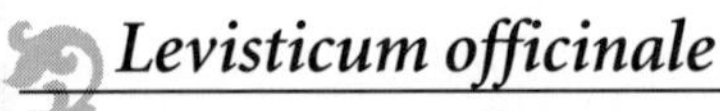

Levisticum officinale

COMMON NAME ■ Lovage

This plant is a member of the carrot family, *Umbelliferae.* The root is used to make medicine, not the leaves. Dr. Bastyr said that *Levisticum* is a gentle diuretic. Give the patient 60 drops of tincture three times daily. As an aside, *Levisticum* contains a psoralen analogue called bergaptene, which has been used in creams to treat psoriasis.

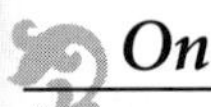

Ononis spinosa

COMMON NAME ■ Spiny restharrow

This plant belongs to the pea family, *Leguminosae.* The root is used for medicine. *Ononis* contains a saponin, which is its diuretic principle. When it is used as a diuretic, herbalists give 60 drops of the tincture twice daily in a glass of water.

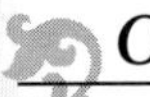

Orthosiphon stamineus

COMMON NAME ■ Indian kidney tea

This plant is a member of the *Labiatae* family. The leaves are used for medicine. They contain a lipophilic flavone called sinensetin.[13] According to Rudolph Weiss, *Orthosiphon* is a diuretic and helps get rid of nitrogenous wastes.[13] Take 2 cups daily. I have no experience with this plant; however, given the recent interest in plants from Australia and other South Pacific areas, *Orthosiphon* may be worth exploring. It does not cure nephrosis but is used rather in the early treatment of developing kidney disorders.

CHAPTER

32

EMETICS

CHAPTER • OUTLINE

Euphorbia corollata
Brassica juncea
Ophioglossum vulgatum
Fomes officinalis
Cephaelis ipecacuanha
Veratrum viride
Eupatorium perfoliatum
Salt

Emetics are agents that induce vomiting. In the 19th century, emetics were used as part of a cleansing therapy to purge the body of toxins. Samuel Thompson (1769-1843), for example, used emetics in what became known as the Thompsonian system of medicine. Thompsonian eclectics believed that plants could be used to cleanse and stimulate the body. The stimulated body would then heal itself. For example, a plant like aconite would be given in nearly toxic doses. The same was true for *Lobelia, Bryonia, Gelsemium,* and other fairly toxic plants. During the crisis of eliminating these toxins by vomiting, the body would become stronger. This is sort of botanical Nietzscheism. Modern naturopathic physicians do not generally practice this use of emetics. Instead, emetics such as ipecac are occasionally used to induce vomiting in a patient who has ingested poisonous materials.

Euphorbia corollata

COMMON NAMES ■ Blooming spurge, Milk purslane

The bark is used to make medicine. *Euphorbia* is only mildly emetic, so a dose of 30 or 40 drops may be needed. Kuts-Cheraux mentions that doses of 1 to 2 drops of *Euphorbia* can be used to treat cholera infantum. I find the plant mildly nauseating even in doses of 10 drops. Dr. Bastyr said that as an expectorant it is similar to *Kali bichromium. Euphorbia* has been used to treat constipation. For this purpose, Dr. Bastyr recommended 10 drops of tincture in 4 ounces of water every hour until results are attained.

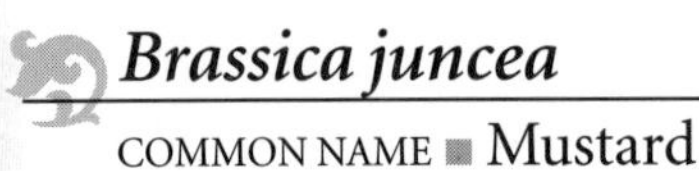

Brassica juncea

COMMON NAME ■ Mustard

The seeds are used for medicine. As an emetic, 1 to 2 teaspoons of the mustard powder in a cup of hot water should be taken. Dr. Bastyr said that small doses stimulate the appetite and the secretion of digestive juices. I have found that placing $\frac{1}{8}$ teaspoon of hot mustard paste on the tongue helps to drain the sinuses.

To make a mustard pack, Dr. Bastyr taught us to use one part mustard powder to three parts flour. Four parts flour can be used if the mustard is particularly active. Add vegetable oil or water until a paste is obtained. Sandwich this between two pieces of 100% cotton fabric and apply it for 10 or 15 minutes, or until the chest appears pink. *CAUTION: If the mustard pack is left on the skin too long, a burn can result.*

Ophioglossum vulgatum

COMMON NAME ■ English adder's tongue

The tops of the plant are used for medicine. This plant is an emetic. Once again, I list this plant for historical reference. Dr. Bastyr taught about it as one of the emetics; however, I have no experience with this particular plant. Nevertheless, it may be worthwhile to learn more about it. Dr. Bastyr said that *Ophioglossum* is helpful as a poultice for scrofulous tumors.

Fomes officinalis

COMMON NAME ■ Lichen

Large doses are purgative and emetic. Dr. Bastyr said to use 3 to 30 grains to produce emesis. Again, this plant was mentioned more as an aside, and I do not recall any further information given about it. I have included it for historical purposes.

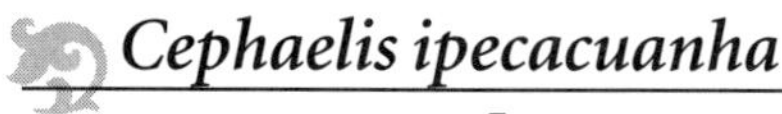

Cephaelis ipecacuanha

COMMON NAME ■ Ipecac

The medicine is made from the root. Ipecac is the most popular emetic worldwide. The active ingredient in ipecac is emetine. The syrup of ipecac is available at any drug store. The dose is listed on the bottle and will be about 2 to 3 teaspoons. This remedy is a reliable emetic. *CAUTION: Do not use ipecac in cases of corrosive poisoning unless advised to do so by the poison center.* Hematemesis can increase in these patients.

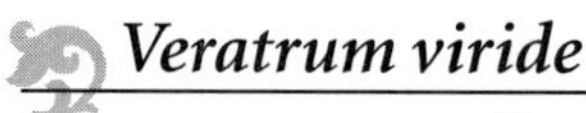

Veratrum viride

COMMON NAME ■ Green hellebore

The root and leaves are used to make medicine. Veratrine, which is a mixture of cevadine, veratridine, and cevine, is a drastic emetocathartic. It is poisonous and is seldom used as an emetic. Dr. Bastyr said that the dose as an emetic is about 10 drops of the tincture per 50 pounds of body weight, although a larger dose may be needed.

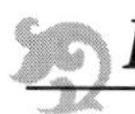

Eupatorium perfoliatum

COMMON NAME ■ Boneset

The flowering tops and leaves are used to make medicine. Large doses of *Eupatorium* are emetic. I have found that at least 150 drops of the tincture may be needed for emesis. Some of the old eclectics used 3 cups of the strong standard tea to induce emesis to clear the upper gastrointestinal tract. Dr. Bastyr reminded us that this remedy also produces diaphoresis.

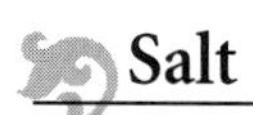

Salt

When using salt as an emetic, dissolve 1 tablespoonful of salt in a cup of warm water and drink the entire amount.

CHAPTER

33

EMMENAGOGUES

CHAPTER • OUTLINE

Emmenagogues are remedies that promote normal and regular menstrual flow. The emmenagogues were explored and used before we had birth control and hormone therapy to regulate periods.

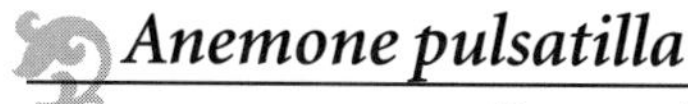

Anemone pulsatilla

COMMON NAME ■ Pasque flower

The aerial parts of the plant are used to make medicine. One main cause of menstrual irregularity is tension. Because *A. pulsatilla* is so specific for nervous exhaustion, it is a particularly good remedy for abnormal cycles produced by excessive tension. Therefore *A. pulsatilla* may be used in amenorrhea associated with tension. To normalize the menstrual cycle, Dr. Bastyr recommended 20 drops of tincture three times daily. For dysmenorrhea, he said to combine *A. pulsatilla* with *Piscidia erythrina* in equal portions and give 60 drops of the tincture every 3 hours until the pain subsides.

In addition to its use as an emmenagogue, *A. pulsatilla* can be used for a variety of other conditions. Dr. Bastyr taught that it could help to maintain the version, or position of the fetus, in pregnancy. He said that this remedy also affects the heart like a low dose of cactus. A useful tea may be made twice daily for dread of calamity. Use 20 drops of the tincture in each cup. *A. pulsatilla* has been used as a douche in leukorrhea caused by *Trichomonas vaginalis.*

Dr. Bastyr taught us about another interesting use for *A. pulsatilla.* He said that it was used for heart consciousness associated with insomnia. This is when the patient is lying in bed and is aware of the heart beating. We cannot usually feel our heart beating in our chest. The dose he suggested was 10 to 20 drops of the tincture twice daily. One of these doses should be taken at night.

Caulophyllum thalictroides

COMMON NAME ■ Blue cohosh

This plant is a member of the barberry family, *Berberidaceae.* The root is used to make medicine. This remedy is an emmenagogue for use in delayed or suppressed menstruation. The dose for this purpose is 10 to 20 drops of tincture twice daily. It is a good uterine tonic for women in their fifties or for any woman with an atonic uterus. Dr. Bastyr used *Caulophyllum* for rigid os uteri. For deficient labor pains (Dr. Bastyr delivered more than 800 babies), he used *Caulophyllum* in doses of 1 to 10 drops two to three times during labor as needed. Although this does not sound like very much, Dr. Bastyr said that it was plenty. I have used *Caulophyllum* on three occasions to help start overdue labor. In all three cases, labor began that day. The dose I used was 30 drops in 2 cups of water, sipped throughout the day.

Polygonum punctatum

COMMON NAME ■ Water smartweed

The medicine is made from the flowering herb. Dr. Bastyr taught us to use 10 to 20 drops of the tincture to reestablish the menstrual cycle after missed periods. He said that *Polygonum* could also be used to treat urinary suppression. Here it acts rapidly. The dose he suggested was 30 drops of the tincture twice daily.

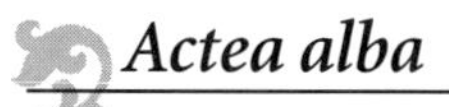

Actea alba

COMMON NAME ■ White cohosh

The roots are used to make medicine. Dr. Bastyr said that this is a dependable emmenagogue and nerve tonic. It is useful for amenorrhea, dysmenorrhea, and ovarian neuralgia. Generally, ovarian neuralgia describes pain in the ovary or ovarian area. As an emmenagogue, Dr. Bastyr recommended a dose of 3 to 6 drops of the tincture given often if needed. For premenstrual syndrome, I mix one part *Actea* tincture with four parts licorice root tincture. The dose of the mixture is 60 drops twice daily. This remedy is frequently successful. Interestingly, Kuts-Cheraux mentions that *Actea* is useful in anorexia nervosa, possibly as a gentle nerve tonic.[28]

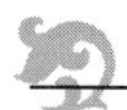

Chamaelirium luteum

COMMON NAMES ■ False unicorn root, Blazing star root

This remedy may be found under the name *Veratrum luteum*. The root is used to make medicine. *Chamaelirium* contains the steroid saponin, chamaelirin. I cannot speak highly enough of this herb's capacity to tonify and strengthen the reproductive system. *Chamaelirium* may be taken daily as an emmenagogue. The dose is 40 drops of tincture for this purpose. My formula for normalizing the menstrual cycle is equal parts of the tinctures of *Chamaelirium luteum*, *Mitchella repens*, *Cimicifuga racemosa*, and *Vitex agnus-castus*. The dose I recommend is 30 drops of the mixture twice daily. I learned a great deal about *Chamaelirium* from Chanchal Cabrera, an excellent British herbalist and friend.

In addition to its use for women, *Chamaelirium* is also useful for men as a genitourinary alterative and strengthener.

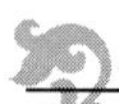

Mentha pulegium

COMMON NAMES ■ Pennyroyal, Tickweed

Also look for this plant under the name *Hedeoma pulegiodes*. Pennyroyal is in the mint family, *Labiatae*. The aerial parts of the plant are used to make medicine. *CAUTION: Avoid this plant altogether during pregnancy*. The main constituent, pulegone, is found in the oil of pennyroyal. When using pennyroyal, the oil should be avoided because its action is too strong. This emmenagogue will help to strengthen uterine contractions during menses. The tincture dose that herbalists recommend is 20 drops twice daily.

Practitioners should avoid using this plant as an abortifacient if asked by the patient about its usefulness in this area. The amount of pennyroyal needed for this purpose can be toxic to the patient. Certainly, pennyroyal's use for the purpose of abortion can be acknowledged as a historical reality and then hopefully discarded. Putting the life of the patient in danger by giving a toxic dose of a botanical remedy is against the time-honored principle of naturopathic medicine to do no harm.

Senecio aureus

COMMON NAMES ■ Life root, Female regulator herb, Golden ragwort, Golden groundseal

This plant is a member of the sunflower family, *Compositae.* Other species of *Senecio* are also used, including *S. vulgaris* and *S. jacobaea.* The dried herb and fresh plant are harvested during the flowering season to make medicine. This plant contains many alkaloids. For example, *S. vulgaris* contains the alkaloids seneciphylline, senecionine, retrorsine, spartioidine, usaramine, and integerrimine.[26,87,88,119]

Senecio's emmenagogue activity is accomplished by increasing the vascularity and tone of the reproductive system. Dr. Bastyr said to think of this remedy to treat lax uterine ligaments in women who have given birth many times. He also said that prolapsed bladder may respond to *Senecio*, especially in elderly patients. The dose of the tincture is 20 drops three times daily.

Vitex agnus-castus

COMMON NAME ■ Chaste berry

The fruit is used to make medicine. *Vitex* contains flavonoids and iridoids and may contain 3-ketosteroids.[26] Aucubin and agnuside are two of the iridoids. I cannot resist adding *Vitex* to the list of emmenagogues. *Vitex*'s action as an emmenagogue is different from that of some of the other plants. It works by normalizing the pituitary gland, which is one of the master glands that, along with the hypothalamus, begins the cascade of hormone signals that keep us in balance.

The hormone system is a very complex system regulated by feedback loops. It is hard to imagine really treating the whole person relative to the endocrine system without addressing the master glands. I think of *Vitex* as a pituitary tonic, alterative, and normalizer. For hormonal imbalances, *Vitex* may simply be added to other formulas. The dose of *Vitex* alone is 30 drops in the morning. I suggest mixing *Vitex* with *Cimicifuga* to achieve hormone balance by means of pituitary normalization.

Gratiola officinalis

COMMON NAME ■ Hedge hyssop

This plant belongs to the *Scrophulariaceae* family. The herb and roots are used to make medicine. *Gratiola* can be found in France and Germany. Rudolph

Weiss says that this plant is considered to be one of the best emmenagogues.[13] I have no experience with this plant, but given that recommendation, it is certainly worth looking into.

CHAPTER

34

EMULSIFIERS

CHAPTER • OUTLINE

Zea mays
Avena sativa
Egg yolk
Acacia senegal
Manihot esculenta

I have opted to include a few emulsifiers in this book because of my belief that one of the important aspects of health is the absorption of fats from dietary sources, including plants. These agents help to emulsify oils so that the oils can be better absorbed. Oil-rich plants may be mixed with or taken with these agents. Dr. Bastyr did not discuss emulsifiers as a group.

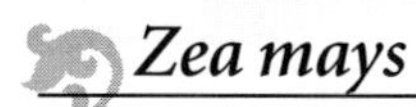

Zea mays

COMMON NAME ■ Corn

I have patients cook the corn kernels and then blend them into a mush. Regular frozen corn works very well. This mush is a good emulsifying agent. Patients who eat salad with high-quality oil will do well to include a corn mush. This will help to enhance the absorption of the oil used on the salad as well as the xanthophylls contained in the green leaves. The xanthophylls are fat-soluble carotenoids, which are particularly good for the eyes, the reproductive system, and the brain.

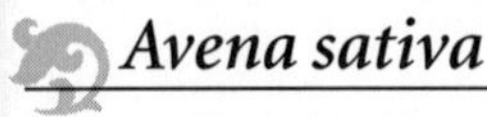

Avena sativa

COMMON NAME ■ Oats

Oatmeal makes an excellent emulsifier. Oatmeal can be used in the same way as corn. I suggest having the patient drink carrot juice rather than orange juice with breakfast. The oatmeal will help in the absorption of the beta-carotene in the carrots.

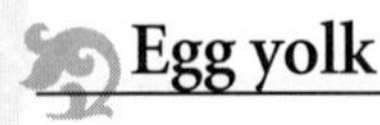

Egg yolk

I encourage my patients to eat eggs with vegetables. The whole egg can be scrambled and eaten with a plate of greens as an emulsifying food. Remember that the egg yolk contains cholesterol, which is the precursor building block of hormones. During menopause, when hormone levels are dropping, and for anyone over 45 years of age, hormone levels may be increased by simply consuming eggs. The white of the eggs is a highly absorbable form of protein.

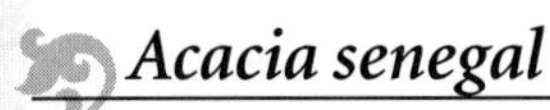

Acacia senegal

COMMON NAME ■ Gum arabic

The gum of the plant is used to make medicine. *Acacia* is a very ancient remedy, discussed in the oldest herbals. The powdered gum arabic may be mixed with fluid and used as an emulsifying agent. Noteworthy is the considerable solubility of this hydrocolloid, making it useful in forming suspensions with other plant medicines. Plants with this characteristic are called suspending agents.

Manihot esculenta

COMMON NAME ■ Cassava

Tapioca pudding is an excellent emulsifier. It is made from the root of the cassava plant. Carrots, either cooked or raw, may be consumed during the same meal as tapioca. This will help to increase the absorption of the beta-carotene in the carrot. I recommend tapioca for my elderly patients, since the elderly often have a difficult time absorbing oils from their foods. Any emulsifier helps, and tapioca tastes pretty good and is easily consumed.

CHAPTER

35

EXPECTORANTS

CHAPTER • OUTLINE

Lobelia inflata
Sanguinaria canadensis
Cephaelis ipecacuanha
Urginea maritima
Grindelia squarrosa
Aspidosperma quebracho-blanco
Oenothera biennis
Sticta pulmonaris
Asclepias tuberosa
Asclepias syriaca
Drosera rotundifolia
Euphrasia officinalis
Momordica balsamina
Potassium bichromate
Pinus palustris
Populus gileadensis
Thymus serpyllum
Viola odorata
Marrubium vulgare
Ribes nigrum
Justicia adhatoda
Tilia europaea
Angelica archangelica
Pimpinella saxifraga
Saponaria officinalis

Expectorants are medicinal materials that encourage the patient to cough up mucus. These remedies are extremely useful when dealing with dry, unproductive coughs. In upper respiratory infections, it is important to support the body's production of mucus and to enhance its expectoration. In doing so, the protective globulins, which are carried in the mucus, are provided to the surface of the mucous membranes to help kill microorganisms.

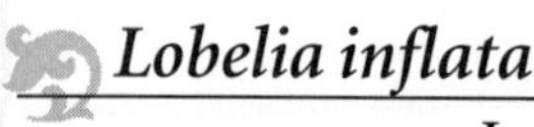

Lobelia inflata

COMMON NAME ■ Indian tobacco

The aerial parts of the plant are used for medicine. This plant contains a number of piperidine alkaloids, the most studied of which is lobeline. *Lobelia* is a systemic relaxant and an antispasmodic, with some respiratory leanings. It has been used historically for asthma. Larger doses are emetic.

As an expectorant, *Lobelia* can be mixed with other plants. Dr. Bastyr used to mix *Lobelia* with *Capsicum* to help offset its sedative effects. Dr. Bastyr's dose for an acute asthma episode was 30 drops of the tincture of *Lobelia* mixed with 10 drops of *Capsicum* tincture. He said that this dose should never be repeated more than twice. He said that *Lobelia* also combines well with *Aspidosperma.* He used *Lobelia* for whooping cough in cases where the membranes were dry and lacking expectoration. The best formula for whooping cough that I have found is one part *Lobelia* tincture, one part *Aspidosperma* tincture, four parts *Glycyrrhiza* fluid extract, and four parts *Grindelia* tincture. Take 60 drops of the formula four times daily. Dr. Bastyr mentioned that *Lobelia* is similar in action to *Grindelia.*

Evidently, *Lobelia* is excellent in a drawing poultice. For this purpose it has been mixed with slippery elm and *Echinacea.* I use Epsom salts with a little *Sanguinaria* and *Hydrastis* added as a typical drawing poultice for an open wound or boil. Drawing poultices are very useful in helping to drain boils once they have been lanced.

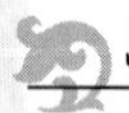

Sanguinaria canadensis

COMMON NAME ■ Blood root

The rhizome is used for medicine. This plant contains several isoquinoline alkaloids, including berberine and sanguinarine. As an expectorant, Dr. Bastyr mixed this plant with other botanicals. I have found that it mixes well with *Glycyrrhiza, Grindelia, Tussilago,* and *Verbascum.* Add to these a little *Hydrastis* and you have an excellent expectorant. I mix the above in equal parts and add a little lomatium isolate. I give the resulting formula in doses of 60 drops four times daily.

For atonic conditions of the lungs or as an expectorant in allergies affecting the upper respiratory tract, I also use 2 capsules of quercetin chalcone three times daily and 2 capsules of *Urtica* three times daily. The Mohegans and the Pillager Ojibwas used the root juice of *Sanguinaria* as a gargle for sore throats. The dose of *Sanguinaria* itself as an upper respiratory expectorant is 15 drops three times daily.

Dr. Bastyr mentioned the use of *Sanguinaria* for sensations in the lower pharynx and midpharynx. I do not know what he meant by sensations; however, I have seen a number of patients each year who have complained of odd feelings in this area.

Cephaelis ipecacuanha

COMMON NAME ■ Ipecac

The root is used to make medicine. Dr. Bastyr used ipecac to treat violent paroxysmal coughing. He said that ipecac is an expectorant for the cough of flu. He also used ipecac for bronchitis and for children with whistling respiration. His dose was 5 to 15 drops of the syrup daily. He taught us that ipecac is also used for the violent cough of pneumonia in small doses of 5 drops of the syrup repeated every hour for up to 5 hours. An 8-hour break should be taken before repeating this regimen.

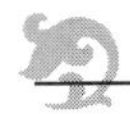

Urginea maritima

COMMON NAME ■ Squill

The bulbs are used for medicine. *CAUTION: Dr. Bastyr taught us that* Urginea *potentiates digitalis, so be careful with patients who are taking heart medication.* This plant contains bioflavonoids, tannins, and fructans. *Urginea* is an expectorant, a diuretic, and an emetic. It helps to increase expectoration in severe bronchial coughs. The dose of the tincture is about 20 drops three times daily.

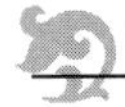

Grindelia squarrosa

COMMON NAME ■ Gumweed

Grindelia is a member of the sunflower family, *Compositae.* The flowers and terminal leaves are used to make medicine. *Grindelia* is an expectorant and an antispasmodic. Dr. Bastyr was very fond of this remedy and included it in many of his cough preparations. He taught its use for harsh, dry, unproductive coughs. He said that you might not get marked action at first, but as you continued to use it, you would see results. Give 30 drops of *Grindelia* extract three times daily as an expectorant.

Grindelia has also been used for allergy cough and hay fever. I use *Grindelia* and *Glycyrrhiza* together. These two plants combine well medicinally for their expectorant action; they are synergistic. Remember the close therapeutic relationship of *Grindelia* and *Glycyrrhiza.* I mix these plants in equal parts and prescribe 60 drops three times daily.

A poultice of *Grindelia* has been used in folk medicine to treat poison ivy. *Grindelia* contains phenolics, which may account for the antimicrobial activity. It also contains grindelic acid and its derivatives.

Aspidosperma quebracho-blanco

COMMON NAME ■ Quebracho

The bark of this plant is used to make medicine. This plant is a respiratory and cardiac stimulant. Dr. Bastyr called quebracho the digitalis of the lungs. It tonifies and encourages expectoration from the lungs and bronchi. It helps to expectorate mucus in patients with dyspnea, emphysema, and bronchitis. It increases oxygen to the tissues by stimulating the respiratory center. Dr. Bastyr gave 10 drops of the tincture several times daily.

In addition to its use as an expectorant and a respiratory stimulant, this plant contains yohimbine, as does *Corynanthe yohimbe.* Yohimbe is a very famous aphrodisiac. Quebracho can be used in the same manner as yohimbe. The alkaloid, yohimbine, is an alpha-2 blocker. It increases norepinephrine availability. Other alkaloids in quebracho include aspidospermine and akuammidine.[25]

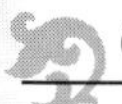

Oenothera biennis

COMMON NAME ■ Common evening primrose

The leaves, twigs, and bark are used to make medicine. Dr. Bastyr included this remedy under expectorants; however, he did not clearly explain how to use this remedy as an expectorant. I have included it here for historical purposes. *Oenothera* is nontoxic, and Dr. Bastyr said that it is specific for nervous, irritable patients. For general respiratory distress, it is a mild sedative to the nervous system supplying the respiratory centers. His dose was 15 drops of the tincture repeated often.

Oenothera oil is a great source of both linoleic acid and gamma-linolenic acid (GLA). In addition, *Oenothera* oil is a useful nutritive botanical for patients who have low delta-6-desaturase levels. Delta-6-desaturase is needed to produce GLA. Given the dietary source of GLA provided by *Oenothera*, simply using *Oenothera* compensates for a delta-6-desaturase deficiency.

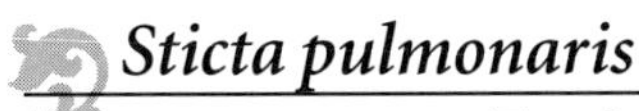

Sticta pulmonaris

COMMON NAME ■ Tree lungwort

Another scientific name for this plant is *Pulmonaria officinalis.* Use the whole upper herb to make medicine. Dr. Bastyr said to use 15 to 20 drops of the tincture three times daily as an antitussive and an expectorant. He mentioned *Sticta* to relieve short, hacking coughs. I have also used it in acute bronchitis, sneezing, and coryza. In addition, *Sticta* helps to relieve the pain of sore pectoral and intercostal muscles caused by excess coughing.

Sticta contains many interesting active ingredients, including allantoin, quercetin, kaempferol, vitamin C, mucilage, and tannins. Allantoin is a vulnerary. Dr. Bastyr told me that allantoin is applied to the lower legs of race horses to help heal and soothe sore legs. Comfrey is another plant that is rich in allantoin.

From the list of active constituents, you can see that *Sticta* is indicated for allergies affecting the gastrointestinal tract. Quercetin is a mast cell stabilizer, mucilage is a demulcent that soothes the intestine, and kaempferol is an excellent liver remedy. The liver is closely linked to the intestine in proper management of food.

Dr. Bastyr said that *Sticta* could also be used in ulcerative colitis. Its tannin content may be helpful in securing the health of the intestinal lining. Two teaspoons of the dried herb are infused into a cup of water for 15 minutes. Several cups of this preparation may be taken daily.

Asclepias tuberosa

COMMON NAMES ■ Butterfly weed, Pleurisy root

The root is used to make medicine. This plant has a long history of use in early American eclectic medicine. Dr. Bastyr spoke about it very fondly. *Asclepias* is an expectorant. It is an upper and lower respiratory herb. It is used to treat bronchitis, pneumonia, intercostal disease, influenza, pleurisy, and colds. Dr. Bastyr used it for tight painful coughs with difficult respiration. I have frequently prescribed it for flu with a tight chest feeling or for painful coughs. The dose I use is 60 drops three times daily. Dr. Bastyr said that *Asclepias* is specific to pleuritis, promoting rapid removal of effusion. Use 20 drops of tincture every 2 hours for all of the above conditions. The powdered dose is 20 grains twice daily. For pleurisy, I also use large doses of bioflavonoids and some vitamin C. The flavonoids are important here.

Asclepias contains rutin, kaempferol, quercetin, isorhamnetin, and other bioflavonoids. The effectiveness of *Asclepias* is probably the result of its flavonoid content. The integrity of the capillary mesh throughout the body is improved with adequate levels of bioflavonoids.

Asclepias tastes how I imagine the forest would taste if it were tinctured. It is very bright tasting and feels green in your mouth.

Asclepias syriaca

COMMON NAME ■ Milkweed

The root is used to make medicine. This is a pain-relieving expectorant and a stimulant. It is useful to treat asthma, bronchitis, and viral pharyngitis. Dr. Bastyr used it especially in painful viral pharyngitis. For all of these conditions, 60 drops of the tincture are given three times daily.

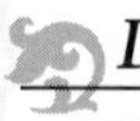

Drosera rotundifolia

COMMON NAME ■ Sundew

The whole plant is used to make medicine. I am overwhelmed by the miniature exquisiteness of *Drosera*. I remember wildcrafting it and sitting for a long while just looking at it. *Drosera* contains several naphthoquinones, including plumbagin and ramentaceone.

Drosera is an expectorant. Dr. Bastyr said that it would help stop whooping cough and that it is a good cure for nervous cough and for the cough of measles. In addition, he used it for children who cough in their sleep. *Drosera* tastes a little bit like sherry. Have the patient take the tincture in doses of 20 drops four times daily. This dose may be increased as needed. After tasting this plant, the patient feels a chest action or presence after about 3 to 4 minutes.

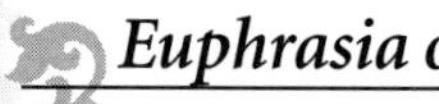

Euphrasia officinalis

COMMON NAME ■ Eyebright

The whole plant is used to make medicine. *Euphrasia* is one of my favorite plants. It is an expectorant, an antiinflammatory, a mild astringent, and a respiratory emollient. I use doses of 30 to 90 drops of the tincture twice daily as an expectorant. *Euphrasia* treats catarrhal diseases of the upper respiratory tract, especially colds and flu. Dr. Bastyr told us to use 15 drops every 2 hours for acute coryza. He said that it was also good for sniffles in young infants. For this purpose, he mixed 10 drops of tincture in $\frac{1}{3}$ glass of water and gave this in doses of 1 teaspoon every 15 minutes. Relief is almost instantaneous. For the itchy eyes of hayfever, make a standard tea and give several cups daily.

Momordica balsamina

COMMON NAMES ■ Wonder apple, Southern balsampear

The fruit is used to make medicine. This remedy is an expectorant that is used for pulmonary congestion and chest distress from acute colds. Use 30 drops of tincture three times daily. Dr. Bastyr said that *Momordica* resembles *Cimicifuga*.

Unfortunately, I do not know what he meant by that. As a vulnerary, the fruit may be applied externally on all types of wounds.

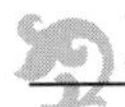

Potassium bichromate

COMMON NAME ■ Kali bichromium

Kali bichromium is used as an expectorant for yellow, ropelike mucus. This remedy is also useful in bacterial pharyngitis. Dr. Bastyr taught the use of a 6X homeopathic tablet for this purpose. He suggested melting 2 tablets in the mouth four times daily. He always used this medicine homeopathically.

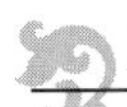

Pinus palustris

COMMON NAMES ■ Long leaf pine, Pitch pine, Southern yellow pine

Turpentine is an oleoresin obtained from pine tree wood by means of steam distillation. It is an anthelminthic, an antiseptic, a stimulant, a counterirritant, a hemostatic, and an expectorant. It is used as an expectorant for acute bronchitis, laryngitis, and pharyngitis. The dose is a couple of drops of turpentine on the tongue three times daily.

Populus gileadensis

COMMON NAME ■ Poplar

The buds are used to make medicine. *Populus* contains salicylates. It is a stimulating expectorant used in chronic bronchitis to help break up and expectorate phlegm. Dr. Bastyr taught us to use this plant to treat laryngitis with aphonia. I suggest infusing 40 grains of the dried buds in a cup of water. The dose is 3 cups per day. The fluid extract is also used at a dose of 4 mL twice daily.

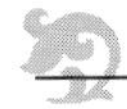

Thymus serpyllum

COMMON NAME ■ Wild thyme

The whole herb is used to make medicine. Dr. Bastyr taught that *Thymus* clears mucous congestion from the lungs and is a good tonic in lingering upper respiratory infections. A standard tea may be used twice daily. Incidentally, herbalists have said that this tea is also a good antiflatulent. The dose of the tincture is 30 drops twice daily.

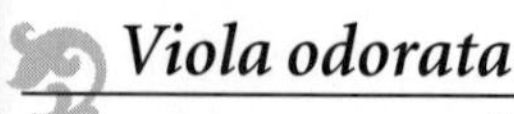

Viola odorata

COMMON NAME ■ Sweet violet

The leaves and flowers are used to make medicine. *Viola* contains saponins, which are often good expectorants. *Viola* is an expectorant used to treat bronchitis, chronic nasopharyngeal catarrh, and coughs. The dose is 30 to 50 grains of the dried herb twice daily. The tincture dose is 30 to 60 drops twice daily.

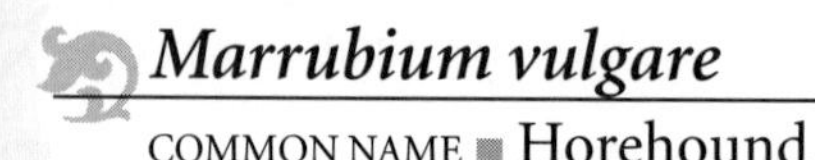

Marrubium vulgare

COMMON NAME ■ Horehound

The flowering tops and leaves are used to make medicine. *Marrubium* contains diterpene alcohols such as marrubiin and phytosterols. These seem to relax the muscles of the bronchial tubes. Dr. Bastyr taught the use of *Marrubium* as a respiratory remedy to promote expectoration. As a cough syrup, he said to mix one part *Marrubium* infusion with two parts honey. Stir this mixture until it is smooth. It makes an effective expectorant and stimulant that will break up pharyngobronchial congestion. Dr. Bastyr taught that *Marrubium* should be considered when the cough is nonproductive and the chest is tight. He suggested 20 to 30 drops of tincture every 3 hours. I have found that *Marrubium* mixes well with licorice and *Grindelia.*

Ribes nigrum

COMMON NAME ■ Black currant

The dried leaves are used to make medicine. Dr. Bastyr said that this plant was a good whooping cough remedy. He said to make a tea of the leaves and drink 3 to 4 cups per day. The fruit of *Ribes* is loaded with anthocyanins. Black currants are a great nutraceutical for the treatment of circulatory problems in which the peripheral circulation is deficient. Incidentally, I have discovered that most of the anthocyanins are effective hypoglycemic agents for the treatment of diabetes.

Justicia adhatoda

COMMON NAME ■ Malabar nut

The bromhexine in *Adhata* is an effective bronchodilator. It is an expectorant as well. Dr. Bastyr taught us to use 3 to 15 drops of tincture twice daily as an expectorant.

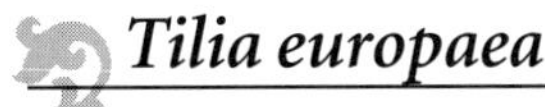

Tilia europaea

COMMON NAME ■ Lime tree

Use the flowers for medicine. Dr. Bastyr said that *Tilia* helps to remove mucus from the lungs and the trachea, especially when it is combined with coltsfoot. *Tilia* is mildly tonic. Make an infusion of the flowers and drink a cup several times daily. Dr. Bastyr said that the tincture should be given in doses of 20 to 40 drops three times daily.

Angelica archangelica

COMMON NAME ■ Angelica root

Angelica is an expectorant, a renal stimulant, and an antiarthritic in gouty arthritis. It is also phytoestrogenic. When it is used as an expectorant, Dr. Bastyr said to use 15 drops of *Angelica* tincture twice daily.

Angelica contains several monocyclic monoterpenoids, including alpha- and beta-phellandrene. Monocyclic monoterpenoids have the basic p-menthane skeleton. The phellandrenes in *Angelica* are somewhat irritating to the tissue, which perhaps accounts for *Angelica*'s ability to stimulate gastric secretions as is mentioned in some literature.

Pimpinella saxifraga

COMMON NAME ■ Burnet saxifrage

This plant is a member of the carrot family, *Umbelliferae.* The root is used to make medicine. *Pimpinella* is a good expectorant. I give 60 drops of tincture twice daily.

Saponaria officinalis

COMMON NAME ■ Soapwort

Saponaria is a member of the *Caryophylaceae* family. The roots and leaves are harvested during the flowering season to make medicine. This plant contains saponins. It is used as an expectorant, although less frequently than the better known plants. Use 60 drops of tincture every 4 hours.

CHAPTER

36

FEBRIFUGES

CHAPTER • OUTLINE

Aconitum napellus
Atropa belladonna
Gelsemium sempervirens
Bryonia alba
Veratrum viride
Toxicodendron radicans
Alstonia constricta
Asclepias tuberosa
Duboisia myoporoides
Eupatorium perfoliatum
Salix nigra
Populus tremuloides
Nepeta cataria

Febrifuges are remedies that reduce fevers. In most cases, naturopathic physicians do not recommend reducing fever. Fevers are part of the body's natural immune response. We use febrifuges only when temperatures are dangerously high. *CAUTION: In all cases of fever, make sure that the patient receives adequate fluids. Remedies are no substitute for water in febrile-induced dehydration.* Before giving any febrifuge, make sure that the febrile patient is properly hydrated.

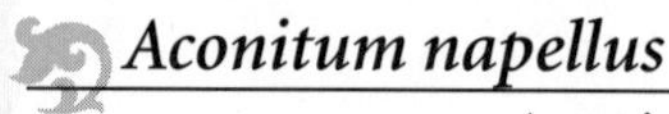

Aconitum napellus

COMMON NAMES ■ Aconite, Monkshood

Use the root to make medicine. *CAUTION:* Aconitum *is poisonous, and therefore its usefulness is primarily limited to external and homeopathic applications.* My classmate, Dr. Powell, noted that Dr. Bastyr contraindicated *Aconitum* in asthenia. *Aconitum* contains nor-diterpene alkaloids, including aconitine and mesaconitine. It also contains aconitic acid. Dr. Bastyr taught us to use this plant in first-stage fevers and for sthenic fevers only. He always used the homeopathic preparation. Do not use this remedy if the patient has a weak pulse or low vitality. Indications for *Aconitum* include a hard, quick, and sharp pulse and dry, hot, and burning skin. The standard homeopathic dose is 3X to 6X, given often if needed. Dr. Bastyr said that 1 to 3 drops of the tincture could also be given in water. *Aconitum* will reduce fever and is somewhat anodynal.

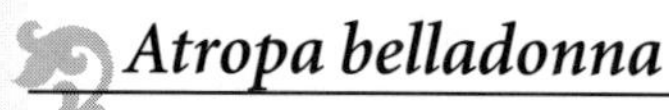

Atropa belladonna

COMMON NAME ■ Deadly nightshade

The medicine is made from the dried leaf and flowering tops of the plant. *CAUTION: Belladonna is a powerful remedy that can be toxic in large doses. It is contraindicated in glaucoma.* There are two main alkaloids in belladonna, hyoscyamine and atropine.

A homeopathic remedy of belladonna is given for fever. As I recall, Dr. Bastyr most frequently used a 6X potency given as often as needed. Fevers that respond best to belladonna are those in which patients have the following symptoms: bright red face, cool extremities, dilated pupils, and excess cerebral congestion.

There are many uses for belladonna. Dr. Bastyr suggested using a 1% solution of atropine sulfate locally to prevent adhesions between the iris and lens of the eye in iritis, iridocyclitis, and keratitis.

Gelsemium sempervirens

COMMON NAME ■ Yellow jasmine

The root is used to make medicine. For fever, *Gelsemium* is generally used in a triturated form. Homeopathically, I use a 6X potency in repeated doses. Fevers responsive to *Gelsemium* are usually associated with flu, muscular weakness, myalgia, flowing pulse, violent headache, remittent fevers, apathy, deliriousness, and hysteria. Obviously not all of these symptoms need to be present; however, fever associated with one or more of these symptoms is likely to respond to *Gelsemium*. *Gelsemium* contains several toxic alkaloids, including gelsemine, gelsedine, and the even more toxic gelsemicin. It also contains sempervirine and scopoletin.

Dr. Bastyr commented that *Gelsemium* tincture could be used for rigid os uteri, which might be slowing labor. He said that several drops of the tincture could be given two or three times to treat the rigid os. In cases of facial neuralgia, where the attack is imminent, he said to use 3 drops of tincture. I treat facial neuralgia with a concentrate of elderberry anthocyanins given in doses of 2 tablespoons twice daily.

Bryonia alba

COMMON NAME ■ White bryony

The root is used to make medicine. This medicine is used for fever in later stages of inflammation. During this fever, the face is flushed and the patient is aggravated by motion or deep inhalation. The medicine is given as a 6X homeopathic preparation. This medicine can help absorb exudate.

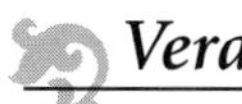

Veratrum viride

COMMON NAME ■ Green hellebore

Use the root or leaf to make medicine. *Veratrum* is used at the onset of sthenic fevers. During these fevers, the pulse is full and there is a fullness of capillary congestion. The patient may have spasms, twitching, or convulsions. A 6X homeopathic dose is given four times daily. For the onset of pneumonia, especially in adults, Dr. Bastyr said to give 1 drop of tincture every 30 minutes for 5 to 6 hours. This increases emptying of the lungs.

Toxicodendron radicans

COMMON NAME ■ Poison ivy

The leaves are used to make medicine. This remedy is known in the natural healing circles as *Rhus toxicodendron* or *Rhus tox*. *Rhus tox* is used in homeopathic preparations. When I was a student of Dr. Bastyr's at the National College of Naturopathic Medicine, the dosage of *Rhus tox* used was a 12X or a 200X homeopathic preparation. *Rhus tox* is used for inflammation with skin involvement, redness, vesicular eruptions, and burning with restlessness. It is used to treat fever associated with any of the above. Dr. Bastyr used to say that the *Rhus tox* patient would have a red-tipped and red-edged tongue. This remedy helps prevent further inflammation in suppurative diseases. It can be used where there are fiery red mucous membranes.

Rhus tox works on connective tissue, tendons, sheaths, and fascia. Dr. Bastyr taught us that it could be used to treat enlarged lymph nodes and body stiffness. He also mentioned its use in the treatment of cellulitis, erysipelas, pruritus ani, and herpes zoster. *Rhus* is very specific for herpes zoster. I have used it for all of these conditions with good results.

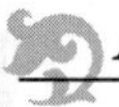

Alstonia constricta

COMMON NAME ■ Fever bark

The bark of the root and trunk is used to make medicine. Dr. Bastyr said that the fluid extract may be used at a dose of 10 drops every 2 hours in a large glass of water until the fever comes down. Besides being a tonic and a febrifuge, this remedy is also an antirheumatic. Dr. Bastyr said that the dose of the dried bark should be 2 to 8 grains of the powder twice daily or more often if needed. *Alstonia* has a number of very interesting constituents, including yohimbine, astonidine, reserpine, deserpidine, and alstonine.

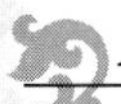

Asclepias tuberosa

COMMON NAMES ■ Pleurisy root, Butterfly weed

The root is used to make medicine. Dr. Bastyr said to take 2 drops of the tincture in a cup of water for fevers associated with toxic conditions. This plant is also used as a diuretic.

Duboisia myoporoides

COMMON NAME ■ Corkwood elm

You can also use *Duboisia leichardtii.* The leaves and berries are used to make medicine. This plant is rich in the alkaloid atropine. As a febrifuge, Dr. Bastyr taught us to use a 6X potency, much like you would use belladonna.

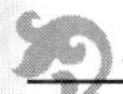

Eupatorium perfoliatum

COMMON NAME ■ Boneset

The leaves and flowering tops are used to make medicine. Dr. Bastyr used to say that for fevers, take a wine glass dose of the standard tea and sip it until the fever reduces. You can also use 15 to 40 drops of the tincture. *Eupatorium* is also a good diaphoretic, so make sure that the patient is drinking extra fluid with each dose.

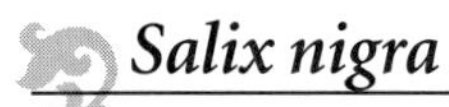

Salix nigra

COMMON NAME ■ Black willow

The bark is used to make medicine. *Salix* contains salicin, and is an antirheumatic and a febrifuge. It is an age-old folk remedy used to treat fevers. Take 10 to 30 grains of the powdered bark several times daily for this purpose. If *Salix* is taken at mealtime, its tendency to upset the stomach is reduced.

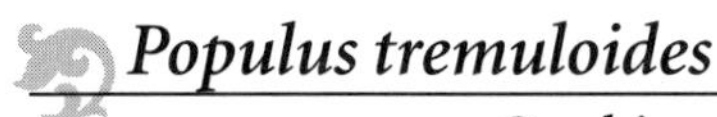

Populus tremuloides

COMMON NAME ■ Quaking aspen

The buds are used to make medicine. Quaking aspen is a very effective febrifuge. It contains tremendous amounts of salicylic acid. Tea can be made of the dried buds, or a tincture may be taken. I recommend 30 drops of tincture every 4 hours as a febrifuge.

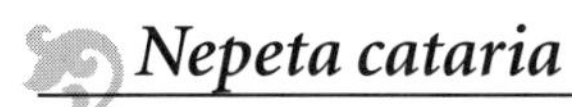

Nepeta cataria

COMMON NAME ■ Catnip

Catnip is part of the mint family, *Labiatae.* The leaves are used to make medicine. The chief constituent in its volatile oil is nepetalactones. A tea or tincture of this plant will produce diaphoresis and help to assuage fevers. Catnip is also a mild diuretic, so it is important to drink plenty of water when using catnip. Use 60 drops of the tincture three times daily as a febrifuge, as an antispasmodic, or as a gallbladder stimulant.

. . .

Having written about these remedies, I want to again emphasize that I don't ever reduce a fever unless the fever is 105 degrees or higher. Obviously, fluid must be given to make sure that the patient is well hydrated. Remember, most microorganisms do not do well in a febrile environment, which is why the body produces fever in the first place. Fever should be monitored but basically left alone. To this day, people are still trying to take down fevers any time they occur. This practice should stop.

CHAPTER

37

FUNGICIDES

CHAPTER • OUTLINE

Melaleuca alternifolia
Thuja occidentalis
Grindelia squarrosa
Coal tar
Thymus vulgaris
Cinnamomum species

Fungicides are agents that are destructive to fungi or their spores. Fungal infections can be tenacious, and frequently several different medicines must be tried to achieve relief.

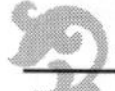

Melaleuca alternifolia

COMMON NAME ■ Tea tree

The leaves are used to make medicine. The tea tree is a small tree that is native to the northeast coastal region of New South Wales, Australia, where it has been used for thousands of years by the Bunkjalung aborigines who roam that area.[120] The oil obtained from the leaves is used topically as a fungicide. It is useful for infections caused by *Tinea* species, *Alternaria* species, and *Trichophyton* species. Apply two or three times daily.

Tea tree oil can be added to vaginal pack preparations that are inserted on a cotton pessary into the vagina to kill microorganisms that cause vaginal infection. Tea tree has demonstrable effect against *Trichomonas vaginalis* and *Candida albicans.*[121]

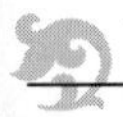

Thuja occidentalis

COMMON NAME ■ Cedar

The needles and young branches and twigs are used to make medicine. This plant is a fungicide and an antiseptic. The principal constituent of *Thuja* is thujone. *Thuja* oil can be applied externally to treat warts, although its success is variable. Dr. Bastyr used a 200X potency of *Thuja* to treat warts. I've seen *Thuja* work occasionally on *Trichophyton* species.

Thuja is also a diuretic and a urinary antiseptic. Dr. Bastyr suggested taking 3 drops of tincture several times daily for this purpose.

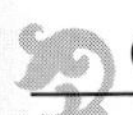

Grindelia squarrosa

COMMON NAME ■ Gum weed

The flowers and dried terminal leaves are used to make medicine. Dr. Bastyr said to apply the tincture locally on *Tinea* twice daily. I have had more success in treating *Tinea* infections using topical applications of *Grindelia* tincture than I have using *Thuja* oil.

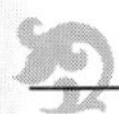

Coal tar

Historically, coal tar has been used to treat fungal diseases. Using coal tar preparations has many drawbacks, not the least of which is the strong odor and link to cancer. Coal tar preparations are good on toenail fungus if one does not mind smelling like a railroad tie all day long.

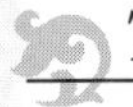

Thymus vulgaris

COMMON NAME ■ Thyme

The whole flowering plant is used to make medicine. Dr. Bastyr said that *Thymus* is probably a stronger fungicide than either tea tree or *Thuja*. It is applied topically on fungal infections. Its phenolic content ranges from 20% to 45%, which is very high. *Thymus* contains a number of constituents, including volatile oils such as thymol, p-cymene, borneol, flavonoids, and triterpenes.[122-124] My experience with this remedy is very limited.

Cinnamomum species

COMMON NAME ■ Cinnamon

The medicine is distilled from the leaves and twigs of the plant. There are a number of cinnamons. Cinnamon contains cinnamaldehyde and cinnamic acid, as well as several flavonoids. Dr. Bastyr taught that cinnamon oil is a potent antifungal. It is applied topically. As with *Thymus*, I don't have very much experience with this oil.

CHAPTER

38

GALACTAGOGUES

CHAPTER · OUTLINE

Lactuca virosa
Gaultheria procumbens
Polygala vulgaris
Borago officinalis
Anethum graveolens
Foeniculum vulgare
Silybum marianum
Galega officinalis

Galactagogues are medicinal agents that stimulate or increase the secretion of milk. Historically, Europeans have used carrot juice as a milk substitute when galactagogues failed. Goat milk has also been used as a substitute for breast milk if the mother is unable to nurse. I always encourage mothers to breast feed! Breast milk is the ideal food for a baby. Breast milk contains antibodies and other nutrients that a baby needs to ward off disease and grow.

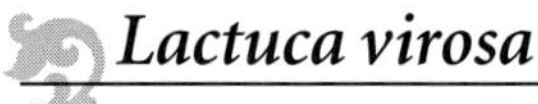

Lactuca virosa

COMMON NAME ■ Prickly lettuce

The dried latex and leaves are used to make medicine. *Lactuca* contains a number of sesquiterpene lactones, including lactucin and lactucopicrin, and several triterpenes such as taraxasterol and beta-amyrin.[125,126] The Meskwaki Indians used this plant in tea form as a galactagogue. The tincture may be taken in doses of 30 drops three times daily.

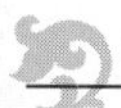

Gaultheria procumbens

COMMON NAME ■ Wintergreen

The dried leaves are used to make medicine. Herbalists suggest using *Gaultheria* tea to promote milk secretion. The tincture may be used in doses of 10 to 30 drops twice daily. Wintergreen oil may also be used. *Gaultheria* is also a febrifuge. For this purpose, 10 to 40 drops of tincture are taken three times daily.

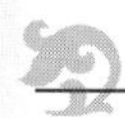

Polygala vulgaris

COMMON NAMES ■ Rogation flower, Milkwort

One may also use *Polygala amara.* The root is used to make medicine. *Polygala* contains the saponin, senegin, and the bitter principle, polygalin.[25] To increase the milk supply, Dr. Bastyr recommended 10 drops of the tincture every 4 hours. He also mentioned *Polygala* as an expectorant. For this purpose, take 30 drops of tincture three times daily.

Borago officinalis

COMMON NAME ■ Borage

The leaves and seeds are used to make medicine. Traditionally, herbalists have used the leaves and seeds to stimulate milk flow in nursing women. Make a standard tea for this purpose. Dr. Bastyr said to discontinue *Borago* after the establishment of normal milk flow.

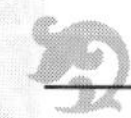

Anethum graveolens

COMMON NAME ■ Dill

The medicine is made from the aerial parts and from the dried ripe fruits. Dill oil contains carvone and limonene.[42] Dr. John Lust suggests the following combination for stimulation of milk flow: dill, coriander, anise, fennel, and caraway. A tea is prepared from equal parts of these remedies, and 1 cup is given daily.

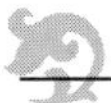

Foeniculum vulgare

COMMON NAME ■ Fennel

The roots and seeds are used to make medicine. Herbalists say that *Foeniculum* tincture may be taken in doses of 10 to 30 drops three times daily as a galactagogue. Dr. Bastyr suggested putting the tincture in barley water, which is an even more effective galactagogue.

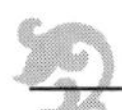

Silybum marianum

COMMON NAME ■ Milkthistle

The seeds are used to make medicine. This is a great liver medicine, and it is also a very worthy galactagogue. I learned about the use of this plant as a galactagogue from Molly Linton, ND, LM. The tincture dose is 60 drops twice daily. Higher doses of the tincture may be used safely as indicated, up to 120 drops twice daily. Capsules may also be used. I recommend 300 to 500 mg of powdered milkthistle twice daily.

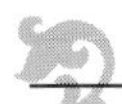

Galega officinalis

COMMON NAME ■ Goat's rue

The leaves and tips of the flowering branches are used to make medicine. *Galega* contains a guanidine derivative called galegine and a quinazoline alkaloid called (+)-peganine.[127] It is a very good galactagogue. It promotes milk production and stimulates development of the mammary glands. Dr. Bastyr's recommended dose was 40 drops of tincture three times daily.

CHAPTER

39

GASTROINTESTINAL TONICS, ASTRINGENTS, AND STIMULANTS

CHAPTER • OUTLINE

Geranium maculatum
Quercus alba
Melaleuca leucadendra
Abies canadensis
Myrica cerifera
Geum urbanum
Chelone glabra
Bidens tripartita
Ajuga reptans
Prenanthes alba
Strychnos nux-vomica
Collinsonia canadensis
Robert's formula
Fragaria virginiana
Berberis aquifolium
Brassica oleracea
Allium sativum

These remedies improve the function or performance of the gastrointestinal tract. They have been very important in previous generations of naturopathy and today. This is in keeping with our philosophy that good health begins with a healthy intestinal tract.

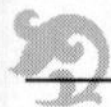

Geranium maculatum

COMMON NAME ■ Cranesbill

The dried aerial parts are used to make medicine. The high tannin content of *Geranium* makes it a good astringent for gastrointestinal bleeding and ulcers. Dr. Bastyr spoke highly of *Geranium* as a plant that stimulates the production of hydrochloric acid (HCl). By stimulating HCl, the digestion of proteins is improved. For this purpose, I use 10 drops of *Geranium* per meal.

Geranium has been used by eclectic physicians for ulcers, gastritis, occult intestinal blood, hematuria, and diarrhea. Dr. Bastyr said that when there is blood in the stool, a good diagnosis is required rather than symptomatic therapies.

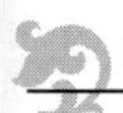

Quercus alba

COMMON NAME ■ White oak

The bark is used to make medicine. It is an astringent and can be used for dysentery, hemorrhoids, and leukorrhea. It is of some value in proctitis and anal fissures. The dose of the tincture is 10 drops twice daily. I remember Dr. Bastyr talking about using 40 drops of *Quercus* tincture in a pint of liquid as an enema. I have found that 90 drops works better. In addition, *Quercus* can be made into a gargle for sore throat.

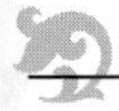

Melaleuca leucadendra

COMMON NAME ■ Cajeput

The oil is distilled from the fresh leaves and twigs. *Melaleuca* contains about 50% cineole, alpha-terpineol, and various sesquiterpenes.[128] It is a diaphoretic, a stimulant, and a carminative. It stimulates digestion while helping to relieve gas. Dr. Bastyr briefly discussed its use for laryngitis and bronchitis. He also mentioned mixing it with olive oil for ear infections. I have done this on a number of occasions for otitis media and *Candida* infections in the ear with good effect.

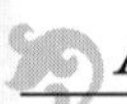

Abies canadensis

COMMON NAME ■ Hemlock spruce

The leaves are used to make medicine. *Abies* is an astringent, a mild antiseptic, and a stimulant. It may be used in gastritis. The tincture dose of *Abies* is 5 to 20 drops three times daily. Topically, *Abies* can be used for eczema and pruritus.

In speaking about this dermatologic use of *Abies,* especially for eczema, Dr. Bastyr said that herbal infusions can be used by soaking a small towel in the infusier and applying it to the skin. Dr. Bastyr had a number of "favorite" herbal wraps, among them chamomile tea, comfrey tea, and witchhazel tea. To use *Abies*, simply add 90 drops of *Abies* tincture to a cup of chamomile tea and soak a cloth with the resulting mixture. Apply the cloth to the worst areas of the eczematous rash. Since chamomile is antiseptic, it is a good choice as the basis of a combination herbal infusion.

Myrica cerifera

COMMON NAMES ■ Bayberrry, Wax myrtle

The root bark is used to make medicine. Bayberry is a tonic and an astringent. I use it to treat mucous colitis and chronic diarrhea in doses of 60 drops three times daily. I have found it effective for these conditions. In addition, herbalists have recommended its use to treat liver problems with jaundice. For this purpose, use 20 drops of bayberry tincture three times daily combined with equal parts of *Quercus.*

I have frequently used bayberry to treat bleeding and spongy gums. Patients take 30 drops of the tincture directly in the mouth three times daily, and they swish it around their teeth and gums for 30 seconds before spitting it out.

Geum urbanum

COMMON NAMES ■ Avens, Bennet's root

The dried aerial parts are used to make medicine. *Geum* contains eugenol. *Geum* is an antidiarrheal, a hemostatic febrifuge, and an astringent. Dr. Bastyr taught its use in cases of catarrhal and ulcerative colitis. He said that the tincture could be taken in doses of 20 to 60 drops three times daily.

The eclectics and herbalists historically used Bennet's root for the treatment of hemorrhoids. Dr. Bastyr suggested applying herbal solutions to the anal area to treat hemorrhoids. For this purpose, add 1 teaspon of *Geum* tincture and 1 tablespoonful of *Hamemelis virginiana* (witchhazel) to $\frac{1}{4}$ cup of water, soak a cotton pledget in the resulting solution, and apply to the anus.

Chelone glabra

COMMON NAME ■ Balmony

The whole flowering herb is used to make medicine. I think of *Chelone* as a stimulant to the entire digestive system and an aid to absorption. It is a cholagogue, a laxative, and a hepatic tonic. According to Dr. Bastyr, *Chelone* is used to treat gallstones where there is jaundice. He combined *Chelone* with equal parts of *Hydrastis* and *Gentiana* for hepatic jaundice. I use 60 drops of this combination twice daily. Herbalists have given *Chelone* as a tincture in doses of 1 to 2 milliliters twice daily or as a powder using 15 to 30 grains twice daily. Dr. Bastyr said that high doses of *Chelone* have been used to treat worms.

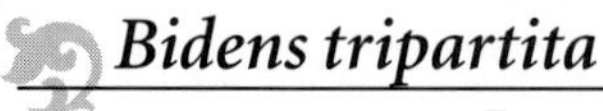

Bidens tripartita

COMMON NAME ■ Burr marigold

The dried aerial parts are used to make medicine. *Bidens* contains tannins, which are its principal astringents. It is an astringent and an antihemorrhagic for the treatment of peptic ulcers. In addition, Dr. Bastyr suggested using *Bidens* for essential hematuria. For this purpose, I suggest combining it with an equal part of *Symphytum*. The dose of the tincture combination is 60 drops twice daily. The dose of *Bidens* alone is 20 to 40 drops of the tincture or 30 grains of the powder, twice daily.

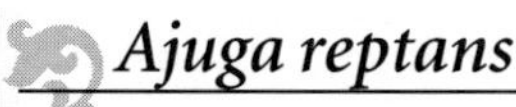

Ajuga reptans

COMMON NAME ■ Common bugle

The aerial parts of the flowering plant are used to make medicine. This medicine is an astringent and a tonic to the gastrointestinal membranes. Herbalists have recommended taking a standard tea three times daily for this purpose. Dr. Bastyr recommended bugle as a useful mouthwash in gingivitis. Use 60 drops of a 1:5 extract of bugle in 2 tablespoons of water and swish around the mouth for 30 seconds.

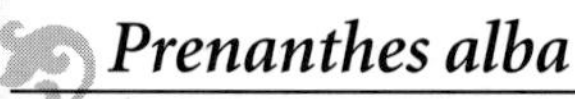

Prenanthes alba

COMMON NAME ■ Rattlesnakeroot

The whole plant is used to make medicine. This plant is a bitter astringent used to treat diarrhea and dysentery. For this purpose, add 1 teaspoon of the dried root to 1 cup of water to make a tea. Give the patient 1 cup of tea twice daily. In addition to its use for diarrhea and dysentery, herbalists have taught that the leaves of *Prenanthes* may be used as a poultice on wounds to expedite the healing process.

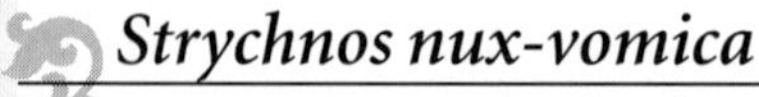

Strychnos nux-vomica

COMMON NAME ■ Quaker buttons

The seeds are used to prepare the medicine. I primarily use *S. nux-vomica* as a gastrointestinal stimulant. *S. nux-vomica* is used for gastrointestinal atonicity.

It contains several powerful indole alkaloids, including strychnine and brucine. Strychnine increases sensory excitability and heightens muscular excitability. This includes excitation of the muscles involved in peristalsis. I use *S. nux-vomica* with other gastrointestinal medicines as an activator. For example, *S. nux-vomica* may be combined with *Gentiana* or *Corydalis*. The dose of *S. nux-vomica* is 2 drops of the tincture twice daily. The dose of *S. nux-vomica* is 2 drops of tincture and no more unless the patient has greater than normal body mass. In the same breath, I would not discourage its use. It is a very useful medicine when used carefully. Dr. Bastyr mostly used *S. nux-vomica* homeopathically.

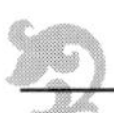

Collinsonia canadensis

COMMON NAME ■ Stone root

The whole plant is used to make medicine. *Collinsonia* contains the sesquiterpenoid, caryophyllene. It also contains rosmaric acid. *Collinsonia* is a tonic and an astringent to the gastrointestinal tract. I recommend 30 drops of the tincture before meals. Dr. Bastyr highly recommended *Collinsonia* as an anodyne in proctologic problems. It is a good ingredient for suppositories in rectal hemorrhoid treatment. *Collinsonia* may be used for laryngeal and pharyngeal viral disease, or as Dr. Bastyr would say, for Parson's sore throat.

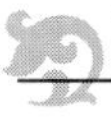

Robert's formula

Robert was a British seaman in the 19th century. He was also a very fine herbalist who created this formula to treat his own case of colitis. To make this formula, combine equal parts of *Hydrastis, Echinacea, Althea, Phytolacca*, and *Geranium*. I give two double-ought capsules four times daily for the treatment of duodenal ulcers, gastrointestinal bleeding, peptic ulcers, Crohn's disease, and ulcerative colitis. Robert's formula also stimulates digestion. A liquid form of the formula might be better as a digestive bitter. I have prescribed Robert's formula for many years and have found it to be helpful in colitis, especially when used with quercetin and deglycyrrhizinated licorice root in doses of 1000 mg twice daily.

Fragaria virginiana

COMMON NAME ■ Wild strawberry

The whole plant is used to make medicine. *Fragaria* is an astringent, a diuretic, and a tonic, and it is useful in dysentery, diarrhea, and hematuria. Dr. Bastyr suggested a dose of 5 to 15 drops of tincture twice daily. Clearly, a causal diagnosis is needed for these disorders.

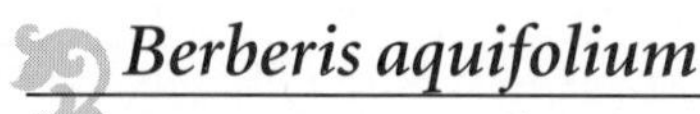

Berberis aquifolium

COMMON NAME ■ Oregon grape

The root is used to make medicine. *Berberis* is one of the best gastrointestinal stimulants and astringents. I have found that this remedy works well in hypotonic bowel syndromes where the patient may have gas or bloating, belching, constipation, or just plain lethargy with frequent sour stomach. I recommend that my patients take 15 drops of tincture per meal. Rest assured, the patient needs more exercise. *Berberis* is probably best taken while walking a mile. *Berberis* is also an antibacterial; therefore, I use it in enteric bacterial disease. For this purpose, I recommend a dose of 60 drops four times daily.

When considering *Berberis*, think in terms of the skin–digestive system connection. Most cases of acne, eczema, and psoriasis are eased symptomatically by using *Berberis*. Patients report that they have more well-formed bowel movements when using this remedy. Naturopaths believe that the gastrointestinal tract is functionally improved, thus aiding the health of the skin. The dose I recommend for tonifying the bowel to treat the skin is 30 drops of tincture three times daily taken with meals.

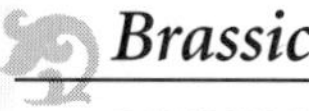

Brassica oleracea

COMMON NAME ■ Cabbage

The whole edible vegetable is used. Cabbage is a member of the mustard family. Research as far back as the 1950s indicated that cabbage juice speeds the healing of gastric ulcers.[129] According to Dr. Rudolph Weiss, the active ingredient in cabbage juice is methylmethioninesulfonium bromide.[13] Herbalists and folk healers recommend a dose of 1 pint of raw cabbage juice daily. I have frequently recommended 1 cup of cabbage juice twice daily to patients with gastic and duodenal ulcers. Patients report good results.

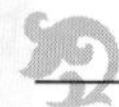

Allium sativum

COMMON NAME ■ Garlic

The bulb is used for medicine. Garlic is a mild digestive stimulant. It helps with protein digestion when taken with meals. Dr. Bastyr instructed us to insert a peeled bulb of garlic rectally for hemorrhoids. It takes the soreness right out. Garlic also slightly lowers serum triglycerides, thus helping to prevent heart disease. It tends to lower serum glutamic-oxaloacetic transaminase and serum glutamic-pyruvic transaminase levels and to increase adenosine triphosphate activity.

CHAPTER

40

GENITOURINARY AGENTS

CHAPTER • OUTLINE

Barosma betulina
Arctostaphylos uva-ursi
Triticum repens or *Agropyron repens*
Eupatorium purpureum
Althaea officinalis
Eryngium aquaticum
Galium aparine
Petroselinum sativum
Agrimonia eupatoria
Chondrodendron tomentosum
Blatta orientalis
Solidago odora
Parietaria diffusa
Aphanes arvensis
Vaccinium vitis-idaea
Sambucus ebulus
Polygonum aviculare
Adonis vernalis
Peumus boldo
Chimaphila umbellata
Abies canadensis
Berberis vulgaris
Achillea millefolium
Lespedeza capitata
Cantharis vesicatoria

Genitourinary agents benefit the genitourinary system in various ways. I am presenting genitourinary agents in the format that Dr. Bastyr taught them. He taught two separate categories of these agents, which he called genitourinary agents and genitourinary sedatives and stimulants. I am unable to discern any clear distinction between the two groups.

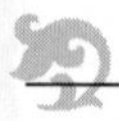

Barosma betulina

COMMON NAME ■ Buchu

The leaves are used to make medicine. Buchu is a diuretic, a renal tonic, an antiseptic, a carminative, and a circulatory stimulant. It contains a constituent called barosma camphor, which is also termed diosphenol. The flavonoids in buchu include rutin and diosmetin.[130,131]

I have found that buchu is useful in cystitis, pyelitis, and chronic irritable bladder. This plant renders the urine somewhat antiseptic. I prescribe 1 teaspoon of the tincture or 60 drops of the fluid extract three times daily. Buchu should always be taken with a glass of water. Most urinary tract remedies are taken with a glass of water to facilitate their action. Herbalists and naturopathic physicians frequently mix buchu with other urinary tract remedies as needed.

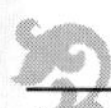

Arctostaphylos uva-ursi

COMMON NAMES ■ Bearberry, Uva-ursi

The leaves are used to make medicine. In the history of botanical literature, uva-ursi has been used to decrease the irritation of stone passage through the ureters. For patients who are passing stones, I use uva-ursi in combination with marshmallow, *Hydrangea,* and *Ammi visnaga.* Uva-ursi helps to eliminate the cause of mucus in the urine. I have used uva-ursi for patients with irritation of the genitourinary tract and for those with Bright's disease. I use 120 drops of the tincture three to four times daily. If using the powder, 10 to 60 grains is appropriate. Uva-ursi is useful against *Escherichia coli* infections in the genitourinary tract. In many cases I have found that frequent doses, as high as six to seven times a day, may be needed. Dr. Bastyr praised uva-ursi as one of our finest genitourinary agents.

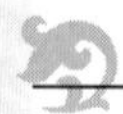

Triticum repens or *Agropyron repens*

COMMON NAME ■ Couch grass

Couch grass is in the grass family, *Gramineae.* The stem or rhizome is used to make medicine. Couch grass is a diuretic, an aperient, a demulcent, and an antimicrobial. Dr. Bastyr noted that couch grass relieves tenesmus and dysuria of both prostatitis and strangury. The very best remedy I have ever found for treating strangury is made by combining equal parts of *Hydrangea* and *Ammi visnaga*. I give 90 drops of the botanical extract combination four times daily.

Couch grass contains triticin, which is a fructosan polysaccharide. Historically, herbalists have used couch grass to treat gonorrhea, cystitis, pyelitis, and dysuria. It can also be used to treat phosphate urine. The general dose of couch grass is 90 drops of the botanical extract three times daily. I think of couch grass as a soothing diuretic that is mildly antiseptic. Couch grass is a remarkable-tasting remedy. Try 10 drops of the tincture, and see how it feels in your body. It is so important for practitioners to experience plant medicines directly.

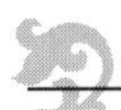

Eupatorium purpureum

COMMON NAME ■ Gravel root

The root is used to make medicine. *Eupatorium* dissolves gravel as the patient urinates. Dr. Bastyr used it to treat patients who experienced brick dust deposits in their urine. He said that it was useful in hematuria and empties the pelvis from the kidney on down. *Eupatorium* is used by botanical medicine practitioners for the nauseating backache that frequently accompanies kidney problems. For genitourinary conditions, I have found that a dose of 60 drops of the botanical extract four times daily is effective. In addition, an infusion or decoction of this plant works well. Eclectics and herbalists have recommended 1 cup every 2 hours for excess uric acid. By this I assume they meant uric acid crystals in the urine. *Eupatorium* contains arbutin, which is a hydroquinone glycoside.

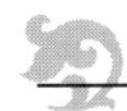

Althaea officinalis

COMMON NAME ■ Marshmallow

The whole plant is used to make medicine. This plant is an excellent demulcent. Marshmallow contains mucilage and pectin. It is an astringent and a diuretic. Its mucilaginous component soothes both the gastrointestinal and the genitourinary tracts. Dr. Bastyr taught us to use it to treat cystitis, ammonia urine, and dysuria. I have found *Althaea* to be very synergistic with *A. uva-ursi.* The dose of the powder is 10 to 30 grains. The dose I have settled on is 90 drops of the tincture three times daily. If needed, it may be used more frequently and in higher doses.

Eryngium aquaticum

COMMON NAME ■ Button snakeroot

One may also use *Eryngium yuccafolium.* The root is used to make medicine. This plant is a diuretic, a diaphoretic, and an emetic. *Eryngium* is useful in treating urethral irritation and gravel in the urine. Dr. Bastyr commented that it is also useful in chronic laryngitis, influenza, and irritation in the upper respiratory tract. The eclectics mention its use for the lingering effects of gonorrhea. The dose that botanical practitioners typically give is 15 drops of the tincture or 5 to 20 grains of the powder three times daily.

Galium aparine

COMMON NAME ■ Cleavers

The whole aerial parts are used to make medicine. This remedy is a diuretic, a tonic, and a laxative. To prevent the recurrence of kidney stones, I use *Galium* and magnesium. The dose of *Galium* is 90 drops three times daily; the dose of magnesium is 200 mg twice daily. *Galium* contains several nutritive antioxidants such as hesperidin and isorutin. It also contains tannins, coumarins, umbelliferone, scopoletin,[20] and several iridoid glucosides, including monotropein and asperuloside.[132] The iridoid glycosides are mildly laxative.

For prostate irritation, dysuria, or tenesmus, use 30 to 40 drops of the tincture three times daily. My good friend David Winston, a remarkable herbalist and Cherokee medicine keeper, says that *Galium* is great for treating lingering *Chlamydia* infections and the damage that they can cause to the urinary tract. He recommended the use of *Galium* daily for urinary strictures and Peyronie's disease. He suggested 30 drops of tincture twice daily for up to a year. Dr. Bastyr taught that this remedy was useful in lymphadenitis and psoriasis. For psoriasis, I recommend 3 cups of tea per day. Each cup is made by adding 90 drops of cleavers botanical extract to 1 cup of water.

Petroselinum sativum

COMMON NAME ■ Parsley

The root and seeds are used to make medicine. *CAUTION: Large doses of parsley should be avoided during pregnancy because parsley tends to stimulate the uterus.* This remedy is an emmenagogue, a diuretic, and a mild expectorant. The classical herbal use of *Petroselinum* is for cystitis with high specific gravity, for strangury, and for burning during urination. In my practice, *Petroselinum* has been particularly effective as a diuretic. For this I use half *Petroselinum* tincture and half *Usnea* tincture. The dose is 90 drops of the formula in 1 cup of water four times daily. One may eat the fresh plant. The dose of the tincture is classically given as 30 to 60 drops four times daily. The dose I have settled on is 120 drops four times daily.

Agrimonia eupatoria

COMMON NAME ■ Agrimony

The leaves or root are used to make medicine. This plant is an astringent and a bitter tonic. *Agrimonia* contains catechin and tannin, both of which are mildly astringent.

As a genitourinary tonic, we are taught to use 30 drops of the tincture three times daily. It acidifies alkaline urine. The general rule is that to acidify the urine, eat protein. To alkalinize the urine, drink vegetable juices such as carrot juice. Eclectic literature discusses using *Agrimonia* for chronic cystic inflammation and dropsy.[133] Dr. Bastyr recommended this remedy for dribbling urine in elderly patients.

Chondrodendron tomentosum

COMMON NAME ■ Pareira

The bark and the dried roots are used to make medicine. This plant is a diuretic and an antipyretic. It contains tubocurarine and chondocurarine, which are isoquinoline alkaloids.[134]

Dr. Bastyr used this remedy primarily for chronic diseases of the kidneys and bladder. Eclectic medicine texts reported its use for ulceration of the kidneys and bladder or for painful urination. It was also used for pyelitis, cystitis, phosphate urine, and lithemia, which is excess uric acid or its salts in the blood. The dose reported by the eclectics was 5 to 10 drops of the tincture. My experience with this plant is very limited. I have included it because it was discussed briefly in Dr. Bastyr's class.

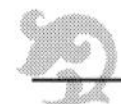

Blatta orientalis

COMMON NAME ■ Cockroach

The whole, dried bodies are used for medicine. Dr. Bastyr mentioned that *Blatta* is a good diuretic. His suggested dose is one capsule of the dried body of *Blatta* three times daily. He taught us to use this remedy in a 3X potency for asthma. I have no experience with this insect remedy, however. It is listed here for historical purposes. Perhaps someone in the pest control division would be happy to know that there is a use for the cockroach after all.

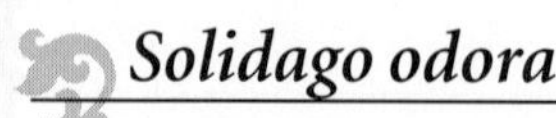

Solidago odora

COMMON NAME ■ Goldenrod

The flowering tops and leaves are used to make medicine. This remedy is used to treat kidney disease. Dr. Bastyr specified its use for patients with painful or scanty urination with backache. He recommended 5 to 15 drops twice daily. I have not personally used *Solidago* as a single remedy. Rather, I have combined it with other genitourinary remedies such as *Parietaria, Chimaphila,* and buchu. *Solidago* contains flavonoids, carotenoids, triterpene saponins, and phenolic glucosides including leicarposide. The contents vary with the species.

Rudolph Weiss, in his fine book *Herbal Medicine,*[13] writes about *Solidago virgaurea,* another species of goldenrod. He states similar uses for this species of *Solidago.* Weiss mentions the high quantity of flavonoids in this plant. Either *S. odora* or *S. virgaurea* can be used as a genitourinary agent.

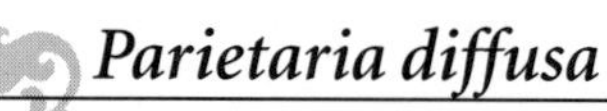

Parietaria diffusa

COMMON NAME ■ Pellitory of the wall

Medicine is made from the dried aerial parts of the plant. *Parietaria* contains a load of flavonoids, including quercetin and kaempferol. Dr. Bastyr reported that the eclectics used *Parietaria* in pyelitis and recurrent cystitis, as well as in edema of renal origin. I use it for urinary lithiasis in doses of 60 to 90 drops three times daily in water. The flavonoids may be part of the reason that this plant is effective for cystitis. Bioflavonoids tend to improve the integrity of the capillary mesh in the bladder wall.

Aphanes arvensis

COMMON NAME ■ Aphanes, Parsley piert

This plant is also called *Alchemilla arvensis.* The dried aerial parts are used to make medicine. In folk medicine, *Aphanes* has been used to treat renal calculus and as a diuretic. For this purpose, make a standard infusion. Drink 1 cup of the tea twice daily. *Aphanes* contains tannins, which are well represented when the tea is consumed. Historically, the tea has been used rather than the tincture. If a tincture is chosen, the dose is 120 drops three times daily.

Vaccinium vitis-idaea

COMMON NAME ■ Alpine cranberry

The dried leaves and ripe dried fruit are used to make medicine. The leaves are an antiseptic, an astringent, and a diuretic. I use *Vaccinium* primarily for bacterial cystitis. I use 60 drops of the tincture three times daily for this purpose. Herbalists use an infusion made of the dried leaves for bladder problems. The dose is 1 cup of standard tea taken three times daily. Remember that the leaves are antibacterial. Dr. Bastyr said that the berries, in addition to being an astringent, are edible and help increase the appetite.

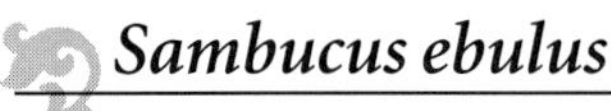

Sambucus ebulus

COMMON NAME ■ Dwarf elder

The flowers, leaves, and inner bark are used to make medicine. *Sambucus* contains a number of iridoid monoterpene glycosides including ebuloside. According to Dr. Bastyr, *Sambucus* helps with the elimination of waste material through the kidneys. When the kidneys are not functioning properly, the result is often edema. This is why eclectic physicians used *Sambucus* to treat dropsy or edema. As a kidney remedy, I suggest a dose of 30 drops of tincture three times daily.

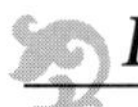

Polygonum aviculare

COMMON NAME ■ Knotgrass

The flowering herb is used to make medicine. Dr. Bastyr taught the use of *Polygonum* for the prevention and removal of renal calculi. The tincture is taken in doses of 15 to 30 drops four times daily. *Polygonum* contains quite a number of flavonoids, including avicularin, hyperoside, quercetin, and vitexin. It also contains several hydroxycoumarins, notably umbelliferone and scopoletin. *Polygonum* is an acetylcholinesterase inhibitor and an astringent.[25]

Adonis vernalis

COMMON NAME ■ Pheasant's eye

The whole plant is used to make medicine. Dr. Bastyr used *Adonis* for nephrosis found in cardiorenal affectations in which albumin urea is present. He suggested a dose of 1 to 5 drops of the tincture three times daily. In some cases it is a tremendous diuretic. An *Adonis* 30X homeopathic potency may be used. Dr. Bastyr related several amazing cases of the use of this remedy to treat edema resulting from heart weakness and/or tachycardia. He told us the story of an elderly patient who had cardiac failure with massive edema of the ankles. He prescribed *Adonis* 200X potency, which was all he had in his bag for her at the time. He returned the next day to check on her and she looked completely different. She said that she had urinated frequently during the night, and he noticed that almost all of the edema in her ankles was gone.

Many patients have come to me who had gone to Dr. Bastyr when he was alive. Amazing accounts such as the one that I have just given are more the rule than the exception among these patients.

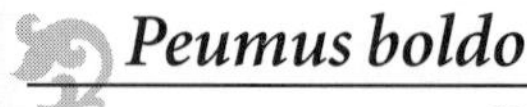

Peumus boldo

COMMON NAME ■ Boldo

The dried leaves are used to make medicine. *P. boldo* contains the isoquinoline alkaloid, boldine. The volatile oil contains p-cymene, cineol, and ascaridole. This urinary tract remedy is a good diuretic, a mild urinary demulcent, and an antiseptic. I prescribe 20 to 40 drops of tincture four times daily. It is also useful to treat cystitis. *P. boldo* has a completely unique flavor, that I would describe as biting and delightful. I use boldo as a liver medicine; however, it is a good plant to add to cystitis formulas.

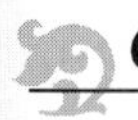

Chimaphila umbellata

COMMON NAME ■ Pipsissewa

The root is used to make medicine. *Chimaphila* is a urinary tract antiseptic, a diuretic, and a tonic. It helps to flush the renal and urethral structures and is often used for urinary tract infections. Dr. Bastyr said that it is most useful in early pyelitis and nephritis, especially with accompanying mucous discharge and the usual detritis of pus, erythrocytes, and leukocytes. He pointed out that *Chimaphila* is useful where there is albumin urea and urethritis. Fairly high doses of this tincture should be given. Use 90 drops in a large glass of water three times daily. I use *Chimaphila* frequently in many urinary disorders. For urinary tract infections, I prescribe 120 drops of the botanical extract four times daily. I often mix it with *A. uva-ursi*, parsley, or buchu as a urinary tract antiseptic. Other times I use two parts *Chimaphila umbellata* tincture mixed with one part *A. uva-ursi* fluid extract, one part *Berberis aquifolium* tincture, and one part *Usnea* species tincture. For bladder infections, I give 90 drops of this mixture five times daily in water.

Dr. Bastyr, eclectics, and herbalists have all recommended using *Chimaphila* to remove catabolic wastes from the kidneys. In the past, eclectic physicians used *Chimaphila* to help treat gonorrhea. Today, you can use *Chimaphila* for patients who are concurrently using antibiotic treatment for gonorrhea.

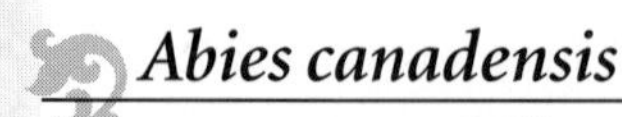

Abies canadensis

COMMON NAME ■ Hemlock spruce

The leaves are used to make medicine. A decoction of *Abies* is useful in treating vaginitis, leukorrhea, and cervical erosions. Historically, herbalists have used

Abies to treat bladder infections in cases where there is excessive mucous production. Dr. Bastyr was very confident in *Abies* in a decoction form as an effective douche for vaginitis and cervicitis. The decoction is made from the needles of the tree. It is rich in pycnogenol bioflavonoids. Dr. Bastyr suggested that *Abies* be used as a remedy for prolapse of the uterus or bladder. I cannot recall his exact dose, but 60 drops of tincture in a cup of water would be appropriate.

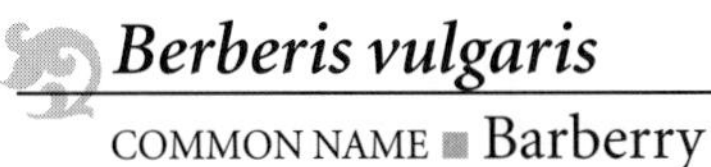

Berberis vulgaris

COMMON NAME ■ Barberry

The root, berries, and bark are used to make medicine. This plant contains various acids, notably malic, acetic, and chlorogenic acids. It also contains isoquinioline alkaloids and is useful as a urinary antiseptic. *Berberis* is a genitourinary tonic that is useful in catarrhal urethritis. Dr. Bastyr suggested 20 to 30 drops of tincture three times daily for this purpose. In my practice, I prefer to use doses of 60 drops three times daily.

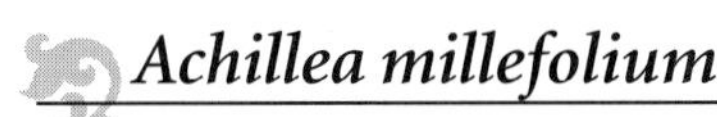

Achillea millefolium

COMMON NAME ■ Yarrow

The whole flowering top is dried and used to make medicine. Dr. Bastyr suggested using *Achillea* as a douche to tonify the vaginal mucous membranes. An interesting use of *Achillea*, which was also suggested by Dr. Bastyr, is as an antispasmodic in the treatment of parametrial pain. I gave a patient *Achillea* as a digestive bitter, and she mentioned that it also relieved pelvic pain that she had been experiencing slightly lateral to the uterus. I came across the same spasmolytic effect mentioned by Weiss in *Herbal Medicine.*[13] When it is used as a spasmolytic, the dose is 30 drops of the botanical extract three times daily.

Achillea mixed with goldenseal is one of the best preparations for congestive prostatitis in which infection is present. The two tinctures are mixed in equal portions. A dose of 90 drops is taken four times daily for 10 days. *Achillea* oil has a blue color similar to that of chamomile oil, which is partly because of the presence of chamazulene. Chamazulene is an antiinflammatory,[20] which may account for the antiinflammatory effect of both *Achillea* and chamomile.

An interesting aside on *Achillea* is that archeologists have found remnants of this plant in the gravesites of the Neanderthals. *Achillea* is very bitter and not likely used as a food, which suggests that it was included in the burial site as a medicine to be used in the afterlife. *Achillea* has very wide application in pathologic conditions affecting most body systems. It would have helped with bacterial digestive disorders that might have been common to these people. It is also a great plant to use as a poultice against infection in skin wounds. If indeed the

Neanderthals used this plant medicinally, it would be the earliest record of the medicinal use of a plant (40,000 years ago).

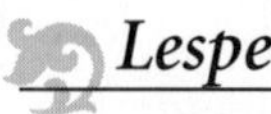

Lespedeza capitata

COMMON NAME ■ Roundhead lespedeza

This plant is a member of the *Papilionoifeae* family. Weiss[13] mentions that Obrowski reported its effectiveness in treating acute and chronic renal insufficiency. Obrowski's dose is 50 drops of tincture three times daily for the first 3 days. This is followed by 100 drops three times daily for another 20 days.[135] I have a feeling that the therapy should be continued in smaller doses for a prolonged period of time. Dr. Bastyr did not discuss this remedy, and I have no experience with this particular plant. However, any plant that appears to be effective in renal insufficiency is worth our attention, especially when it is suggested by as noteworthy a botanical practitioner as Rudolph Weiss.

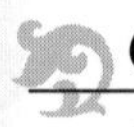

Cantharis vesicatoria

COMMON NAME ■ Spanish fly

Most of the literature on *Cantharis* discusses its use for urinary tract problems. Dr. Bastyr taught us to use it homeopathically for irritation of the urinary tract. Dr. William Turska, a contemporary of Dr. Bastyr, used *Cantharis* botanically. His formula for urinary tract problems was 10 drops of *Cantharis* tincture and 10 drops of *Apis* tincture in 4 ounces of water. He gave 1 teaspoon of the tea four times daily.

CHAPTER

41

Genitourinary Sedatives and Stimulants

CHAPTER • OUTLINE

Zea mays
Eupatorium purpureum
Equisetum arvense
Cucurbita
Juniperus communis
Piper methysticum
Hydrangea arborescens
Strychnos nux-vomica
Fabiana imbricata
Xanthium spinosum
Polytrichum juniperinum
Apis mellifera
Delphinium staphisagria
Serenoa serrulata, Sabul serrulata, or *Serenoa repens*
Turnera aphrodisiaca
Piper cubeba
Copaiba langsdorfii
Santalum album
Daucus carota
Atropa belladonna
Polygala verticillata
Achillea millefolium

Following are 22 remedies that principally affect the urinary tract. Several of the botanicals also help the prostate, which is an important and often affected part of the male urinary tract. Infections passed back and forth between the reproductive and urinary systems within a patient's body are relatively common. For this reason, Dr. Bastyr taught this category, titled *genitourinary remedies.* Some of these remedies are sedative in their actions, and others are stimulatory.

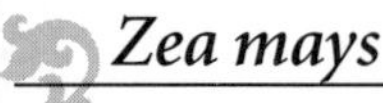

Zea mays

COMMON NAME ■ Corn

The corn silk is used to make medicine. *Zea* is calmative to the genitourinary tract. According to Kuts-Cheraux, *Zea* is useful for phosphate urine and for urine with mucus in it.[28] Nongonococcal urethritis can be helped with this remedy. I use the tincture to treat catarrhal cystitis. For this purpose, I mix it with equal parts of *Chimiphilla* and *Berberis.*

In addition to being calmative to the genitourinary tract, *Zea* is also a diuretic. These seemingly contradictory indications for this plant are actually complementary. *Zea* is a tonic to the cardiovascular system and therefore improves the hemodynamics of the kidneys, which stimulates diuresis. This soothing diuretic can help in urinary tract irritations. When treating genitourinary conditions, I prescribe 60 to 120 drops of the tincture four times daily in a glass of water. Higher doses may be used as necessary. I often mix *Zea* with marshmallow to soothe the urinary tract. Try eating raw corn silk. It is very good.

Eupatorium purpureum

COMMON NAME ■ Gravel weed

The root is used to make medicine. *Eupatorium* is a mild tonic to the urinary system. It is used for prolapse of the bladder, burning urination, hematuria, cystitis, and gravel in the urine. *Eupatorium* helps to relieve the feeling of a constant urge to urinate. Dr. Bastyr taught that *Eupatorium* helps to keep urates and uric acid crystals in solution and thereby prevents stone formation. The dose of the tincture is 20 drops four times daily. I would add that vitamin K is also necessary for calcium stone prevention. Vitamin K matures kidney protein, which is what prohibits calcium from coalescing into stones.

Equisetum arvense

COMMON NAMES ■ Horsetail, Shave grass, Scouring rush

One may also use *Equisetum hyemale. Equisetum* is from the horsetail family, *Equisetaceae.* The whole plant is used to make medicine. *Equisetum* contains flavonoids, quercetin glucosides, luteolin, and protogenkwanin glucosides, as well as salicylates and silicates. The silica content gives *Equisetum* its gritty texture, making it good for scouring pots and pans when camping.

Dr. Bastyr underscored *Equisetum* as a urinary astringent. In addition, he said that it aids in the expulsion of accumulated detritus and in the passage of small gravel from the bladder. The eclectics used this plant to treat renal inflammation, acute nephritis, and hematuria. The dose that I recommend for the above problems is 60 drops three times daily. Dr. Bastyr said that it could be made into a douche for leukorrhea as well.

Cucurbita

COMMON NAME ■ Watermelon

Use the whole plant and seeds to make medicine. Watermelon is a diuretic. The fresh fruit or the tincture can be used. The tincture of the plant is useful in cystitis. I recommend 90 drops three times daily. Nephritis has been cured using watermelon fasts. Since we are on the subject of nephritis, another remedy, nettle seeds, should be mentioned. Nephritis and even autoimmune kidney disease can be treated using nettle seeds. I've seen some remarkable results using nettle seed tinctures. The dose is 60 drops of tincture three times daily. Usually a diet consisting of watermelon, water, and vitamin C at a dose of 1000 mg four times daily was used to treat cystitis.

In allopathic medicine, diuretics are often used to combat hypertension. In the same vein, many herbal remedies used to lower blood pressure are also diuretics. This is true of watermelon, which can be used as an antihypertensive.

Juniperus communis

COMMON NAME ■ Juniper

Juniper is a member of the cypress family, *Cupressaceae.* The berries are used to make medicine. Juniper is a gentle diuretic and has antimicrobial properties useful in treating cystitis. The dose is 20 drops three times daily. Pyelonephritis is another condition for which Dr. Bastyr used juniper. I cannot remember his dosage for this purpose. Juniper contains essential oils such as pinenes; beta-myrcene; terpinenes; terpines; beta-cadinenes, which are sesquiterpenes; flavonoids; flavan-3,4-diols; and a number of diterpenes.

Piper methysticum

COMMON NAME ■ Kavakava

The rhizome is used to make medicine. Kavakava is a sedative and an antispasmodic. It has been used to treat edema caused by renal problems. It is used to treat decreased flow in the glomeruli and nocturnal enuresis. When using it as a genitourinary sedative, I recommend using 30 drops twice daily.

Kavakava is a safe and useful remedy when not abused. Recently it has drawn some attention as a potentially toxic remedy. If taken in huge doses, it is. So is aspirin.

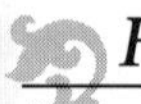

Hydrangea arborescens

COMMON NAME ■ Seven barks

The root is used to make medicine. *Hydrangea* contains saponins and a number of isocoumarin derivatives, one of which is hydrangenol.

Hydrangea is a calmative to the genitourinary system. Dr. Bastyr especially used *Hydrangea* for frequent urination with heat, burning, acute sharp pains in the urethra, and phosphate urine. The dose I would suggest is up to 90 drops four times daily. The infusion of the dried root is equally good. I have used *Hydrangea* extensively with my patients to help relax the ureter for the passage of stones. *Hydrangea* is a nontoxic remedy; therefore, I often increase the dose for patients with severe renal lithiasis. Khella also helps for this purpose. Passing kidney stones is painful business. For this reason, I like to use a demulcent together with *Hydrangea.* Marshmallow is one demulcent that comes to mind.

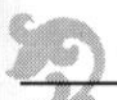

Strychnos nux-vomica

COMMON NAME ■ Quaker buttons

The seeds are used to make medicine. *CAUTION:* S. nux-vomica *contains strychnine, which is a very toxic alkaloid. Be precise in your dosing. S. nux-vomica* is a stimulant to the genitourinary system. Dr. Bastyr said that it increases the tone of the trigone and internal sphincter of the bladder detrusor muscle. He used it for urinary incontinence of aged people and children.

This remedy may be added to *Agrimonia* to treat urinary incontinence in the elderly. I mix ten parts of *Agrimonia* with one part *S. nux-vomica* and prescribe 20 drops twice daily. The eclectics used 1 drop of tincture twice daily for urinary incontinence in adults. I remember Dr. William Turska, an eclectic physician and the longest-practicing naturopath in history, speaking about the use of this remedy for this purpose. I prescribe *S. nux-vomica* in small doses, 1 to 2 drops twice daily, for urinary bladder muscle tone. Do not use it over a prolonged period.

I check patients with bladder problems for difference in leg length. Leg length discrepancies can cause chronic cystitis because of tension of the low back resulting from an unbalanced gait. This can overstimulate the nerves that handle communication between the low back and the bladder. If there is a big discrepancy in the length of the legs, two things need to be done. First, adjust the back to relieve pressure. Second, put a lift in the shoe of the short leg. A 3-mm lift should be used initially, regardless of the leg length discrepancy.

Fabiana imbricata

COMMON NAME ■ Pichi pichi

The leaves are used to make medicine. This plant is a diuretic and an astringent. It is a mild stimulant and tonic to the genitourinary system. Dr. Bastyr taught that *Fabiana* is used to treat cystitis caused by uric acid deposits. It can help vesicle tenesmus and acute dysuria. Dr. Bastyr cautioned against using this remedy for nephritis. He used it only in lower urinary tract problems, especially where pyuria and mucus are present. The general dose used by the eclectics was 10 to 20 drops four times daily.

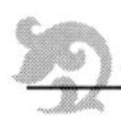

Xanthium spinosum

COMMON NAME ■ Spiny cockleburr

Also use *Xanthium strumarium*, or broad burrweed. This plant is a diuretic, a diaphoretic, and a sialagogue. Dr. Bastyr primarily spoke about *Xanthium* as a sialagogue; however, he also mentioned it for chronic cystitis. It can be used for passive hematuria and irritated chronic cystitis, especially where there is frequent urination. The dose that Dr. Bastyr recommended was 5 to 30 drops three times daily. I have very little experience with this particular plant. I have included it for historical purposes.

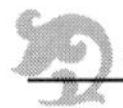

Polytrichum juniperinum

COMMON NAME ■ Hair cap moss

The whole plant is used to make medicine. *Polytrichum* is a renal stimulant used to treat edema and ascites. It contains the stilbenoid lunularic acid. This compound is of some interest in its inhibition of thromboxane synthase, 5 lipoxygenase, and calmodulin.[26]

According to Dr. Bastyr, *Polytrichum* is especially useful in helping to allay urethral pain during urination. In addition, he taught its use in dysuria of pregnancy. He said to use a dose of 5 to 60 drops of tincture three times daily.

Apis mellifera

COMMON NAME ■ Honeybee

The venom of the bee is used as medicine. *Apis* relieves acute swelling and can treat edema of cellular tissue with or without vesicles. Dr. Bastyr reported that the eclectics used *Apis* for urinary incontinence and nephritis that follows scarlet fever. Classically, it is used for right-sided ovarian cysts. Also consider this remedy for peritonitis, pleuritis, and burning and stinging that accompanies tissue swelling. The tincture is used in a dose of 1 drop twice daily. Frequently, and probably more effectively, the 6X homeopathic preparation is used. Dr. Bastyr preferred the homeopathic remedy.

One patient I treated, a 6-year-old girl, had a huge cyst that was seen as an internal tumor pushing her eye out. This was a slow-growing cyst that had increased over 2 months. *Apis* 6X homeopathic strength given twice daily produced full resolution of the cyst in 1 month. Quite a bit of the cystic enlargement was reduced after only 1 week.

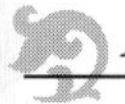

Delphinium staphisagria

COMMON NAME ■ Stavesacre

The seeds are used to make medicine. *Delphinium* is a stimulant and tonic to the central nervous system. This plant has a similar action to aconite, probably because the actions of the alkaloids delphinine and aconitine are similar.

It is a mild tonic to the genitourinary system. I use it to treat inflammation of the seminal vesicles and prostate. Dr. Bastyr frequently used this remedy for the treatment of prostatitis. I have found it effective in the treatment of sexual disorders, especially those accompanied by depression or hypochondriasis, and for somatoform or dissociative disorders. Naturopathically, it is generally used in homeopathic potencies, especially 6X and 12X.

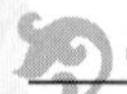

Serenoa serrulata, Sabul serrulata, or *Serenoa repens*

COMMON NAME ■ Saw palmetto

This small palm tree is native to the West Indies and the southeastern coast of the United States. The fruit is used to make medicine. Saw palmetto strengthens the male reproductive system. It contains a variety of flavonoids, but of chief importance are the sterols, notably beta-sitosterol. This plant contains a number of sterols that consist largely of esters and glucosides of beta-sitosterol. Also noteworthy is an impressive array of fatty acids.

Saw palmetto is a tonic and an anticatarrhal, and it also has a variety of odd uses. Eclectics used it variously in enlarged prostate, epididymitis, orchitis, orchalgia, some impotence, undeveloped mammary glands, and of course laryngitis. Many studies have shown that saw palmetto is helpful in treating and preventing benign prostatic hypertrophy. The mechanism of action appears to be in the prevention or inhibition of dihydrotestosterone from binding to cellular receptors. It also inhibits prostate estrogen receptors.

As men get older, their estrogen level goes up and their testosterone level drops. Remembering that the prostate and the uterus are embryologically analogous tissue, which differentiates upon development, estrogen may be the hormone most responsible for prostate enlargement, much as it is responsible for uterine fibroids and various problems in women. I recommend about 150 mg of saw palmetto twice daily. If I use the tincture, I generally prescribe 90 drops twice daily.

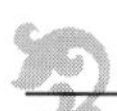

Turnera aphrodisiaca

COMMON NAME ■ Damiana

This plant may also be found under the name *Turnera diffusa*. The dried leaves are used to make medicine. Damiana contains arbutin and a variety of sesquiterpenes, such as delta-cadinene and alpha-copaene, and a number of monoterpenes. Beta-sitosterol is also found in this plant.

Turnera is tonic to the genitourinary system and is a well-known aphrodisiac. I have used it to treat impotence, sexual neurasthenia, and female sexual dysfunction. For any of the aforementioned problems, 30 grains of powder should be taken twice daily. The tincture may also be used in doses of 10 to 30 drops, but Dr. Bastyr seemed to prefer the powder. It is a stimulant and a laxative as well; as a stimulant, I recommend one double-ought capsule of the powder twice daily.

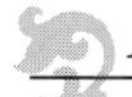

Piper cubeba

COMMON NAME ■ Cubeb

The fruit of the plant is used to make medicine. Cubeb contains a lignan called cubebin. This plant is an astringent, a diuretic, a carminative, and a stimulating expectorant. Dr. Bastyr taught its use as a restorative after urinary tract infections. He recommended 5 to 15 drops of the oil daily. I have little personal experience with this plant and have included it for historical purposes.

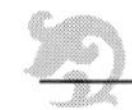

Copaiba langsdorfii

COMMON NAME ■ Copaiba

This plant is also listed as *Copaifera langsdorffi*. The medicine is obtained from a diterpenoid oleoresin in the bark. *Copaiba* medicine is an oleoresin, not a balsam. It is a stimulating antiseptic, an astringent, an expectorant, and a tonic. Eclectic physicians used *Copaiba* in treating chronic urethritis, cystitis, pyelitis, indolent ulcers, fissures, and fistulas. Dr. Bastyr taught that the oil should be taken internally in doses of 2 drops twice daily for 3 days. This plant is also a diuretic and is moderately effective at disinfecting the urinary tract.

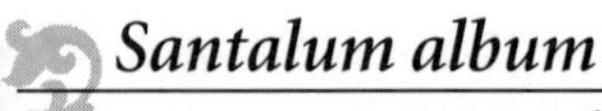

Santalum album

COMMON NAME ■ Sandalwood

The medicine is from the oil in the wood. *Santalum* contains a number of volatile oils called santalols.

Santalum is a calmative. It is a urinary antiseptic useful in treating chronic urethritis and prostatitis. Dr. Bastyr suggested 10 minims of the oil given in capsule form twice daily. *Santalum* is used to help pass kidney stones. Dr. Bastyr said that it coats the genitourinary tract from the kidneys down to and including the urethra.

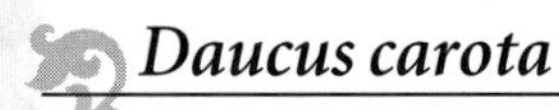

Daucus carota

COMMON NAME ■ Carrot

The whole edible vegetable is used. This is a general alterative. The carotene content of carrots is beneficial to the renal and lower urinary mucous membranes. Carotenes quench free radicals, thereby lowering inflammation in the tissues. For this protective effect, I have patients eat two carrots per day and drink six glasses of water in addition to other foods.

Atropa belladonna

COMMON NAME ■ Deadly nightshade

The roots and leaves are used to make medicine. *CAUTION: Belladonna is a powerful remedy that can be toxic in large doses. It is contraindicated in glaucoma.* *A. belladonna* is a genitourinary sedative. Dr. Bastyr taught that this remedy is useful in urethral colic. It may be used in gastric ulceration and spasmodic bladder conditions. *A. belladonna* decreases intravesicular pressure and the frequency of bladder contractions. Naturopathically, we use a dose of 5 to 10 drops twice daily. For intestinal obstruction that is life threatening, give 1 mg or more subcutaneously.

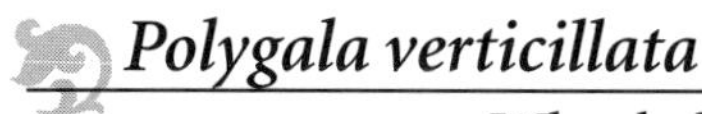

Polygala verticillata

COMMON NAME ■ Whorled milkwort

The root is used to make medicine. *Polygala* is a diuretic and a mild tonic. Dr. Bastyr favored this remedy as a kidney flush. He said that a standard tea could be made from the root and taken in a dose of 1 cup daily. The eclectic physicians recommended a dose of 20 drops of the tincture three times daily. Dr. Bastyr also used this remedy as an alterative in pleurisy.

Achillea millefolium

COMMON NAME ■ Yarrow

The aerial parts of the plant are used to make medicine. *Achillea* is a genitourinary calmative. An interesting use of this plant is for spasm of the uterine area, especially just lateral to the uterus in the region of the parametrium. I gave a patient *Achillea* as a digestive bitter, and she mentioned a decrease in this type of pelvic cramping. I prescribe 30 drops of tincture three times daily for this purpose. In addition, I think very highly of *Piscidia erythrina* for excessive cramping of the uterus.

CHAPTER

42

GLANDULARS

CHAPTER • OUTLINE

Historically, glandular agents have been defined as medicines that primarily affect the lymphatics. I have taken the liberty of expanding this category to include a few plants that affect other glands such as the adrenals, pituitary, thyroid, and hypothyroid. The male and female reproductive glands are addressed in other sections.

Phytolacca decandra

COMMON NAME ■ Pokeroot

One can also use *Phytolacca americana.* Use the whole plant to make medicine. *Phytolacca* contains a number of triterpene saponins, including the phytolaccosides A-G.[136] *Phytolacca* is an alterative and a slow-acting emetic. It was one of Dr. Bastyr's favorite glandular agents. It is used for inflammation and induration of the glands, including the glandular part of the breasts. We also use it for eustachian tube inflammation and chronic tonsillitis. I have used it to treat mononucleosis. A typical dose of *Phytolacca* for general glandular congestion is 7 drops of tincture three times daily.

Dr. Bastyr used to talk about lymphatic stasis in which the lymph nodes are palpable or mildly palpable. The tincture formula for lymphatic stasis is two parts *Iris,* one part *Phytolacca,* one part *Lobelia,* and two parts *Taraxacum* leaf and root. Mix 30 drops of this formula into a large glass of water. Drink 1 glass three times daily between meals.

Phytolacca tends to increase both the number and effectiveness of white blood cells. I often combine it with *Echinacea* to enhance the immune system. I have found a useful immune-enhancing formula to be one part *Phytolacca* tincture combined with three parts *Echinacea* tincture and three parts *Astragalus* tincture. The dose I recommend is 60 drops three times daily.

Stillingia sylvatica

COMMON NAME ■ Queens delight

The root is used to make medicine. *CAUTION: An overdose of* Stillingia *can produce gastroenteritis. Stillingia* contains several diterpenes, including prostatin. The eclectics listed *Stillingia* as a glandular, an alterative, and an astringent. We use it for irritation of the bronchial tubes, larynx, or nasal cavity. The dose is 1 to 20 drops of tincture twice daily. I tend to mix *Stillingia* with other plants such as *Iris* as a glandular.

Corydalis formosa

COMMON NAME ■ Turkey corn

The root is used to make medicine. This plant can also be found under the name *Corydalis cava* or *Corydalis turtschaninovii. C. turtschaninovii* contains a tetra-hydroprotoberberine called tetrahydropalmatine, which is a sedative.[26]

Corydalis is an alterative. Dr. Bastyr instructed us to use this plant to treat nodules on the bones, blood dyscrasias, ulcerations, and breakdown of soft tissues, especially of the lymphatics. He said that it is most often used to treat lymphatic diseases, especially where the female system is involved, such as vaginal infections with some lymph swelling. According to Dr. Bastyr, *Corydalis* has even been used in gynecologic problems such as amenorrhea, dysmenorrhea, and leukorrhea. He suggested a dose of 150 drops of tincture twice daily. *Corydalis* may have an effect on the immune system since it has been shown to stimulate interferon in vitro. Dr. Bastyr made the comment that this plant is almost always mixed with other plants; however, I do not recall him citing specific plants for this purpose.

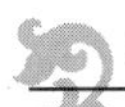

Chimaphila umbellata

COMMON NAME ■ Pipsissewa

The whole plant is used to make medicine. *Chimaphila* is an alterative, a diuretic, a tonic, and an antiseptic. Naturopaths use it to treat prostatitis and inflammation of the cervical lymph plexus. I recommend 120 drops three times daily for this purpose.

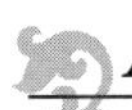

Arctium lappa

COMMON NAMES ■ Burrdock, Cocklebur

Arctium belongs to the sunflower family, *Compositae.* The root is used to make medicine. *Arctium* contains lignans, polyacetylenes, and various organic acids such as acetic and isovaleric acids. These organic acids stimulate the immune and detoxifying systems of the body. It is an alterative, a diuretic, an aperient, a cholagogue, a diaphoretic, and a depurative. *Arctium* is a first-choice remedy for infection of the glandular system. For this purpose, I recommend 60 drops of the botanical extract in 1 cup of water four times daily. *Arctium* is one of the best remedies for swollen glands. In addition to *Arctium*, two of Dr. Bastyr's favorite remedies for swollen glands were *Phytolacca* and *Iris.* Each combines well with *Phytolacca* for lymph stasis or lymphatic enlargement.

I use the concentrated extract of *Arctium* to improve the effectiveness of the Hoxey formula. For the treatment of cancer I use 90 drops or more of tincture twice daily, depending on the constitution and needs of the patient. In addition to being an anticancer formula, the Hoxey formula is also useful for stimulating the immune system. When taken internally, *Arctium* stimulates complement and tonifies the immune system. I have found that *Arctium* and *Echinacea* combine well as an immune enhancer. I also use *Arctium* for psoriatic arthritis.

The young shoots of the *Arctium* plant are edible and nutritious, containing calcium, iron, silicon, and vitamins A, B, and C. Dr. Bastyr told us to simply dig up the burrdock root, clean it, and cook it as a vegetable.

One interesting note on *Arctium* is that its inulin content evidently helps to improve liver storage of glycogen.

Rumex crispus

COMMON NAME ■ Yellow dock

Rumex obtusifolius may also be used. The root is used to make medicine. *Rumex* contains anthracene and naphthalene derivatives. One of the anthracenes is emodin, which is a cathartic. Taken in therapeutic doses, *Rumex* is generally not considered cathartic because it only contains a small amount of emodin.

As a glandular, *Rumex* improves lymphatic flow and function. The dose commonly recommended by naturopaths for this purpose is 30 to 60 drops of the tincture three times daily. *Rumex* is a good source of iron and so is a tonic for iron deficiency anemia. Dr. Bastyr mentioned its use in ulcerative stomatitis. In addition, he made the interesting comment that the 6X homeopathic remedy is good for sinus headache. Herbalists report the use of *Rumex* as a poultice for skin disorders and wounds. They also recommend its use as a topical application for poison ivy and poison oak.

Kalmia angustifolia

COMMON NAME ■ Sheep laurel

Use the leaves to make medicine. *Kalmia* has been used for glandular disorders, including inflammation. Eclectics recommend a tincture dose of 2 to 15 drops twice daily for this purpose. In addition to its use as a glandular, *Kalmia* is an anodyne in myalgic and rheumatic disorders and a sedative in tachycardia. Dr. Bastyr said that it is somewhat similar to *Veratrum viride* when used in potency for tachycardia.

Fucus versicolor

COMMON NAME ■ Kelp

The whole plant is used for medicine. There are many forms of kelp. Herbalist Ryan Drum is a great resource for more information about kelp. I use kelp to treat low-functioning thyroids, especially as the result of iodine deficiency, where there is some thyroid enlargement. I have found that low thyroxine levels often increase when patients have been taking six kelp tablets at lunchtime.

Kelp has the highest mineral content of any botanical and also contains a number of trace minerals and micronutrients. Some types of kelp are mucilaginous and can be soothing to the gastrointestinal tract. Tinctures are made from kelp and can be dosed at 20 drops two to three times daily; however, I prefer the capsulated powders. I really prefer going on field trips with Ryan Drum and listening to stories as we gather kelp from the ocean.

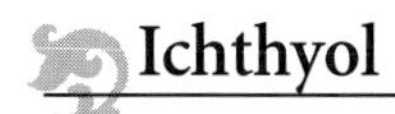

Ichthyol

Ichthyol is a mixture of sulfonated hydrocarbons. Dr. Bastyr said that glycerin can also be used. Ichthyol can be applied topically to help resolve glandular swellings. It was used by naturopaths of old to soften skin in psoriasis. It is an antiphlogistic and can help decrease scarring in pitting skin diseases such as smallpox and sebaceous acne. Historically, ichthyol was used as a local skin antiinfective. I remember Dr. Bastyr talking about this remedy, but I haven't used it in my practice.

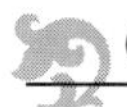

Colchicum autumnale

COMMON NAME ■ Autumn crocus

The bulbs and seeds are used to make medicine. *Colchicum* is an antimitotic and is being explored as a possible drug for use in childhood acute lymphoblastic leukemia. I do not know what the effective dose is for this purpose.

My good friend, Dr. Davis Lamson, knows a lot about *Colchicum.* He mentions its use in treating Peyronie's disease and its reputation in the treatment of gout. Dr. Bastyr used to use a 3X homeopathic preparation for gout. *Colchicum* has been useful in treating diarrhea. The eclectics used a dose of 3 to 5 drops of the tincture twice daily for this purpose. Most practitioners don't use this plant enough. This is one of the plants that converted E.B. Nash to homeopathy.

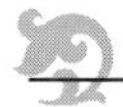

Gaultheria procumbens

COMMON NAME ■ Wintergreen

The leaves are used to make medicine. As a glandular agent, this plant stimulates the ovaries. The eclectics also used it for dysuria and for the treatment of painful hemorrhoids. *Gaultheria* is also a febrifuge. The classic tincture dose used is 5 to 10 drops twice daily. The oil can be given in doses of 3 to 6 drops or higher.

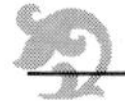

Trifolium pratense

COMMON NAME ■ Red clover

The blossoms are used to make medicine. This plant is an alterative, an antispasmodic, and an expectorant. As a glandular agent, I use *Trifolium* to treat cancer of the lymphatic system. I had a patient who mixed *Trifolium* and chaparral to treat her own breast cancer. She was successful. For cancer involving the glandular system, I recommend 90 to 120 drops of the botanical extract of

Trifolium, or 20 to 40 grains of the powder, four times daily. Herbalists frequently include *Trifolium* in anticancer teas.

Both clover and alfalfa are good sources of vitamin B_{17}. *Trifolium* contains a number of isoflavones, including genistein and daidzein. It also contains several coumarins and so is thought of when thinning of the blood is needed. However, there are more effective blood thinners available.

Trifolium is a famous blood purifier. The term "blood purifier" refers to plants that improve the function and quality of the blood. The blood provides nutrients to tissue and picks up metabolic wastes and disease products from the body. Blood purifiers can work by improving kidney and liver function, improving lymphatic drainage, or improving capillary integrity. I make a blood-purifying formula by combining equal parts of the tinctures of *Trifolium pratense, Arctium lappa, Iris versicolor, Chimaphila umbellata,* and *Euonymus atropurpurea.* The dose I recommend is 30 drops of the formula three times daily.

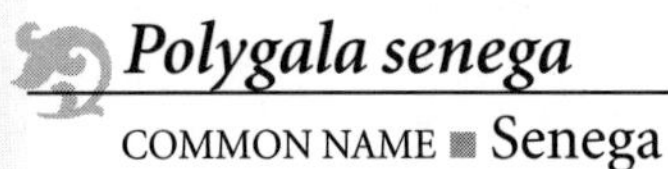

Polygala senega

COMMON NAME ■ Senega

The medicinal part is the dried root. Dr. Bastyr taught *Polygala* as one of the glandular agents. It is included in this section for historical purposes; however, I cannot recall any specific information presented by Dr. Bastyr pertaining to its glandular action.

Polygala contains senegin. It is a stimulant, an expectorant, and a diaphoretic. It affects mucous membranes of the respiratory system. According to Dr. Bastyr, *Polygala* can be used to treat bronchitis and pneumonia, especially in geriatric patients.

In addition, there are a variety of other conditions that *Polygala* may help, including skin diseases of the exfoliative type, eye strain, strabismus, amenorrhea, and laryngitis. The standard eclectic dose is given as 5 to 20 drops twice daily.

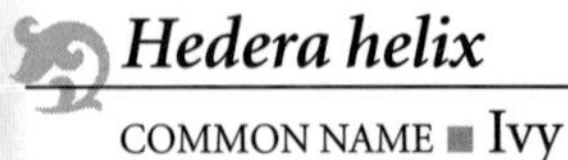

Hedera helix

COMMON NAME ■ Ivy

The leaves or berries are used to make medicine. Dr. Bastyr said that *Hedera* is used to reduce glandular swellings. His dose was 1 to 5 drops taken twice daily. I have had no experience using *Hedera* in my practice.

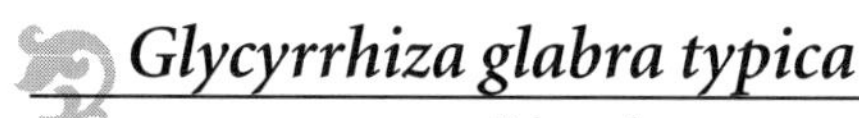

Glycyrrhiza glabra typica

COMMON NAME ■ Licorice

The root is used to make medicine. *Glycyrrhiza* is specific to the adrenal gland. It prolongs the half-life of cortisol, thus easing the effort that the adrenal gland must put out to supply the necessary cortisol to the body. I prescribe 30 drops of the fluid extract once daily at lunchtime. Licorice is mentioned often in this book, since it has dozens of applications in many body systems.

Lycopus virginicus

COMMON NAME ■ Bugleweed

The hormonal activity that *Lycopus* exhibits may be the result of the oxidation of the caffeic acid derivatives rosmarinic acid or lithospermic acid.[137] Dr. Bastyr used *Lycopus* to treat hyperthyroid conditions. I use 90 drops of the tincture twice daily for this purpose. I have accompanied the *Lycopus* with cold packs applied to the throat, which also calms the thyroid. Hyperthyroid conditions are difficult to treat. The dose needed for *Lycopus* to be effective in hyperthyroid conditions may be higher than what I am using. In recent years I have been trying to determine the best dose.

Lycopus inhibits the peripheral deiodination of thyroxine and lowers prolactin levels.[25] Given its prolactin-lowering capability, it is no wonder that *Lycopus* has been used to treat mastodynia. The old eclectics used this remedy to treat Graves' disease with cardiac involvement.

Corynanthe johimbe

COMMON NAME ■ Yohimbe

Also look for this plant under the name *Pausinystalia johimbe.* This plant has several remarkable actions on the hypothalamic communication system. The alkaloid yohimbine blocks the alpha-2 receptor site on the paraventricular nucleus in the central nervous system and thus inhibits the feeling of hunger. As an alpha-2 blocker, my colleague Dr. Ed Madison recommends a starting dose of 5 mg twice daily. This dose may be increased slightly as needed. Yohimbine also increases the amount of norepinephrine available to stimulate the medial preoptic nucleus, thus increasing libido. The dose is the same for this. The alkaloid yohimbine also blocks alpha-2 receptor sites on adipocytes, thus encouraging fat cells to burn rather than to store fat.

CHAPTER

43

HEMOSTATIC AGENTS

CHAPTER · OUTLINE

Hemostatics are remedies that stop bleeding.

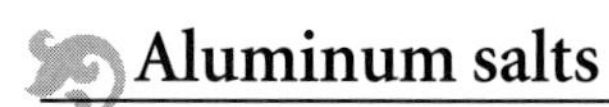

Aluminum salts

COMMON NAME ■ Alum

This medicine is used for small open cuts. It is primarily useful for people who have low fibrinogen levels and may have difficulty with the clotting process. Do not take this remedy internally. It is for external use only. To stop bleeding, apply alum directly to the wound.

Capsella bursa-pastoris

COMMON NAMES ■ Shepherd's purse, Case weed

The whole plant is used to make medicine. *Capsella* contains chlorogenic acid and a beta-glucopyranoside called sinigrin. It is also rich in vitamins C and K. The vitamin K content may be one of the principal hemostatic constituents in *Capsella.*

Capsella is an antihemorrhagic, a diuretic, a styptic, a vasoconstrictor, and an antiinflammatory. Dr. Bastyr taught us that *Capsella* is especially useful in hematuria accompanied by phosphaturia and alkaline uria. *Equisetum* will also stop this type of bleeding. The standard eclectic dose of *Capsella* is 20 to 40 drops of the tincture three times daily, or you can make an infusion by using 1 teaspoon of the herb in $\frac{1}{2}$ cup of water. The infusion is taken a mouthful at a time throughout the day. A time-honored field use of *Capsella* is in the treatment of nosebleed. Pound the plant into a moist pulp and insert a pledget into the nostril.[36]

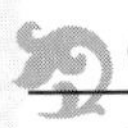

Cinnamomum saigonicum

COMMON NAME ■ Cinnamon

The bark of the shoots is used to make medicine. One may also use *C. zeylanicum.* Cinnamon is a hemostatic, a carminative, and an astringent. Historically, many physicians and herbalists have used a strong infusion of cinnamon to stop hemorrhage. Dr. Bastyr said that cinnamon acts in harmony with *Terebenthinum* and *Erigeron.* It restores tone to the uterine musculature. For this purpose, use a hot infusion twice daily. The tincture can also be used at a dose of 5 to 30 drops three times daily. Cinnamon is used to treat colds and flu and is also a useful home remedy for treating diarrhea. Be aware that the cinnamic acid in cinnamon is being researched in the treatment of diabetes: $\frac{1}{2}$ teaspoon twice daily lowers blood sugar! Cinnamon is part of a diabetes protocol that I use.

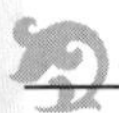

Erigeron canadensis

COMMON NAME ■ Canadian fleabane

The whole plant is used to make medicine. Dr. Joe Boucher introduced this plant to me in the early 1970s on a hike into the Garibaldi provincial park in British Columbia. Dr. Boucher practiced naturopathy for many years in Vancouver, British Columbia. Dr. Bastyr taught that *Erigeron* could be used for passive capillary bleeding, postpartum hemorrhage, hematuria, epistaxis, and uterine hemorrhage. It is also useful in ulcerative colitis. I use 60 drops of the tincture twice daily to help stop excessive bleeding. When *Erigeron* is used as a hemostatic, Dr. Bastyr suggested a dose of 20 to 30 drops of tincture three times daily, or 2 to 3 drops of the oil taken no more often than hourly. The oil is oxytocic. Dr. Bastyr said that *Erigeron* could be used to treat infant diarrhea caused by soybean allergy. In addition, *Erigeron* has antifungal action against *Helminthosporium turciccin.*

Urtica dioica

COMMON NAME ■ Nettle

One may also use *Urtica urens.* The flowering plant and roots are used to make medicine. *Urtica* contains phenolics and several sitosterols, including 7-alpha- and 7-beta-hydroxysitosterols.[138] It also contains quercetin, isoquercetin, and rutin.[139]

Dr. Bastyr spoke of *Urtica* as a hemostatic to treat bleeding hemorrhoids and bleeding ulcers. A strong decoction of the dried leaves is used in doses of 1 cup twice daily. The eclectics used the powdered leaves to make a good expectorant. They also used *Urtica* as a diuretic and to flush the kidneys, ureters, and bladder of accumulated detritus. Their dose of the tincture was 10 to 40 drops four times daily. Dr. Bastyr mentioned that the seeds of this plant produce a lethargic sleep. Two other uses of *Urtica* in my practice are the roots for prostatitis (1000 mg twice daily) and the leaves for the treatment of migraine (very effective) or allergic sinusitis (1000 mg twice daily).

Achillea millefolium

COMMON NAME ■ Yarrow

The tops are used to make medicine. *Achillea* contains achilleine, which has hemostatic action.[140] It also contains sesquiterpene lactones, azulene, and flavones, including pectolinarigenin and 3,6,4′-methylquercetagetin.[26] Dr. Bastyr spoke of *Achillea* as a hemostatic agent.

Apply a poultice of *Achillea* to a wound to help stop bleeding. The Native Americans of the Southwest use *Achillea* for most diseases. One can even use it for bleeding hemorrhoids. Hoffmann makes mention of *Achillea* for treating Bright's disease in its early stages.[46] Another name for *Achillea* is soldier's milfoil. According to legend, Achillea used yarrow to stop the bleeding wounds of his soldiers.

Achillea is a diaphoretic, an antipyretic, a hypotensive, an astringent, and a urinary antiseptic. I have found that 20 to 40 drops of the tincture two to three times daily, or 20 to 70 grains of the dried plant twice daily, may be used safely.

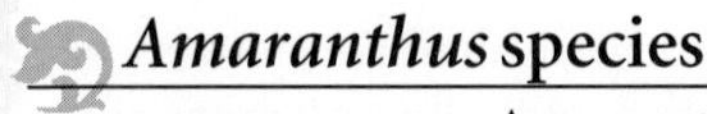

Amaranthus species

COMMON NAME ■ Amaranth

The whole plant is used to make medicine. This is an astringent medicine that can be used to treat bloody stools or, according to Dr. Bastyr, for excessive menstrual bleeding. The eclectics gave a dose of 15 to 30 drops three times daily. One cup of the standard tea may be given twice daily. Dr. Bastyr mentioned that this plant has also been used as a douche for leukorrhea.

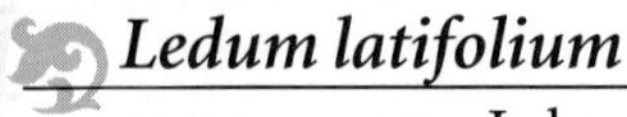

Ledum latifolium

COMMON NAME ■ Labrador tea

The leaves and small twigs are used to make medicine. This plant has been used to treat pertussis and respiratory inflammation where mild hemoptysis is present. For this purpose, eclectic physicians used 10 to 20 drops of tincture twice daily. Do not use more than 20 drops of tincture, since *Ledum* is toxic in larger doses because of its sesquiterpene contents. For this reason, a strong decoction of *Ledum* leaves was used by the eclectics, such as Felter and Lloyd, as an external application to treat lice.

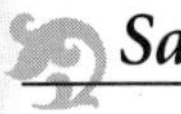

Sanguisorba officinalis

COMMON NAME ■ Burnet

The whole plant is used to make medicine. Burnet contains beta-sitosterol, flavonoids, and triterpene glycosides. It is a hemostatic and a tonic nutritive. It is used on wounds. To stop bleeding, make the herb into a pulp and apply it to the wound on a gauze bandage.

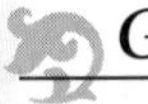

Geranium maculatum

COMMON NAME ■ Geranium

The whole plant is used to make medicine. Historically, naturopaths and herbalists have used *Geranium* for passive bleeding of the stomach, bowels, lungs, and kidneys. It is not for massive internal bleeding. The dose is 20 drops of tincture three times daily. This plant may be used as a gargle for bleeding gums after tooth extraction. For epistaxis, plug the patient's nose with cotton soaked in *Geranium* and bayberry.

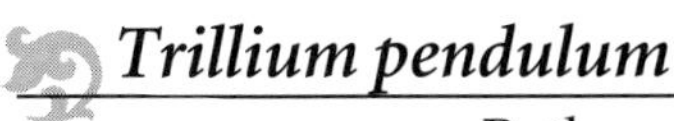

Trillium pendulum

COMMON NAME ■ Bethroot

The root is used to make medicine. Dr. Bastyr used *Trillium* consistently in cases of excessive uterine bleeding. He used a 3X homeopathic potency or up to 60 drops of tincture twice daily. For excessive uterine bleeding, I suggest a mixture of equal parts of *Trillium*, *Erigeron*, and *Mitchella* taken in doses of 30 drops twice daily. In addition, I make sure that my patients are given vitamin K to help stop uterine bleeding. Of course, I rule out fibroids and more serious disease.

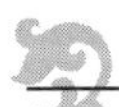

Ceanothus americanus

COMMON NAME ■ New Jersey tea

The root is used to make medicine. *Ceanothus* contains several cyclic peptides, a number of triterpenes, and emmolic acid, which is also called ceanothic acid.

Ceanothus is used both topically and internally as a hemostatic. For mild to moderate internal bleeding, use 1 teaspoon of a strong decoction of the tea every $\frac{1}{2}$ hour for six doses, then decrease the dose to 1 teaspoon every hour until bleeding stops. The dried powder may be applied locally as a hemostatic.

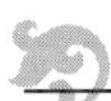

Erodium cicutarium

COMMON NAMES ■ Erodium, Stork's bill

The whole plant is used to make medicine. Stork's bill is used to arrest excessive bleeding, especially uterine bleeding accompanied by inflammation. Eclectics and herbalists suggest a strong infusion. Take 1 cup every 4 hours.

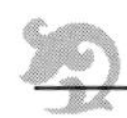

Sanicula marilandica

COMMON NAME ■ Sanicle

The leaves are used to make medicine. Sanicle contains a number of triterpene saponins and flavonoids, including rutin and astragalin. Eclectic physicians used it to treat internal wounds, ulcers, hemorrhage, sore throat, and sore and bleeding gums. The dose I use for these conditions is 5 drops of tincture three times daily. Herbalists use an infusion of sanicle to remove mucous congestion from the bronchi.

CHAPTER

44

HYDRAGOGUE CATHARTICS

CHAPTER • OUTLINE

Ecballium elaterium
Ipomoea jalapa
Helleborus niger
Croton tiglium
Magnesium sulfate
Lime water
Magnesium citrate
Veratrum viride
Ipomoea orizabensis

Hydragogue cathartics are remedies that cause water purgation of the intestines. These remedies were considered part of the naturopathic armamentarium to assist in detoxification of the body by emptying the intestinal tract and thereby eliminating toxins that were thought to be stored there. Before food processing and refrigeration, incidents of food poisoning were more common than we see in modern times. The cathartics were often life saving, and so held a more important place in early medicine.

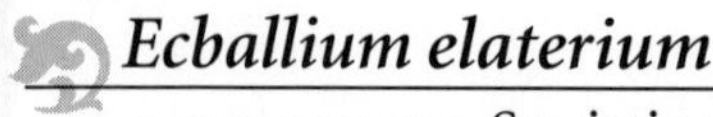

Ecballium elaterium

COMMON NAME ■ Squirting cucumber

Use the juice of the fruit to make medicine. This plant is a hydragogue cathartic and quite a violent remedy. Dr. Bastyr cautioned that *Ecballium* tends to irritate the stomach. The purging principle is alpha-elaterin. The eclectic dose is 1 to 10 drops of tincture per day or per event.

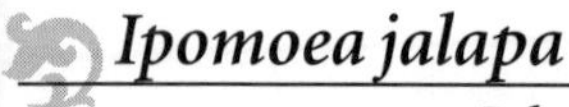

Ipomoea jalapa

COMMON NAME ■ Jalap

The root is used to make medicine. Jalap is a hydragogue cathartic and a drastic purgative. The dose recommended by Dr. Bastyr was 1 to 5 drops of tincture per day. It is used in many laxative tablets. To offset intestinal gripping, Dr. Bastyr combined jalap with *Lobelia* and *Dioscorea.* Dr. Bastyr did not recommend a dose for this mixture. I recommend mixing one part jalap with five parts *Lobelia* and five parts *Dioscorea.* As a hydragogue cathartic, I recommend a dose of 20 drops of this tincture combination per day.

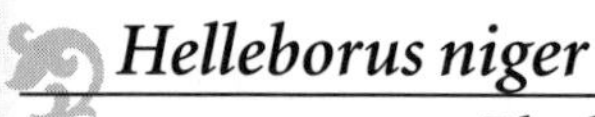

Helleborus niger

COMMON NAME ■ Black hellebore

The roots are used to make medicine. This remedy is a cardiac stimulant and a hydragogue cathartic. If a remedy is a cathartic, you can bet there is a toxic principle that the body is trying to eliminate. In the case of *Helleborus*, one of the toxic principles is protoanemonin.

Helleborus is a purgative and a narcotic, as well as a diuretic. Dr. Bastyr used to say, “Good old Epsom salts is a much less harmful hydragogue.” As a cathartic, he recommended a 2X homeopathic potency of *Helleborus.* For patients who are paralyzed, use higher potencies such as a 30X potency.

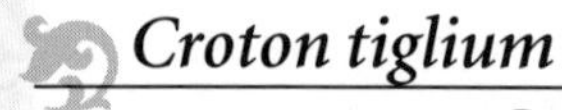

Croton tiglium

COMMON NAME ■ Croton

Use the oil from the seeds to make medicine. *Croton tiglium* is an irritating drastic purgative. The extremely toxic constituent is a phorbol ester. To produce substantial catharsis and purgation, use 1 drop of the tincture or 1 drop of the oil on a sugar cube. Do not use more than this. Larger doses will produce potentially dangerous, drastic purgation.

Per the law of opposites, Dr. Bastyr emphasized the effectiveness of this remedy homeopathically to prevent diarrhea. Use a 6X potency to stop acute enteritis. I give a vial of 6X potency tablets to patients who are going on vacation to help them if they come down with traveler's diarrhea.

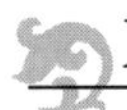

Magnesium sulfate

COMMON NAME ■ Epsom salts

This is a remedy that has been used over the years by many healers. Dr. Bastyr preferred this remedy as a hydragogue because it is gentler than many of the alternatives. For catharsis, use a $\frac{1}{2}$-ounce hot solution. Dr. Bastyr recommended using a 20% solution to treat eclampsia. He also used Epsom salts to treat claudication in the legs. For claudication, I recommend the use of niacin, magnesium, and bromelain as well. Eclectics, herbalists, and naturopaths use external applications of Epsom salts for arthritic and muscular pain.

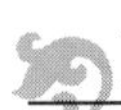

Lime water

Lime water is also called calcium oxide. I have included this remedy for historical purposes; I have no experience with this medicine. Dr. Bastyr spoke about this remedy as a hydragogue cathartic; however, I do not recall what he said about it. The dose that Dr. Bastyr gave was 1 to 2 teaspoons, probably for catharsis. He said that lime water helps to treat canker sores, and that small doses will help diarrhea.

Magnesium citrate

COMMON NAME ■ Pluto water

As a cathartic, Dr. Bastyr recommended that patients take this remedy in cupful doses. He told us that we should warn patients that they would need to use the bathroom right away. His exact words were: "Then remain in the throne room for an hour."

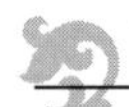

Veratrum viride

COMMON NAME ■ Green hellebore

The root and leaves are used to make medicine. This is a drastic cathartic. I do not recommend this remedy as a cathartic. It is listed here for historical documentation, because Dr. Bastyr taught about it as a cathartic.

Ipomoea orizabensis

COMMON NAME ■ Ipomoea

The roots are used to make medicine. The glycoresins present in this plant are responsible for the cathartic action. Dr. Bastyr taught that *Ipomoea* is used as a hydragogue cathartic in doses of 1 gram. He cautioned us against using this remedy when intestinal bleeding is present. I have yet to use this remedy in my practice.

CHAPTER

45

HYPNOTICS

CHAPTER • OUTLINE

Humulus lupulus
Piper methysticum
Valeriana officinalis
Lactuca virosa
Scutellaria lateriflora
Verbena officinalis

Hypnotics help induce a state of healthy sleep. This category has nothing to do with hypnosis. Sleep deprivation remains a serious medical condition that affects work performance and safety when driving. I encourage practitioners to try these herbs themselves. Too often in my teaching and lecturing, the audience is found wanting in personal experience with the plants. The study of the plants is the study of one's feelings about the plants and one's relationship with them. This is not a simple process but a long and exquisite one.

Humulus lupulus

COMMON NAME ■ Hops

Most of the medicine from hops is derived from the glandular hairs that contain volatile oils, including beta-myrcene and humulene. Hops is an excellent calmative and hypnotic. It has a long history of aiding patients who have trouble sleeping. In the Middle Ages, estate owners observed that hops pickers tired easily. This led to the concept that this plant might be useful to aid sleep. It can be used to treat insomnia and restless tension. The dose that I recommend as a hypnotic is 150 drops of tincture before bedtime. The patient may need to repeat this dose if he or she is still unable to sleep. It is safe to do so.

Dr. Bastyr mentioned stuffing pillows with hops strobili as a sleep aid. I have read this in many other herbals. As a calmative, I recommend using 40 drops of the tincture sweetened with $\frac{1}{2}$ teaspoon glycine in $\frac{1}{2}$ cup of water. This makes a nice bedtime drink.

Piper methysticum

COMMON NAME ■ Kavakava

The rhizome and roots are used to make medicine. This plant contains kava pyrones, which are relatively potent, centrally acting skeletal muscle relaxants.

Kavakava is a fair hypnotic. The neurologic effects of kavakava have not been entirely sorted out; however, Gary Piscopo did a nice job summarizing and speculating about the actions of kavakava based on what is currently known.[141] If using kavakava alone as a hypnotic, I recommend 60 drops of the tincture at bedtime. However, I often mix it with equal parts of other hypnotics, especially *Scutellaria.* The dose of the mixture I recommend is 90 drops of the tincture close to bedtime.

Valeriana officinalis

COMMON NAME ■ Valerian

Valeriana sitchensis is also used. The rhizome and roots are used to make medicine. *Valeriana* is a nervine, a hypnotic, and an antispasmodic. I have patients take four capsules 30 minutes before bed for the hypnotic activity.

Lactuca virosa

COMMON NAME ■ Wild lettuce

The dried latex and leaves are used to make medicine. *Lactuca* calms the mind and body. For insomnia and restlessness, I suggest 120 drops of the tincture of *Lactuca* 30 minutes before bedtime.

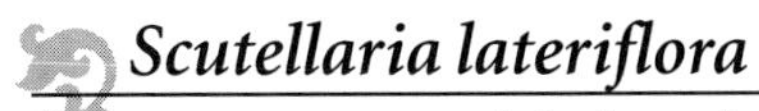

Scutellaria lateriflora

COMMON NAME ■ Madweed, Skullcap

The whole herb is used to make medicine. It contains a flavonoid glycoside, scutellarin, which is responsible for its nervine qualities. The hydrolysis of scutellarin yields scutellaraine. Herbalists have used *Scutellaria* for hundreds of years to help relieve nervous tension, which can help the patient sleep.

I recommend a dose of *Scutellaria* that is often greater than that recommended by the eclectics or early naturopaths. I recommend 150 drops of the tincture shortly before bedtime. *Scutellaria* may be combined with other relaxants and hypnotics, such as *Valeriana* and *Piper.* A combination that I have recommended for stubborn insomnia is 500 mg GABA (gamma-amino-butyric acid), 100 mg 5HPT (5′-hydroxytryptophane), 2000 mg glycine, and a combination of equal parts of *Scutellaria* and *Passiflora* botanical extracts (1 teaspoon). This has worked most of the time.

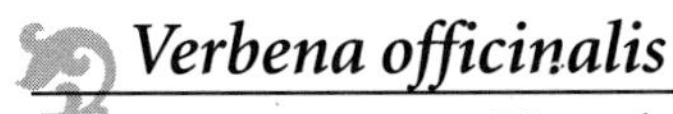

Verbena officinalis

COMMON NAME ■ Vervain

The dried aerial parts are used to make medicine. *Verbena* contains a number of iridoid monoterpenes, including verbenalin, and a large number of flavonoids.[142] This plant is a nervine tonic and a sedative/hypnotic. Dr. Basytr said that it is especially useful to treat restlessness during convalescence. The dose I recommend is 90 drops of tincture in the evening.

CHAPTER

46

HYPOGLYCEMICS

CHAPTER • OUTLINE

Hypoglycemics are used to lower blood glucose levels. They are especially useful in the treatment of type 2 diabetes, notably in the formative stages of the disease. I have also used these remedies for insulin-dependent type 1 diabetes and found that occasionally the blood glucose levels can be lowered. Patients taking these remedies should monitor their blood sugar levels carefully, and insulin adjustment should be coordinated with their endocrinologist. Dr. Bastyr did not cover these remedies as a group.

Camellia sinensis

COMMON NAME ■ Tea

The leaves are used to make medicine. Theaflavins isolated from black tea and galloyl catechins from green tea have shown potent inhibitory effects on salivary alpha-amylase, intestinal sucrase, and maltase. Research has shown that the administration of tea polyphenols causes suppression of the increase in intestinal alpha-amylase activity caused by starch. Tea polyphenols have also been shown to lower blood glucose levels.[143] The gallated polyphenols were far more effective inhibitors than the nongallated ones.

I suggest that my diabetic patients drink a combination of green and black tea daily. This is prepared by combining one tea bag of green tea with one tea bag of black tea in 2 cups of boiling hot water. Let this brew for 15 minutes. Squeeze excess fluid from the tea bags into the tea when removing the bags from the cup to enrich the flavonoid content of the tea. When you do this, you will notice a slight darkening of the tea. I recommend that my diabetic patients drink 2 cups of tea per day.

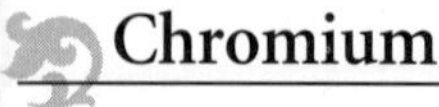

Chromium

COMMON NAME ■ Chromium

Supplementing the diet with 200 to 400 μg of chromium per day helps lower the blood sugar level. Chromium plays a role in increasing the cell's sensitivity to insulin. This allows for improved cellular absorption of the insulin sugar complex, which improves glucose tolerance and decreases fasting blood sugar levels.[92] Chromium-rich foods include brewer's yeast, beef, calf's liver, wheat bran, and potatoes.

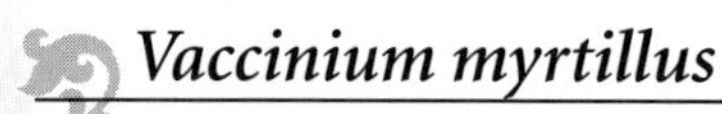

Vaccinium myrtillus

COMMON NAMES ■ European blueberry, Bilberry

The dried leaves and ripe fruit are used to make medicine. *Vaccinium* has lowered blood sugar levels in diabetic patients by as much as 100 points. This is a fairly consistent finding in my practice. I have used a very concentrated extract of the berry anthocyanins in doses of 1 to 3 teaspoons daily for the treatment of diabetes. The extract is added to a large glass of water and drunk slowly. Blueberries themselves may be used, adding 1 cup of blueberries to cereals or yogurt and consumed daily. The blueberries are better when frozen. The freezing breaks cell walls in the berry and frees more of the anthocyanin.

CHAPTER

47

INTESTINAL ASTRINGENTS

CHAPTER • OUTLINE

Epilobium angustifolium
Rubus villosus
Coto bark
Areca catechu
Pterocarpus marsupium
Vaccinium myrtillus
Polygonum bistorta
Vinca major
Krameria triandra

Intestinal astringents are agents used to alleviate bleeding in the gastrointestinal tract. This category also includes plants that alleviate diarrhea caused by disordered mucosa of the gastrointestinal tract.

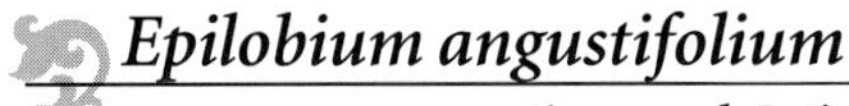

Epilobium angustifolium

COMMON NAMES ■ Fireweed, Wickup

Epilobium palustre may also be used. The leaves are used to make medicine. *Epilobium* contains a large number of flavonoids, including a number of quercetin derivatives. It also contains tannins and several steroids, including the ever-popular beta-sitosterol. Dr. Bastyr told us that *Epilobium* is useful for the entire intestinal tract. This astringent is especially useful for diarrhea. It is an emollient and a tonic demulcent and is good for enteritis and mucous enteritis. I have found it useful for intestinal inflammation with bleeding, especially when used with *Geranium.* For enteritis, Dr. Bastyr said to use an infusion of 1 ounce of the dried herb per pint of water and to take this in doses of 1 teaspoon every 20 minutes. If gathering the herb, be sure to dry it before making the tea or tincture. Dr. Joe Boucher originally taught me the use of this remedy.

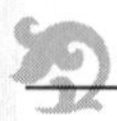

Rubus villosus

COMMON NAME ■ Raspberry

Use the root to make medicine. Another species is *Rubus idaeus.* This medicine is a tonic astringent. Dr. Bastyr said that *Rubus* is particularly helpful in infant diarrhea. For genitourinary hemorrhage, he told us to combine one part *Rubus* with two parts *Myrica cerifera.* The dose of the mixture is 15 drops twice daily. *Rubus* leaves can be dried and used to make a standard tea that herbalists say is a good tonic for women.

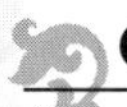

Coto bark

Coto is used to treat diarrhea, nausea, and vomiting associated with great distress. It is also an antiseptic and an astringent. The tincture dose is 20 to 30 drops twice daily. Coto aids in absorption from the alimentary canal. It also slightly dilates the abdominal vessels. It is usually given before meals.

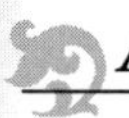

Areca catechu

COMMON NAMES ■ Catechu, Betel nut palm

It may also be found under the name *Terra japonica.* The medicinal part is the nut. *Areca* contains tannin and several pyridine alkaloids, including arecoline and guvacine. The arecoline is a parasympathomimetic.[25]

This intestinal astringent treats intestinal bleeding and diarrhea. The eclectics used it to treat menorrhagia. The dose reported by Dr. Bastyr was 40 drops of tincture twice daily. A very interesting use of *Areca* is to mix it with the leaves of *Piper betle* or gambir. It is a stimulant masticatory known in India as "punsupari." *Areca* is also an anthelminthic.

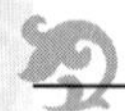

Pterocarpus marsupium

COMMON NAME ■ Kino

Pterocarpus is an intestinal astringent. This astringent can also be used in polyuria, epistaxis, and night sweats. Dr. Bastyr reported a diverse number of ways in which kino has been used, including pharyngitis, nonspecific vaginitis, edematous uvula, gonorrhea, and leukorrhea. He said that the tincture dose is 1 to 2 drams twice daily. The powdered dose is 10 to 30 grains twice daily. I have not used this remedy in my practice. I have included it for historical purposes because Dr. Bastyr mentioned it in his lectures.

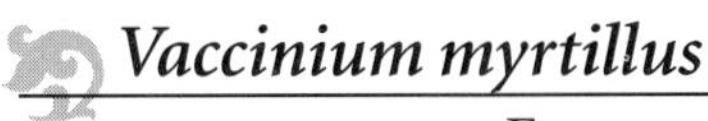

Vaccinium myrtillus

COMMON NAMES ■ European blueberry, Bilberry

The dried leaves and ripe fruit are used to make medicine. Make a tea of the leaves to use as an intestinal astringent. As usual, the tea is best made from dried leaves. Thirty to sixty drops of the tincture three times daily may also be used as an astringent.

Blueberries or blueberry extracts also help to prevent macular degeneration, vein weakening that can lead to strokes, and oxidation of LDL cholesterol and subsequent arterial disease.[144] In addition, they help to improve peripheral circulation.[144] I use blueberry extract daily in my practice as a health-providing nutrient for nearly all of my patients.

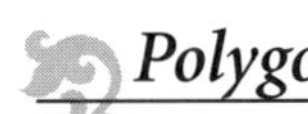

Polygonum bistorta

COMMON NAME ■ Bistort

Also look for this plant under the name *Polygonum bistortoides.* Bistort is a member of the buckwheat family, *Polygonaceae.* The root is used to make medicine. This is an intestinal astringent and a vermifuge. Bistort contains tannins and gallotannins. Dr. Bastyr told us of its use for prolonged dysentery and for ulcers. He recommended making a strong infusion and giving 2 tablespoons of the resulting tea four times daily. He also said that *Polygonum* is even useful where there is bleeding from the lungs or stomach. When applied topically, *Polygonum* is a strong styptic. I often give doses of 5 drops of tincture to patients just to help tonify the mucous membranes of the intestinal tract.

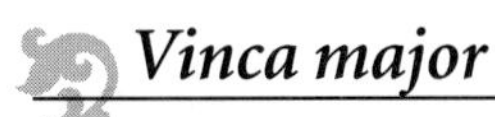

Vinca major

COMMON NAME ■ Greater periwinkle

Use the dried aerial parts of the plant for medicine. Dr. Bastyr recommended using a strong decoction or infusion as an enema for ulcerative proctitis. He said that *Vinca* is an intestinal astringent and a hemostatic, and it can be used to treat hemorrhoids as well. The dose as an astringent is 10 drops of tincture three times daily.

Krameria triandra

COMMON NAME ■ Rhatany

The roots are used to make medicine. This is an astringent, a diuretic, a hemostatic and a styptic. Rhatany contains tannins, procyanidins, and a number of benzofuranoids. Dr. Bastyr used *Krameria* to treat most inflammatory gastrointestinal problems, including enteritis, gastritis, proctitis, diarrhea, and bloody stools. He recommended a dose of 10 to 20 drops twice daily. It may be used in higher doses at the discretion of the practitioner. In addition, Dr. Bastyr mentioned its use in hematuria and as a gargle.

CHAPTER

48

INTESTINAL TRACT SEDATIVES AND ANTISPASMODICS

CHAPTER • OUTLINE

These remedies quiet the activity of the smooth muscles of the intestinal tract. They are used for overactive bowel conditions such as spastic colitis and abdominal gripping.

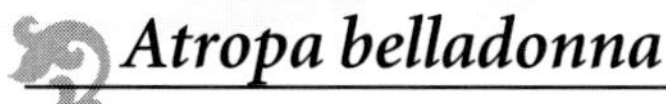

Atropa belladonna

COMMON NAME ■ Deadly nightshade

The leaf yields most of the alkaloids. *CAUTION:* A. belladonna *is a powerful remedy that can be toxic in large doses. It is contraindicated in glaucoma. A. belladonna* has been used to decrease gastrointestinal secretions in acute ulcerative conditions of the alimentary tract. It decreases stomach secretions and decreases motility and peristalsis of the bowel. Dr. Bastyr said that both amplitude and frequency are decreased. It is also useful in spastic colitis. I have treated a number of cases of spastic colitis with *A. belladonna* as part of the therapeutic regimen. The dose that I use is 15 drops of the tincture twice daily. *A. belladonna* is a parasympathetic depressant, which explains its effectiveness in quieting the smooth muscles of the intestinal tract. In addition, it is an antisialagogue.

Datura stramonium

COMMON NAME ■ Jimsonweed

D. stramonium contains atropine and scopolamine. The leaves and the flowering tops are used to make medicine, although the seeds are even slightly higher in alkaloid content. *D. stramonium* is a sedative and an antispasmodic. It is an anticholinergic that acts much like *A. belladonna.* Eclectics used a dose of 5 drops of tincture twice daily. *CAUTION: Do not use jimsonweed in any higher doses, since it is a powerful psychotropic plant.*

Strychnos castelnaei

COMMON NAME ■ Curare

Curare is also extracted from *Chondrodendron tomentosum.* The bark is used to make medicine. The most important active ingredient in curare is (+)-tubocurarine, which is a quaternary compound containing a bisbenzylisoquinoline structure. Curare is primarily a skeletal muscle relaxant used to quiet the abdominal muscles during surgery. To quiet the intestine, Dr. Bastyr recommended $\frac{1}{4}$ drop of the tincture twice daily. A 2X homeopathic potency of *S. nux-vomica* acts in a similar manner and was used by Dr. Bastyr and other naturopathic physicians for the same purposes.

Magnesium

Intenstinal gripping and spasm can be relieved by administering 200 mg of magnesium three times daily. It can be taken in capsule form for this purpose.

Potentilla anserina

COMMON NAMES ■ Cinquefoil, Silverweed

Also look under the names *Potentilla reptans* and *Potentilla canadensis. Potentilla* is a member of the rose family, *Rosaceae.* The medicinal parts are the leaves and flowers. This plant is a mild-acting antispasmodic, a nervine, and a diuretic. Herbalists have used *Potentilla* to treat dysentery. *Potentilla* contains tannin and is also a mild astringent. For dysentery, a cup of the standard tea may be given twice daily. I use 30 drops of the tincture three to four times daily for the treatment of any of the above-mentioned conditions. Dr. Bastyr told us about making a sore throat medication from the leaves. He said to macerate the leaves with a little honey and coat the throat. He said that the tincture could be used as a gargle as well.

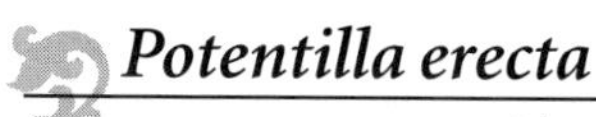

Potentilla erecta

COMMON NAMES ■ Tormentil root, Bloodroot

Potentilla erecta is also called *Potentilla tormentosa.* The rhizome is used to make medicine. The uses of tormentil are similar to those of cinquefoil, as are many of the constituents. Tormentil root contains catechin polymers, gallotannins such as agrimoniin and pedunculagin, single catechins, and proanthocyanidins. It also contains quite a few flavonoids such as kaempferol, which is similar in action to quercetin.

Dr. Bastyr spoke of *Potentilla erecta* specifically for the intestinal tract. I use it for ulcerative colitis, Crohn's disease, and spastic colitis. *Potentilla* is given in doses of 60 drops of tincture three times daily. For all of these diseases, I also prescribe 500 mg of quercetin three times daily in conjunction with other botanicals. I have used *Potentilla pacifica* as well for intestinal upset. I also like chamomile for these disorders.

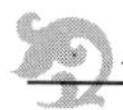

Amaranthus hypochondriacus

COMMON NAME ■ Amaranth

Amaranth cereal may be obtained from the health food store and is a tasty wheat substitute for breakfast. Fresh leaves of amaranth may be boiled to soothe the gastrointestinal tract and to remedy diarrhea.[112] One ounce of leaves, or about a handful, is added to 8 ounces of water and boiled. Sip the tea slowly. In addition, a tablespoon of the powdered dry leaf can be used to make an infusion of amaranth. The tincture dose of amaranth is 60 drops three times daily.

CHAPTER

49

LAXATIVES

CHAPTER • OUTLINE

Cascara sagrada
Rheum officinalis
Aloe barbadensis or *Aloe vera*
Alexandria senna
Ricinus communis
Olea europaea
Rhamnus frangula

Laxatives promote evacuation of the bowels. Laxatives should be used on a temporary basis to prevent laxative dependency. A well-balanced diet that is high in fiber and fluids will help to assure good bowel patterns. Salads with a good dressing made of the essential fatty acids found in olive and safflower oils may be helpful in maintaining bowel regularity. Flaxseed oil goes very well on brown or wild rice, which also helps to prevent constipation. Vitamin C and magnesium are both gentle laxatives. A supplement of both or either will promote bowel activity. Laxatives may be very useful in older patients in whom normal regular bowel movement is lacking because of poor parasympathetic tone related to age. Laxatives should always be taken with several cups of water. Cathartics are strong laxatives.

Cascara sagrada

COMMON NAME ■ Sacred bark

The bark is used to make medicine. This medicine is a cathartic, increasing peristalsis and alleviating constipation. The active ingredients are hydroxyanthraquinone glycosides, chiefly the cascarosides.[26]

Dr. Bastyr suggested that we tell our patients to use *Cascara* in the morning to create the habit of a bowel movement at that time. The general eclectic dose of the tincture is about 50 drops for a cathartic, although more may be needed. Initially, one may give 5 to 10 drops of tincture as a laxative and then decrease the dose to 3 to 4 drops three times daily to regulate bowel movements. In class, we discussed combining *Cascara* with *S. nux-vomica* to increase effectiveness. The flavor of *Cascara* is absolutely delicious.

Rheum officinalis

COMMON NAMES ■ Chinese rhubarb, Turkey rhubarb

One may use *Rheum palmatum.* Do not confuse this with *Rheum rhaponticum,* which is the variety grown in gardens as food. The rhizome is used to make medicine. *Rheum* has an ancient herbal history dating back to 2700 BC.[145] It contains anthraquinone glycosides as do *Cascara,* buckthorn, senna, and other famous laxatives. The anthraquinones include rhein and glucorhein.

According to Dr. Bastyr, *Rheum* is a good remedy for sour stomach and acid vomiting. The dose he gave for this was 5 to 35 drops as a laxative. I have found that small doses such as 5 drops may be used as a tonic. *Rheum* combines well with goldenseal or cinnamon. It is an astringent and as such can have a healing effect on the intestinal lining. I think of *Rheum* for atonic constipation. A dose of 30 drops of the tincture is about right for this purpose.

Aloe barbadensis or *Aloe vera*

COMMON NAME ■ Aloe vera

Aloe is a member of the lily family, *Liliaceae.* Use the dried latex from the leaves for the laxative medicine. The principal active laxative ingredient in aloe is an anthraquinone glycoside called barbaloin. Also worth noting is aloe-emodin, or aloe-emodin anthrone C-10 glucoside, which is also a cathartic principle. As a strong laxative, the dose of aloe tincture is 5 drops. Aloe has also been used to help expel worms.

The antiinflammatory effects of aloe may be attributed to a number of active ingredients contained in the plant, including gamma-linolenic acid (the same fatty acid contained in evening primrose and black currant oils), salicylates (found in willow bark and chemically related to aspirin), and several antibradykinin glycoproteins.

Aloe's antibacterial activity against a number of *Staphylococcus, Streptococcus, Klebsiella, Candida,* and *Enterobacter* species has been noted.[110] McDaniel et al. did an interesting study on the effect of acetylated mannose on retroviral infections.[146,147] The acetylated mannose may hold some promise for AIDS and feline leukemia virus treatment. Time will tell.

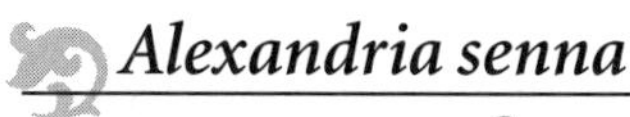

Alexandria senna

COMMON NAME ■ Senna

It is also called *Cassia acutifolia* and *Cassia senna. CAUTION: Use this plant cautiously in nursing mothers, since the cathartic action is imparted to the milk.* The medicine is derived from the leaves. The chief hydroxyanthraquinone glycosides in senna are the sennosides.

When using senna as a laxative, begin by giving 20 drops of the tincture or 30 to 60 grains of the powder. This remedy works to treat chronic constipation by increasing peristalsis. Dr. Bastyr mentioned this as a good duodenal purgative. The pods have a milder laxative action than the leaves.

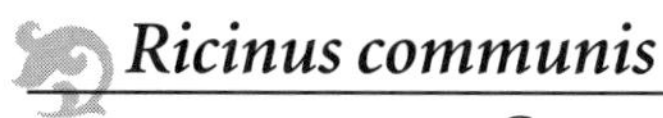

Ricinus communis

COMMON NAME ■ Castor oil

This oil is obtained from the seed. *CAUTION: The castor bean itself is a deadly toxin. The bean contains ricinine, which is a powerful toxin. Do not ingest the bean.*

This plant is a stimulant cathartic and a laxative. A major constituent of castor oil's fatty acid makeup is ricinoleic acid, which may account for the laxative effect of the plant. It is steamed to destroy albumins. Dr. Bastyr suggested that we give 1 teaspoon of the oil to patients as a starting dose. If results are not obtained within several hours, give another teaspoon of the oil. Castor bean oil is somewhat toxic and is usually reserved for external use.

In my opinion, olive oil is safer to use internally as a laxative. I suggest a dose of 3 tablespoons of olive oil as a gentle laxative. However, different people require different doses.

Historically, an excellent poultice has been made to relieve abdominal pain by applying castor oil to the abdomen and covering it with a hot towel. Dr. Bastyr used castor oil as an emollient eyewash, applying 1 drop of castor oil in the eye to wash out foreign objects.

Olea europaea

COMMON NAME ■ Olive oil

As a gentle laxative, I recommend 3 tablespoons of olive oil; 1 to 2 fluid ounces is certainly laxative. Dr. Bastyr taught us the use of olive oil as an enema for fecal impaction. Olive oil can be used to protect the stomach when poisoning has occurred from caustic alkalis. Olive oil is rich in oleic acid, which is an omega-9 fatty acid.

Rhamnus frangula

COMMON NAME ■ Buckthorn

Buckthorn is a member of the *Rhamnaceae* family. The dried or fresh bark is used to make medicine. One may also use the dried ripe fruits of *Rhamnus cathartica.* Buckthorn bark contains hydroxyanthraquinones, which cause the laxative effect. The dried plant contains a monosidic anthraquinone glycoside, glucofrangulin A.[148] Buckthorn has been used as a laxative by eclectics, herbalists, and naturopaths. Buckthorn has an action similar to that of *Cascara sagrada.* When using buckthorn as a laxative, use the powder in level teaspoon doses for adults and have them drink a lot of water.

CHAPTER

50

LAXATIVES (BULK)

CHAPTER • OUTLINE

Chondrus crispus
Gelidium cartilagineum
Gracilaria confervoides
Furcellaria fastigiata
Cydonia oblonga
Pectin
Sterculia urens
Plantago afra
Linum usitatissimum
Cyamopsis tetragonolobe

Bulk laxatives provide material to help form stool. In so doing, they promote movement of the stool through the colon. Laxatives should always be taken with several cups of water.

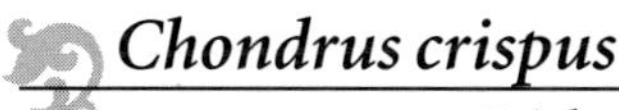

Chondrus crispus

COMMON NAME ■ Irish moss

The whole plant is used to make medicine. Irish moss contains carrageenin and is high in minerals. It is used in the laxative preparation kondremul. Irish moss is more often used as an ingredient in bulk laxatives than alone. It is often mixed with plants that provide a mucilaginous lubricant to aid in the bowel movement.

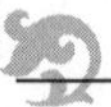

Gelidium cartilagineum

COMMON NAMES ■ Japanese isinglass, Agar

The whole plant is used to make medicine. Agar hydrates are used to form a smooth bulk, which aids normal peristalsis. It is also used as a base material for suppositories.

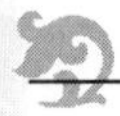

Gracilaria confervoides

COMMON NAME ■ Red algae

The whole plant is used to make medicine. These algae are used in a manner similar to that of *G. cartilagineum*. The algaes and seaweeds are extremely nutritive because they are high in minerals.

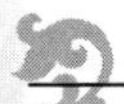

Furcellaria fastigiata

COMMON NAME ■ Danish agar

The whole plant is used to make medicine. The hydrocolloids found in this plant are similar to k-carrageenin, which is found in *C. crispus*.

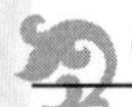

Cydonia oblonga

COMMON NAME ■ Quince

The seeds are used to make medicine. The seeds have a mucilaginous epithelium equivalent to 20% of their weight. As a bulk laxative, the crushed seeds may be eaten with food. I have no experience using quince seed.

Pectin

Pectin is derived from citrus fruits and apples. There is pectin in beet roots as well. A lot of pectin is derived from lemon peels. Like many of the bulk laxatives, pectin is composed of sugar complexes.

Pectin helps absorb toxins. The polysaccharide complexes in the fruit can be found in the middle lamellae of the cell walls. Pectin is more of a bulking agent than a laxative, used to form and firm up the stool. Pectin is used in making gelatin.

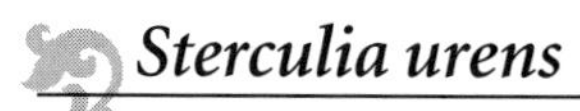

Sterculia urens

COMMON NAME ■ Karaya

The gum from the trunk is used to make medicine. One may also use *Sterculia villosa* and *Sterculia tragacantha*. This tree belongs to the *Sterculiaceae* family and is native to India. The gum is extracted by making incisions into the trunk of the tree, although it is exuded naturally. Karaya gum consists of an acetylated branched heteropolysaccharide that contains a large amount of D-galacturonic acid and D-glucuronic acid residues.[33]

Because karaya gum is not very soluble and because it is hydrophilic, it absorbs water well and swells to several times its original bulk size. The resulting mucilage residue helps form the bulk of the stool. Generally, naturopathic physicians have suggested 1 teaspoon several times during the day as a bulk laxative.

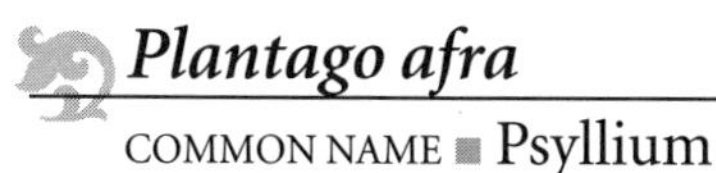

Plantago afra

COMMON NAME ■ Psyllium

The seeds are used to make medicine. This is a bulk laxative. Many commercial products are available that contain psyllium seed. The usual dose given is 7.5 g in water. This may be repeated four times daily. This is the most popular bulk laxative in use today.

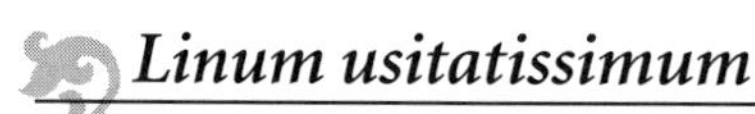

Linum usitatissimum

COMMON NAME ■ Linseed, Flaxseed

The seeds are used to make medicine. For a laxative effect, I use 1 tablespoon of crushed or ground linseeds. Be sure to store linseeds in a tightly sealed container in a cool, dark place. They do not keep long because the omega-3 oils oxidize.

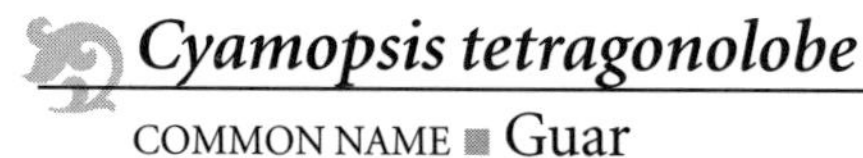

Cyamopsis tetragonolobe

COMMON NAME ■ Guar

The medicine is made from the endosperm of the seed of this annual plant. This endosperm is powdered and can be taken in guar gum capsules. Guar gum is a bulk laxative consisting of a galactomannan hydrocolloid. It is made up of 1,4-linked D-mannopyranosyl units in a linear chain. Single 1,6 linked D-galactonatopyranosyl residues are attached to alternate mannose moieties. One will find guar gum on the label of many processed foods. Dr. Bastyr said that a good starting dose is two capsules twice daily taken with a glass of water.

CHAPTER

51

LESSER LIVER REMEDIES

CHAPTER • OUTLINE

Taraxacum officinale
Polymnia uvedalia
Ceanothus americanus
Euonymus atropurpurea
Yerba delaflecca
Carduus marianus
Phyllitis scolopendrium
Oxalis montana
Erythraea centaurium
Gentiana lutea
Linaria vulgaris
Atropa belladonna
Agrimonia eupatoria

It is unclear why Dr. Bastyr included a section called lesser liver remedies. Probably the eclectic physicians who wrote the books that Dr. Bastyr lectured from considered these remedies less active than the liver stimulants and general liver remedies covered in the next section. I think that Dr. Bastyr was simply following their format. I am presenting these remedies as he gave them in his lectures.

This category of remedies was covered in my original lecture and field notes from my studies with Dr. Bastyr. It has been slightly modified and added to since my 1983 book entitled *Naturopathic Applications of the Botanical*

Remedies, which was a compilation of notes from Dr. Bastyr's lectures and, at that time, my 5 years of practice experience and field notes.

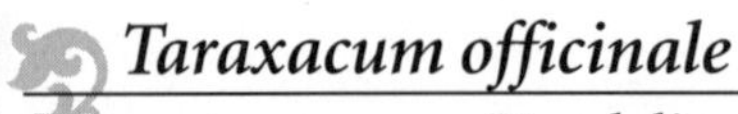

Taraxacum officinale

COMMON NAME ■ Dandelion

The roots are used to make liver medicine. The leaves are used as a diuretic. *Taraxacum* is a cholagogue, a choloretic, and a gastrointestinal tonic. It is a source of choline and is high in iron and trace minerals. I use *Taraxacum* to treat jaundice and autointoxication. This medicine has a mild laxative effect. Dr. Bastyr emphasized the value of *Taraxacum* as an aid for elderly patients with flagging digestion. The dose I recommend is 40 to 60 drops of tincture four times daily in water, or 2 to 8 grains of the dried root daily. For liver complaints or sluggish liver, I combine *Taraxacum* with either balmony or *Chelidonium.*

The whole *Taraxacum* plant tinctured makes a great spring tonic drink. I suggest 90 drops of the tincture in a glass of water twice daily for 2 weeks. This drink is both a tonic to the liver and a mild diuretic that flushes toxins out of the body.

Eclectics have written about the use of *Taraxacum* in cirrhosis, xanthomatosis, hypercholesterolemia, atherosclerosis, and cystinuria. In addition, it can be used for simple nervous exhaustion. This root is edible, incidentally. It can be chopped and steamed like any vegetable.

Polymnia uvedalia

COMMON NAME ■ Bearsfoot

Use the root to make medicine. Dr. Bastyr liked this remedy and used it often. *Polymnia* is an alterative, a digestive stimulant, and a good spleen remedy. Dr. Bastyr taught this remedy in the lesser liver section, although he emphasized its value primarily in treating problems of the spleen.

In addition to its use as a liver remedy, Dr. Bastyr taught that *Polymnia uvedalia* was one of the best hair tonics available. His recipe was two parts of the extract of *Polymnia* combined with three parts castor oil, three parts lanolin, and one part glycerin. He had his patients apply this mixture to the scalp as a hair tonic.

One specific use of *Polymnia* given by Dr. Bastyr, and presented for historical purposes, is its use for decreased granulocytes, decreased neutrophils, increased lymphocytes, and increased eosinophils. His dose was 20 drops of the tincture twice daily. Herbalists have used *Polymnia* as an external application for indurated swellings. I recall that Dr. Bastyr said that he had used this as a poultice as well.

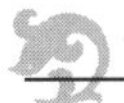

Ceanothus americanus

COMMON NAME ■ New Jersey tea

The dried bark of the root is used to make medicine. This plant is a hemostatic, an astringent, a tonic expectorant, a mild antiseptic, and a liver stimulant. As a liver tonic, I use 60 drops of *Ceanothus* tincture two to three times daily. This medicine is used to treat inactivity of the liver with sluggish circulation and doughy skin. We also use it for pain and hypertrophy of the liver or spleen.

Euonymus atropurpurea

COMMON NAMES ■ Wahoo, Indian arrowwood

The bark of the root is used to make medicine. Wahoo is a tonic and an alterative that increases bile flow. Naturopaths use it for indigestion with biliousness. In hepatomegaly, I use 30 drops of tincture three times daily. Vary this prescription depending on the seriousness of the case and the size of the patient. I use wahoo with *Hydrastis* to promote gastric and duodenal secretions. I like this remedy and use it frequently. Unfortunately, it is not well known.

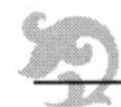

Yerba delaflecca

COMMON NAME ■ Poison wood

Yerba is a purgative. Dr. Bastyr used a 3X homeopathic potency for bilious colic. He said to repeat this dose every hour until the pain is gone. Today, bilious colic is referred for hospitalization and diagnosis to determine whether the gallstone will pass or whether it is obstructive and will need to be surgically removed. In cases of severe bilious colic, I refer my patients to the hospital for a diagnostic work-up. When Dr. Bastyr practiced rural medicine, immediate hospitalization was not an option, in which case relying on plant medicines was crucial.

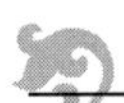

Carduus marianus

COMMON NAME ■ St. Mary's thistle

The leaves and seeds are used to make medicine. The flavonoid structure contained in *Carduus* is hepatoprotective. Dr. Bastyr taught the use of this remedy for congestion of the liver, spleen, and kidney. He also told us that *Carduus* relieves the usual reflex pain in the left shoulder blade caused by liver congestion or gallbladder colic. A tincture dose of 10 to 30 drops is typically used three or four times daily.

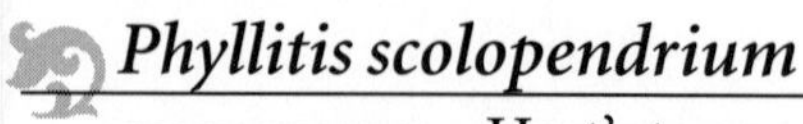

Phyllitis scolopendrium

COMMON NAME ■ Hart's tongue fern

The fronds are used for medicine. This remedy is included as a liver remedy because Dr. Bastyr taught it in this section. Unfortunately, he did not discuss its use as a liver remedy. He did speak of using *Phyllitis* for disorders of the spleen and suggested combining it with *Chionanthus* and *Phytolacca* in patients with colitis and low-grade fever.

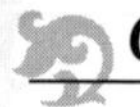

Oxalis montana

COMMON NAME ■ Common woodsorrel

This plant may also be found under the name *Oxalis acetosella.* The whole plant is used to make medicine. To treat mild liver problems such as liver sluggishness caused by overeating, I suggest using 10 to 30 drops of tincture two to three times daily. Woodsorrel contains oxalic acid. It also contains clover acid, which may stimulate gallbladder activity.[25]

Oxalis is astringent. The young leaves may be boiled and used in soups. The leaves may be given to help reduce fever. This plant is also a diuretic. For this purpose, I suggest 90 drops of tincture three times daily. Dr. Bastyr said that a cold infusion might help to relieve heartburn.

Erythraea centaurium or *centaurium erythraea*

COMMON NAME ■ European centaury

Use the flowering herb to make medicine. This is one of the better bitter tonics. Dr. Bastyr used centaury for jaundice, enlarged liver, and biliousness. He said that it helps to clear blood impurities, and he recommended taking 5 drops of the tincture at mealtimes. He said that this dose is quite adequate.

Centaury contains swertiamarin, which is a glucopyranoside that is antibacterial. In the intestine, swertiamarin is metabolized into gentianine, which is a central nervous system sedative.

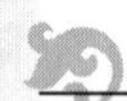

Gentiana lutea

COMMON NAME ■ Gentian

The root is used to make medicine. Dr. Bastyr taught that this remedy is a good mild liver tonic. He said that *Gentiana* is one of the best plants to stimulate hydrochloric acid. Given in doses of 12 drops of tincture, *Gentiana* is an effective digestive stimulant. *Gentiana* contains amarogentin, which is an esterified sweroside. *Gentiana* also contains xanthones such as gentisin and phytosterols.[26]

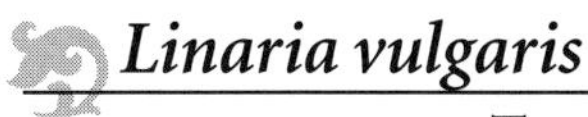

Linaria vulgaris

COMMON NAME ■ Toadflax

The whole plant is used to make medicine. *Linaria* is an excellent jaundice remedy. Historically, the eclectics and herbalists used *Linaria* for intestinal obstructions, lymphatic disorders, and dropsy. The standard tea, or 5 drops of the tincture, can be given two times daily for all of the above conditions. In small doses, this remedy acts as an alterative.

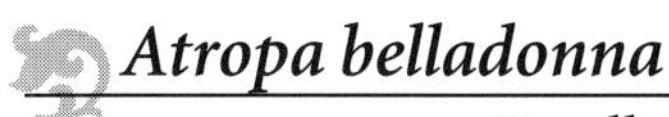

Atropa belladonna

COMMON NAME ■ Deadly nightshade

The leaves and roots are used to make medicine. *CAUTION:* A. belladonna *is a powerful remedy that can be toxic in large doses. It is contraindicated in glaucoma.* I use 15 drops of the tincture to relax the intense spasm of the bile duct for patients who are passing gallstones. This remedy works well. Additional doses of 5 drops may be prescribed every 4 hours until the stone is passed. Decrease the dose at the first sign of dry mouth. Hospitalization may be warranted for patients who have severe pain that does not respond to *A. belladonna.*

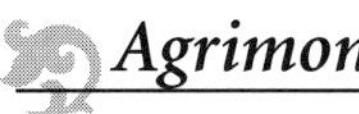

Agrimonia eupatoria

COMMON NAMES ■ Agrimony, Churchsteeples

This plant belongs to the rose family, *Rosaceae.* The flowering aerial parts of the plant are used for medicine. As a lesser liver remedy, it can be used for cholecystopathy. This remedy is a good one to use for the patient who has had a gallbladder episode and is trying to prevent further attacks by making changes in diet and lifestyle. Practitioners such as Jonathan Wright, MD, have suggested that gallbladder disease may be linked to food sensitivities or allergies. In my practice, patients with gallbladder disease often have food incompatibilities. The use of a good digestive aid is well indicated. Agrimony warms the stomach and stimulates hydrochloric acid production. It is a good digestive tonic and is especially indicated in hypochlorhydria associated with gallbladder problems. I suggest a dose of 40 drops of tincture three times daily in a cup of water. In addition, a standard tea may be made of the herb. Agrimony has a peculiar sweet, astringent taste that some patients find pleasant. It may be taken directly after meals. Dr. Bastyr said to use agrimony for at least 2 months.

CHAPTER

52

LIVER STIMULANTS AND GENERAL LIVER REMEDIES

CHAPTER • OUTLINE

Podophyllum peltatum
Leptandra virginica
Iris lacustris
Chionanthus virginicus
Chelidonium majus
Rosmarinus officinalis
Juglans cinerea
Peumus boldo
Cynara scolymus
Raphanus sativus subspecies *niger*
Silybum marianum

Liver stimulants and remedies are plants that improve or increase liver function. They accomplish this by increasing the production of bile, enhancing hepatic enzymatic activity, or increasing blood flow or nerve traffic to the liver. Dr. Bastyr spoke about these remedies as a group under this particular category.

Podophyllum peltatum

COMMON NAME ■ Mayapple

The dried rhizome is used to make medicine. *CAUTION:* Podophyllum *is contraindicated in pregnancy.* The main constituent in this plant is an antimitotic lignan called podophyllotoxin.

Dr. Bastyr used small doses of this plant to treat liver enlargement, congested liver, or mild jaundice. Its specific hepatic use is in constipation with hepatic involvement. He suggested using 5 drops of tincture twice daily. This dose stimulates the production of bile. Larger doses of 20 to 50 drops are purgative. I do not suggest the old use of *Podophyllum* as a purgative because large doses can cause glomerulonephritis. In fact, per the law of opposites, a 6X homeopathic potency of *Podophyllum* has been used to treat glomerulonephritis. In addition to its use as a liver stimulant, the tincture of *Podophyllum* has been used topically on warts. In spite of all this, I use *Podophyllum* frequently as an ingredient in liver tonics. For example, in a 2-ounce bottle of *Chelidonium* and *Chionanthus*, I add 30 drops of *Podophyllum* to the bottle and dose the resulting remedy at 30 drops twice daily.

Leptandra virginica

COMMON NAME ■ Culver's root

Use the rhizome for medicine. *Leptandra* contains tannins and cinnamic acid compounds. This plant is a cholagogue, a cathartic, and an alterative. Dr. Bastyr used *Leptandra* specifically to treat liver-related dull headaches, hepatomegaly, and jaundice. He defined *Leptandra* as a relaxant to the liver. Use doses of 5 to 60 minims of tincture, or 30 grains of powder, twice daily. This plant is a bitter and tastes, in tincture form, almost exactly like the tops of bracken ferns when they are eaten young as the tops are unrolling.

Iris lacustris

COMMON NAME ■ Iris

One may also use *Iris versicolor* or blue flag. The root is used to make medicine. *Iris* contains irone, which is a monocyclic monoterpenoid with a *p*-methane skeleton. This remedy is a cholagogue and a cathartic. I use *Iris* to treat cases of eczema in which the liver is involved in the disease picture. Dr. Bastyr specifically used it to treat liver congestion with lymphatic involvement or swollen lymph nodes. He said that it is a good remedy to use for clay-colored stools, jaundice, or chronic obstruction of the biliary tract. He also noted that this remedy is useful for patients who are experiencing pain around the umbilicus. When using *Iris* as a liver stimulant, I prescribe 10 to 25 drops three times daily. When using it as a cathartic, I suggest 20 grains in a single dose.

Chionanthus virginicus

COMMON NAME ■ Fringe tree

Use the root bark to make medicine. Fringe tree contains lignan glycosides. This plant is a cholagogue, an alterative, and a purgative. It is used for hepatomegaly and jaundice. Dr. Bastyr said that *Chionanthus*, administered over a prolonged period, could be used to help dissolve soft gallstones. It is a good remedy to use in a comprehensive program to help dissolve gallstones. Patients will need to be encouraged to follow a carefully monitored nutritional program. Catastrophic eating can yield catastrophic results. There is little room for irresponsible eating when trying to treat gallstones naturopathically.

I have used *Chionanthus* with other liver remedies to treat hepatitis and cirrhosis of the liver. It is also an excellent spleen remedy. Eclectics and naturopaths have used the tincture in doses of 15 to 20 drops three times daily. It can also be used for incipient nephritis and for painful eyeballs. *Chionanthus* and *Chelidonium* are two of the best and most widely used liver tonics in the naturopathic *Materia Medica.*

Chelidonium majus

COMMON NAMES ■ Tetterwort, Celandine, Greater celandine

The whole plant is used to make medicine. *Chelidonium* is a cholagogue and a liver stimulant. The tincture improves circulation to the liver. Dr. Bastyr described it as a medicine that treats the functional deficiencies of the abdominal glandular organs. Eclectics have used *Chelidonium* to treat clay-colored stools, acid urine, and general ascites. Dr. Bastyr used *Chelidonium* to treat biliary calculi and to aid in the digestion of fats. I suggest a dose of 30 drops three times daily. *Chelidonium* mixes well with *Chionanthus* and *Taraxacum* as a good liver stimulant. I have used it to treat hepatitis C. I use 30 drops of tincture twice daily with promising results. Patients with hepatitis should add the tincture to boiling hot water to evaporate some of the alcohol. It might be useful to try to find *Chelidonium* in capsule form for this purpose.

Rosmarinus officinalis

COMMON NAME ■ Rosemary

The leaves are used to make medicine. This medicine increases liver function and stimulates digestion. I use doses of 10 to 20 drops of tincture twice daily. Dr. Bastyr said that the oil of rosemary could be used in doses of 2 drops to cure general tension headaches or liver colic–related headaches.

Rosemary contains rosmarinic acid, which is an antioxidant.[149,150] Other antioxidants in rosemary include the diterpenoid *o*-diphenols. Diterpenoids are 20-carbon compounds derived from four isoprinoid residues.[97] Rosmarinic acid is an aromatic compound, which in part gives rosemary its odor. Rosmarinic acid potently inhibits the 5-lipoxygenase products 5-hydroxyeicosatetraenoic acid and leukotriene B-4.[151] Rosemary oil also contains camphor, alpha-pinene, and cineole.

Juglans cinerea

COMMON NAMES ■ Butternut, White walnut

The bark is used to make medicine. *Juglans* contains a naphthaquinone, juglone. It also contains tannins.

Juglans is a liver stimulant, an alterative, and a cholagogue. Dr. Bastyr said that it increases the secretion of bile. The dose is 1 to 20 drops twice daily. Large doses of this medicine cause catharsis. It is a good remedy to think of for bile-laden diarrhea. A fresh infusion of the bark is best; however, the tincture may be used as well. The eclectic physicians suggested its use in medium doses to treat clay-colored stools.

Peumus boldo

COMMON NAME ■ Boldo

The leaves are used to make medicine. *Boldo* is a liver stimulant, a sedative, a diuretic, and a mild urinary demulcent and antiseptic. I have found boldo extremely useful in treating liver and gallbladder problems. It is one of my favorite liver remedies. It serves us well in the area of toxic or sluggish liver. It has specific use for cholelithiasis with pain. It is not a bad remedy for fast food eaters, especially if they eat their fast food fast. The dose I recommend as a liver stimulant is 30 to 60 drops of tincture twice daily. Because boldo tastes good, I often have patients take a squirt of tincture directly in their mouths or added to a swallow of water after meals to stimulate a sluggish liver.

Cynara scolymus

COMMON NAME ■ Globe artichoke

The dried or fresh basal leaves are used to make medicine. This plant belongs to the daisy family. Globe artichoke contains cynarin, which is an active principle capable of stimulating choleresis.

Cynara is a good hepatic antioxidant. Use *Cynara* together with equal parts of milkthistle to help regenerate a depleted, deteriorated, and diseased liver. I use *Cynara* specifically for Gilbert's syndrome. This is also a good remedy for sluggish gallbladder, gallbladder colic, and the nausea and pain associated with gallbladder disease. I use 60 drops of *Cynara* twice daily for all of these conditions. More may be used for extreme acute pain. When using the capsules of *Cynara*, give 2 capsules, or about 500 mg, twice daily. This is a safe and effective remedy.

Raphanus sativus subspecies *niger*

COMMON NAME ■ Black radish

The root is used to make medicine. Black radish is a liver detoxifying agent. When I was a student clinician at the National College of Naturopathic Medicine in 1974, we used black radish capsules. Dr. Robert Overton, ND, a teacher of mine who taught naturopathic manipulation, was fond of this remedy. To detoxify the liver, he would start with 1 black radish capsule daily for 3 days, then increase to 2 daily for 3 days, and so on up to 4 or 5 capsules daily. The total program lasts about 15 days. The patients always had a detoxifying reaction, thus ample water consumption was encouraged.

Silybum marianum

COMMON NAME ■ Milkthistle

The seeds are used to make medicine. Milkthistle is a general liver medicine. It works by quenching singlet oxygen and other inflammatory molecules produced when the liver detoxifies substrates. It also helps the liver regrow and replenish new cells. One of the main active components of milkthistle is silybin. The other two main isomers are silydianin and silychristin. These constituents are categorized as flavanolignans, which the plant produces by combining a flavonoid and coniferyl alcohol. Note that silymarin is a term denoting three flavonoids: silybin, silydianin, and silychristin.

I use a lot of milkthistle in my practice. The usual dose for hepatoprotection, especially for protection against damage wrought by the liver's frantic effort to detoxify chemotherapy and other chemical medicines, is 450 mg of standardized milkthistle extract three times daily. It is standardized to 80% silymarin content. Any skin disease that has its root cause in a toxic liver condition may be helped by administration of milkthistle, particularly eczema and psoriatic eczema.[152]

Another bit of good news is that milkthistle increases glutathione content in the liver in healthy people by 35%. Studies have shown that it increases the level of glutathione in rats by more than 50%![153] Glutathione is used to detoxify chemicals, hormones, drugs, and deviant fats.

Liver function can also be improved by drinking more water, about 1 cup every hour and a half, and getting adequate exercise. Exercise improves the circulation of blood through the liver, which helps to flush the tissue.

CHAPTER

53

Male Reproductive System Agents

Chapter • Outline

Chamaelirium luteum
Mitchella repens
Anemone pulsatilla
Citrullus colocynthis
Gaultheria procumbens
Equisetum arvense
Zinc
Phytolacca decandra
Berberis aquifolium
Essential fatty acids
Sabal serrulata
Turnera aphrodisiaca
Corynanthe johimbe
Pygeum africanum
Colchicum autumnale

Male reproductive remedies are used to treat a variety of problems specific to the male reproductive system. This includes problems in both the genital and urinary systems of men. These problems include orchitis, prostatitis, epididymitis, cystitis, and urethritis.

Chamaelirium luteum

COMMON NAME ■ False unicorn root

The old dispensaries may have this plant listed as *Helonius opulus.* The root is used to make medicine. *Chamaelirium* is used to treat the enlarged prostate gland. Dr. Bastyr told us that the man would feel like he was sitting on a ball and must constantly move around on the seat. The tincture dose given by eclectics and herbalists is 10 to 60 drops twice daily. For the treatment of prostatitis and epididymitis, I have found that *Chamaelirium* mixes well with equal parts of pasque flower and saw palmetto. The dose of this tonic mixture is 60 drops twice daily continued for at least 2 weeks. Because this plant has estrogen precursors, I have frequently used it in female reproductive tonification formulas as well.

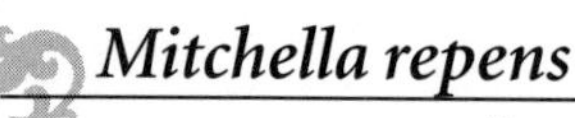

Mitchella repens

COMMON NAMES ■ Squaw vine, Partridgeberry

Use the whole plant to make medicine. *Mitchella* has been used to treat disorders of the female reproductive tract; however, it is effective in treating prostate enlargement as well. I give 30 to 60 drops of tincture twice daily for prostatic enlargement. I also mix *Hydrastis* with *Mitchella* for this purpose. The dose is 90 drops of the tincture combination four times daily. *Hydrastis* is excellent for infections of the prostate such as nongonococcal urethritis. *Mitchella* is used to treat dysuria and is a specific remedy for decreased flow of urine in men. I recommend a dose of 60 drops of *Mitchella* twice daily for this purpose.

Anemone pulsatilla

COMMON NAMES ■ Wind flower, Pasque flower

The whole plant is used to make medicine. *A. pulsatilla* is a premier remedy to treat orchitis and epididymitis. Dr. Bastyr used it especially for epididymitis. In my practice, I have seen several dozen cases of epididymitis respond to *A. pulsatilla.* For men with epididymitis, I prescribe 30 drops of tincture three times daily. In addition, I use *A. pulsatilla* for the treatment of prostate problems, specifically when the prostate is painfully enlarged. I mix equal parts of *A. pulsatilla*, goldenseal, and parsley for this purpose. The tincture is then given in doses of 90 drops three times daily.

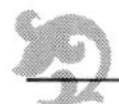

Citrullus colocynthis

COMMON NAME ■ Bitter apple

Medicine is made from the dried pulp. Dr. Bastyr used either a 3X or 6X potency of *C. colocynthis* twice daily to treat orchialgia. According to the eclectics, the tincture of *C. colocynthis* is a potent hydragogue cathartic. In my practice, I have opted not to use this remedy in toxic doses for the purpose of producing catharsis.

Gaultheria procumbens

COMMON NAME ■ Wintergreen

The leaves are used to make medicine. *Gaultheria* is useful in spermatorrhea and priapism caused by prostate enlargement. *Gaultheria* is a febrifuge and tends to decrease inflammation. Herbalists use a standard tea made from the leaves or tea bags at a dose of 1 cup three times daily.

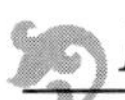

Equisetum arvense

COMMON NAME ■ Horsetail

Use the whole plant to make medicine. Dr. Bastyr used this remedy to treat urethritis and inflammation of the spermatic cord. His dose was 40 drops of the tincture in 1 cup of water six times daily. This remedy is also a diuretic.

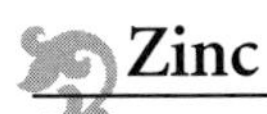

Zinc

This mineral is useful in treating benign prostatitis. The dose is 100 mg per day for a month; then taper back to a 50 mg per day maintenance level. Zinc seems to balance reductase enzyme function in the prostate. It is a key player in DNA-dependent mRNA polymerase enzymes in the body. This enzyme has a lot to do with protein synthesis and management, especially as it concerns the proteinaceous aspects of the immune system. Taking zinc almost always improves immune function.

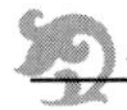

Phytolacca decandra

COMMON NAME ■ Pokeweed

One may also use *Phytolacca americana*. The root is used to make medicine. Dr. Bastyr suggested the use of this remedy to treat lymphogranuloma venereum. He recommended 10 drops of *Phytolacca* tincture four times daily. For treatment of lymphogranuloma venereum, in addition to *Phytolacca*, use vitamin C at a dose of 1 to 3 grams per hour for a day or two, then back down on the dose. In addition, I use *Phytolacca* for fibrosing proctitis, together with up to 2000 IU of vitamin E per day.

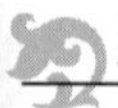

Berberis aquifolium

COMMON NAME ■ Oregon grape

The root is used to make medicine. This remedy has some use in Peyronie's disease, as has *Colchicum* and vitamin E. The dose I recall Dr. Bastyr suggesting is 30 drops three times daily. I mix *Berberis* and *Gentiana* together to aid digestion. I prescribe 30 drops of this mixture at mealtimes. Improving digestion helps to detoxify the body and improve the health of the prostate gland. Patients report an improvement in formation and passage of stools when taking Oregon grape.

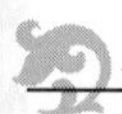

Essential fatty acids

Essential fatty acids are important for health in general, but they certainly seem to be indicated for treatment of prostatitis. Evening primrose oil was recommended by Dr. Bastyr in the 1970s. Safflower and sunflower oil have been used for their linoleic acid content. For treating benign prostatitis, some of the older literature suggested using 2 tablespoons of safflower or sunflower oil daily. More modern thinking has called for the use of at least some omega-3 oil, such as flaxseed, in a dose of 2 teaspoons daily. I give my patients 1 tablespoon per day for 1 week, then maintain them on 1 teaspoon per day. I also include 50 mg per day of zinc in this protocol. I use *Pygeum* and saw palmetto as well.

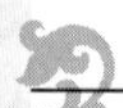

Sabal serrulata

COMMON NAME ■ Saw palmetto

The fruits and seeds are used to make medicine. Saw palmetto contains fatty acids, including lauric acid. It also contains vitamin E and other aliphatic alcohols, several alkanes, and the sterols sitosterol and campesterol.

This tremendous male reproductive herb can be used as a tonic to the male hormone level and to prevent the binding of 25-dihydrotestosterone to the receptor sites in the prostate. This prevents prostate hyperplasia and potentially helps to prevent prostate cancers. For weakened sexual power, I prescribe saw palmetto combined with *Avena sativa*, yohimbe, and damiana in doses of 60 drops of tincture three times daily. The proportions of this tincture mixture are two parts saw palmetto, three parts *Avena sativa*, one part yohimbe, and two parts damiana.

The dose of saw palmetto for the prevention of prostate problems is 60 drops of tincture twice daily. More may be used at the discretion of the physician.

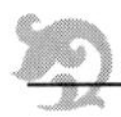

Turnera aphrodisiaca

COMMON NAME ■ Damiana

Also look for this plant under the name *Turnera diffusa*. The leaves are used to make medicine. Damiana is basically a good nerve tonic and an antidepressant. Historically, it has been used in folk medicine to help tonify and strengthen the male reproductive system. Given this, one would suspect a tonic effect on the production of progesterone. Testosterone, like progesterone, is a 3-ketosteroid. I would speculate that perhaps both hormones are increased when using damiana. I suggest using doses of 30 drops two to three times daily. In addition to damiana's effects on the male reproductive system, it also helps with insufficient menstruation.

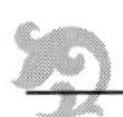

Corynanthe johimbe

COMMON NAME ■ Yohimbe

This plant is an alpha-2 receptor site blocker. As such, it tends to increase norepinephrine, which is then available to activate the medial preoptic center in the midbrain, which increases libido. It has been written about extensively in scientific literature for its use in attaining and especially maintaining erection. The dose I recommend is 10 mg of yohimbine, the active ingredient, about 15 minutes before sexual activity. *C. johimbe* combined with *Pimpinella* is also excellent for increasing libido. Mix three parts of *Pimpinella* tincture with one part of *C. johimbe*. The dose to increase libido is 15 drops twice daily.

Curiously, and importantly, the alpha-2 site is represented on the fat cell. By blocking this site with yohimbine, the fat cell is encouraged to burn rather than store fat. This may aid in weight loss, especially of fat gathered on the thighs and buttocks, where alpha-2 sites predominate.[154]

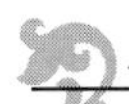

Pygeum africanum

COMMON NAME ■ Pygeum

The bark is used to make medicine. *Pygeum*, which is native to Africa, is a tall evergreen tree reaching heights of up to 150 feet. This plant is useful in treating benign prostatitis. The trials on *Pygeum* have used standardized extract of the plant. Both beta-sitosterol and n-docosanol are constituents of the standardized extract and are two of the active compounds. It has been shown that one of the active constituents, n-docosanol, reduces serum prolactin levels, which is interesting in that elevation of prolactin increases the uptake of testosterone and the levels of dihydrotestosterone. Therapeutically, we want to decrease the latter, since the elevation and accumulation of both testosterone and dihydrotestosterone are thought to be involved in the enlargement of the prostate. In my experience, saw palmetto tends to work better than *Pygeum* both in preventing prostate hypertrophy and in reestablishing better urine flow.

I use *Pygeum*, damiana, and saw palmetto in combination. Equal parts of the tinctures can be given in doses of 60 drops twice daily. This combination works well for benign prostatitis.

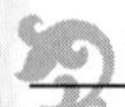

Colchicum autumnale

COMMON NAME ■ Meadow saffron, Autumn crocus

The fresh flowers and dried ripe seeds are used to make medicine. I have included this plant in this section because of its potential use in treating Peyronie's disease. My friend and colleague Dr. Davis Lamson discussed the use of *C. autumnale* to treat Peyronie's disease in one of his lectures at the AANP conference.[78] I recommend 7 drops of the tincture twice daily.

CHAPTER

54

NERVINES

CHAPTER • OUTLINE

Nervines are agents that have a calming, soothing, or strengthening effect on the nervous system. These medicines may also reinforce or nourish the nervous system. Dr. Bastyr did not talk about nervines as much as he did sedatives and stimulants.

I have included a section on nervines for those readers and clinicians who might be more familiar with that term. Herbalists are especially familiar with the term. The remedies I have chosen have a gentle, beneficial effect on the nervous system. For a wider list of sedative remedies, see Chapters 63 through 65; for further information about stimulants, see Chapters 68 and 69; and for additional calmative remedies, see Chapter 20.

Melissa officinalis

COMMON NAMES ■ Balm, Lemon balm

Balm is in the mint family, *Labiatae*. The dried aerial parts are used to make medicine. The volatile oils in *Melissa* act on the midbrain, or limbic system. *Melissa* is useful in treating the autonomic nervous system and can be regarded as a gentle herbal tranquilizer. I prescribe 60 drops of the tincture twice daily in a cup of hot water sweetened with a teaspoon of the amino acid glycine. *Melissa* is a spasmolytic and an antiviral as well.

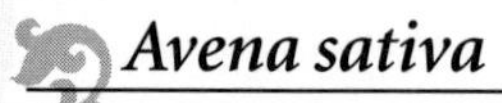

Avena sativa

COMMON NAME ■ Green oat

The whole, young aerial part of the plant is used to make medicine. Green oat seems to be a true nervine. It is nutritive and relaxing to the mind. Dr. Bastyr used *Avena* to treat drug addiction. He advised patients to take 60 drops of the tincture up to six times daily. He even used it for treating heroin addiction. For what it is worth, Dr. Boucher, ND, from Canada suggests 200 mg of vitamin B_1 twice daily for the same thing. I remember both of them specifically talking about heroin addiction; however, I have used both therapies for all types of drug addictions.

CHAPTER

55

NUTRITIVE BOTANICALS

CHAPTER • OUTLINE

Viola papilionacea
Glechoma hederacea
Nepeta cataria
Borago officinalis
Hordeum distichon
Polygonatum multiflorum
Cyperus esculentus
Caltha palustris
Medeola virginiana
Epilobium latifolium
Fritillaria lanceolata
Erythronium grandiflorum
Triticum vulgare
Rosa rugosa

Some of the success in using plant medicines traditionally and in various folk traditions may be attributed to the nutritive value now being discovered in these herbs. Certainly, this is not a complete list, nor could it ever be because the actual list is vast, and frankly, many plants have at least some contributory nutritive value. The following are some of the plants that I have used and found interesting. Dr. Bastyr did not teach about nutritive botanicals as a separate group; however, he did mention the importance of the vitamin and mineral contents of some plants.

Viola papilionacea

COMMON NAME ■ Blue violet

The leaves and blossoms are used to make medicine. The leaves contain 210 mg of vitamin C per 100 g of leaf material. The pro-vitamin A content is 8300 IU per 100 g. The dried plant contains salicylic acid methyl ester. The volatile oils contain zingiberene, curcumene, and isoborneol. Tea may be made from the leaves, and the blossoms can be used in salads.

Glechoma hederacea

COMMON NAME ■ Ground ivy

The whole plant is used to make medicine. The leaves are especially medicinal. *Glechoma* contains several volatile oils, including pulegone and pinocarvone. It also contains the sesquiterpenes glechomafuran, glechomanolide,[25] caffeic acid, and rosmaric acid.

This plant is a bitter tonic and an antiscorbutic. The leaves are a source of vitamin C. An herbalist, whose name I cannot recall, once told me that an infusion of the leaves is helpful for people who are experiencing ringing in the ears.

Nepeta cataria

COMMON NAME ■ Catnip

Catnip is a member of the mint family, *Labiatae.* Use the flowering dried aerial parts of the plant to make medicine. This plant is high in vitamin C. Catnip contains volatile oils, principally nepetalactone.

Catnip is a mild stimulant to appetite and menstrual flow. Herbalists suggest using the dried leaves in an infusion rather than a decoction. Catnip helps to decrease fever and is also widely used for its carminative properties. Dr. Bastyr said that catnip was used for the treatment of scarlet fever and smallpox. I have a reference in my notes from Dr. Bastyr's lectures about mixing catnip with saffron; unfortunately, I don't recall any specifics.

Max Barlow, a botanist from Idaho who wrote *From the Shepherd's Purse,* discusses folklore reports that chewing the root will produce personality changes.[36] The person will change from a docile, meek individual to fierce and courageous. He also mentions combining catnip and saffron in a standard infusion to treat scarlet fever and smallpox. Given that you will probably never see a case of smallpox this is a moot point, but certainly streptococcal infections will be seen frequently. Saffron contains a water-soluble carotenoid that may help to prevent scarring of the skin from the infection.

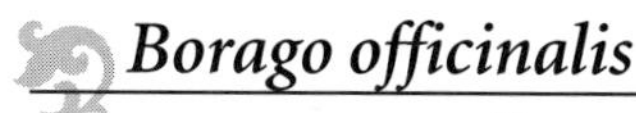

Borago officinalis

COMMON NAME ■ Borage

The seeds and leaves are used to make medicine. This plant is high in minerals and healthy oils. Borage also contains pyrrolizidine alkaloids, including supinine, lycopsamine, and intermedine.[155] It is a good salad herb. I find that having patients use nontraditional wild greens mixed in their salads is both healthy and empowering. Borage is a mild laxative and a galactagogue. Herbalists have found that borage is useful for treating ringworm, insect bites, and stings when applied topically as a poultice. I have found that borage is a great adrenal builder, especially when mixed with licorice and rose hips. This can be used to increase the adrenal strength or to assist in adrenal recovery after adrenal exhaustion. The formula for this purpose is equal parts of the botanical extracts of borage, licorice, and rose hips. The dose I recommend is 60 drops of the mixture twice daily.

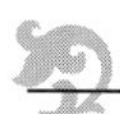

Hordeum distichon

COMMON NAME ■ Barley

The grain is used to make medicine. Dr. Bastyr mentioned the use of barley water for dysentery in his lectures. It is rich in B vitamins and iron.

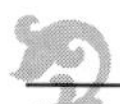

Polygonatum multiflorum

COMMON NAME ■ Solomon's seal

Use the dried rhizomes and roots to make medicine. Traditional Chinese doctors use Solomon's seal to keep their patients physically young. It stimulates sexual potency. Some of its contents are nitrogen, minerals, unsaturated fat, and lecithin. Solomon's seal also contains steroid saponins and mucilages. This plant is a good tonic to the central nervous system. It contains oxymethylanthraquinone, which apparently is a preventive agent for cholesterol deposition in the liver.

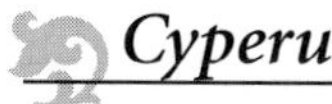

Cyperus esculentus

COMMON NAMES ■ Chufa, Nut grass

The edible tuber is used as medicine. The dried, ground tuber may be used as a coffee substitute. *Cyperus* is high in protein and carbohydrates. It can be cooked and eaten like a vegetable.

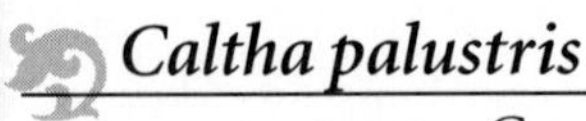

Caltha palustris

COMMON NAME ■ Cowslip

The leaves are used to make medicine. This is a good pot herb. *Caltha* is high in vitamins C and A. Boil the leaves and drain the water, since the leaves are acrid and bitter. Curiously, the aroma of this plant has a sedative effect. According to Dr. Withering,[100] an English physician practicing during the 19th century, cowslip was put in bunches in the room of epileptics and was reported to decrease seizure activity.

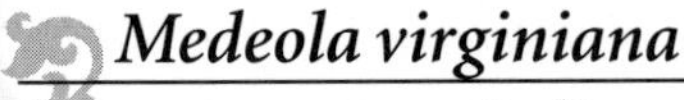

Medeola virginiana

COMMON NAME ■ Indian cucumber root

The young leaves are nutritive and pleasant to add to salads.

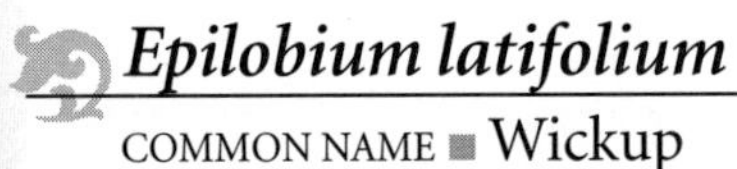

Epilobium latifolium

COMMON NAME ■ Wickup

Most of the species in the *Epilobium* genus contain steroid compounds—in this case, beta-sitosterol. Wickup also contains an abundance of flavonoid compounds, including quercitrin, myricitrin, and isoquercitrin. The Bellacoola Indians ate the inner stems. The leaves and top shoots are used as medicine for the digestive apparatus. This plant is a gastrointestinal astringent that is very safe and effective. Dr. Bastyr suggested $\frac{1}{4}$ cup of the standard tea four times daily. Dr. Joe Boucher of British Columbia introduced me to this plant.

Fritillaria lanceolata

COMMON NAME ■ Chocolate rice root

The root bulbs are used to make medicine. The Indians of the Pacific Northwest steamed or boiled the bulbs. They are tender and delicate, resembling rice except for a slight bitter taste. *Fritillaria* contains carbohydrates.

Erythronium grandiflorum

COMMON NAME ■ Yellow avalanche lily

The Indians of British Columbia used the corms as food. They contain both carbohydrates and protein. The whole plant may be macerated or pulverized with water and applied to scrofula and other skin problems.

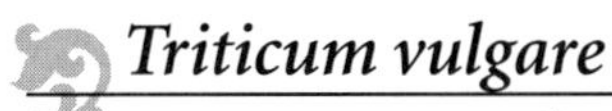

Triticum vulgare

COMMON NAME ■ Wheat grass

One may also use *T. aestivum*. A juice is made from the young shoots of the wheat plant. It is an excellent nutritive botanical that is high in carotenes and minerals. When using it as a general tonic, I recommend one shot of wheat grass juice daily.

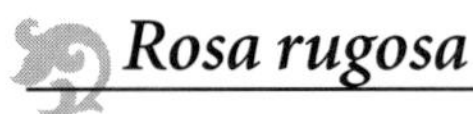

Rosa rugosa

COMMON NAME ■ Rose hips

The hip, the edible fleshy floral receptacle, contains the vitamin C. The average hip contains between 200 and 400 mg of vitamin C, which is substantial. The many species of the *Rosa* genus contain vitamin C. This plant can be used to treat scurvy, connective tissue weakness, and acute upper respiratory problems. Several hips may be consumed daily.

• • •

The list of nutritive botanicals could and should go on and on. With the discovery of nutrients that have implications in human health, the study of the plant and food medicines has become increasingly fascinating. Perhaps Thomas Jefferson's idea that one day food would be our medicine will soon be realized. The sulforaphanes in broccoli, the antiviral compounds in garlic, and the anthocyanins in berries, which are now thought to be cardioprotective, the flavones in russet potato skins are just a few of the many examples of the plant and food medicinals that are currently available. It is very satisfying to break off the end of a small branch of a pine tree, steep it in hot water for an hour, and know that you are drinking a tea rich in vitamin C and bioflavonoids. It is equally satisfying to put flowers and greens that contain sight-saving xanthophylls in your salad. The study of food-medicines is worth our attention for the affordable future health of people everywhere.

CHAPTER

56

Ovarian Neuralgia Remedies

CHAPTER • OUTLINE

These remedies are used to treat pain in the ovaries and surrounding tissue. They have been used to treat painful ovulation and the pain of ovarian cysts. Many of the remedies in this category are also used to treat dysmenorrhea.

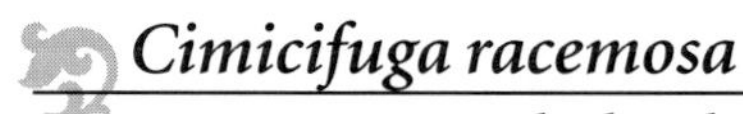

Cimicifuga racemosa

COMMON NAME ■ Black cohosh

The roots are used to make medicine. *Cimicifuga* is a nervine, an antispasmodic, and an emmenagogue. Dr. Bastyr said that this is one of the better remedies for relieving pain in the ovaries. It contains salicylic acid and is therefore useful for muscle pain and intercostal myalgia. It is possible that the salicylates in *Cimicifuga* block the formation of uterine cramping prostaglandins. I use 30 drops of tincture twice daily in these cases.

Cimicifuga affects the reproductive organs through its action on the pituitary gland. Rather than taking my word for this, get a tincture of *Cimicifuga* right now. Take 10 drops in the mouth and quietly sit and feel where this plant is going. There you have it. It can be felt in the emotional body as well as in the midbrain and in the pituitary. The 6th chakra and the 2nd chakra are connected in the Hindu outlook of the balance of life as expressed by the seven chakras or energy centers. Indeed, the pituitary in the 6th chakra is linked to the reproductive apparatus in the 2nd chakra. The great Hindu masters and yogis knew the connection between the various areas of the body long before any "hormone" had been discovered.

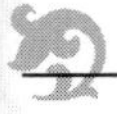

Viscum flavescens

COMMON NAME ■ Mistletoe

The leaves are used to make medicine. *Viscum* is used for postpartum hemorrhage, hypertension, anxiety, and headache where there is hyperemia. Dr. Bastyr recommended a dose of 20 drops of tincture three times daily for ovarian neuralgia. Eclectic physicians have used *Viscum* for amenorrhea, dysmenorrhea, nervous tachycardia, and rheumatic pains. For these conditions, use 30 drops of tincture twice daily.

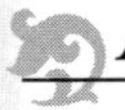

Anthemis nobilis

COMMON NAME ■ Roman chamomile

The flower heads are used to make medicine. A cup of chamomile tea may be taken several times daily for ovarian neuralgia. Chamomile is not only a relaxing tea, it also kills bacteria. Dr. Bastyr emphasized that chamomile is excellent for teething pains in children. He used a 3X potency of chamomile repeated four or five times daily. I have seen this work time and time again. Dr. Bastyr taught us that chamomile is specific for babies who are uncomfortable and stretch out and arch their backs. Again he used a 3X homeopathic preparation. *Anthemis* helps with dyspepsia associated with mental stress.

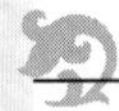

Lilium tigrinum

COMMON NAME ■ Tiger lily

The flowers and leaves are used to make medicine. The naturopaths that I know primarily use *Lilium* in homeopathic potency. It is for neuralgic pains in the breasts, uterus, and ovaries. Dr. Bastyr used *Lilium* for burning pains in the ovaries. For tedious recovery after childbirth, he used a 6X potency of *Lilium tigrinum.*

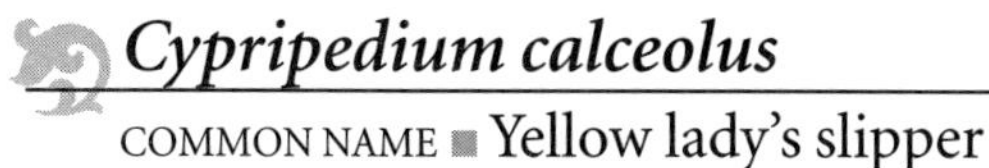

Cypripedium calceolus

COMMON NAME ■ Yellow lady's slipper

Look for this also under the names *Cypripedium pubescens* and *Cypripedium luteum.* Lady's slipper is in the orchid family, *Orchidaceae.* The root is used to make medicine. *Cypripedium* is a uterine tonic. Eclectics, herbalists, and naturopaths have used it to relieve ovarian neuralgia, mental depression, and insomnia. The tincture is taken at a dose of 40 drops twice daily. This plant is now an endangered species, and it should not be used at this time.

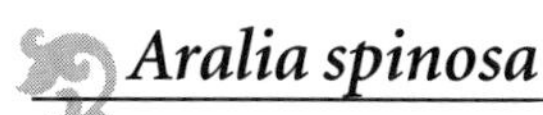

Aralia spinosa

COMMON NAME ■ Dwarf elder

The root is used to make medicine. *Aralia* is used for pain in the uterus and pelvic area, including the ovaries. Dr. Bastyr used *Aralia* for the bearing-down pain caused by uterine prolapse and for the pains sometimes associated with suppression of menses. Eclectics and herbalists tell us that it may help with dysmenorrhea and works as an expectorant in chronic pulmonary complaints. The dose of the tincture is 5 to 20 drops twice daily. The powder is used in doses of 5 to 30 grains twice daily. It has been used as a douche in offensive leukorrhea.

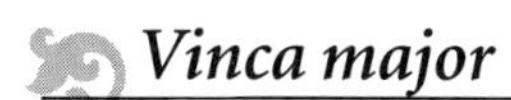

Vinca major

COMMON NAME ■ Greater periwinkle

The dried aerial parts are used to make medicine. For ovarian neuralgia, use 20 drops of the tincture twice daily. *Vinca* can be used to treat menorrhagia; as an antihemorrhagic, use 1 to 3 milliliters. Dr. Bastyr said that *Vinca* could be used as a low bowel retention enema in ulcerative proctitis. For this purpose, he suggested making a strong decoction or infusion.

Piscidia erythrina

COMMON NAME ■ Jamaican dogwood

The bark is used to make medicine. Large doses of *Piscidia* are given for ovarian neuralgia. I have seen this work consistently both in ovarian pain and in uterine cramping pain during menses. Initially, I give two 500-mg capsules. After an hour, if the pain persists, a second dose of two capsules is given.

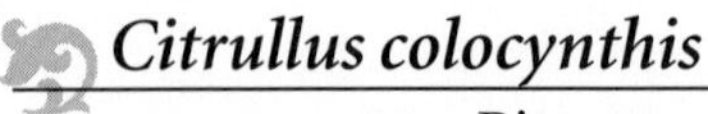

Citrullus colocynthis

COMMON NAME ■ Bitter apple

The dried pulp is used to make medicine. *CAUTION: This plant is a potent hydragogue cathartic, and therefore the homeopathic potency is the only dose that should be given. Even $1\frac{1}{2}$ teaspoons of the powder will cause death by severe gastroenteritis. C. colocynthis* contains cucurbitacins, which are tetracyclic triterpenes, and a caffeic acid derivative called chlorogenic acid.

Dr. Bastyr used *C. colocynthis* to treat ovarian cysts and ovarian neuralgia. He taught us to use a 6X potency of *C. colocynthis* three times daily. A 30X potency is often useful in abdominal pain. He taught us to use *C. colocynthis* in a 6X or higher homeopathic potency to treat a baby or young child who bends forward in a ball or fetal position. He said to use *C. chamomila* 6X potency if the baby arches the back in discomfort.

CHAPTER

57

OXYTOCICS

CHAPTER • OUTLINE

Oxytocin
Ustilago maydis
Claviceps purpurea
Erigeron canadensis
Paeonia officinalis
Gossypium herbaceum
Aristolochia clematitis

Oxytocics are agents that promote rapid labor by promoting contractions of the myometrium.

Oxytocin

Oxytocin is a hormone used to induce labor. Dr. Bastyr discussed this remedy as an emergency medicine for the induction of labor; 10 units are given by intravenous infusion. Oxytocin is formed by the neuronal cells of the hypothalamic nuclei and stored in the posterior lobe of the hypophysis. Oxytocin stimulates contraction of the uterine musculature and is used to induce active labor or to cause contraction of the uterus after delivery of the placenta. To control postpartum hemorrhage, give 3 to 10 units intramuscularly.

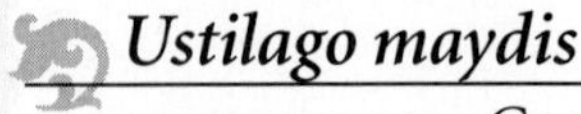

Ustilago maydis

COMMON NAME ■ Corn smut

The medicine is obtained from the parasitic fungus *Ustilago* species, which grows on the stems and flowers of *Zea mays.* It is an oxytocic and a cerebrospinal stimulant. Dr. Bastyr used this remedy for involution following delivery and for postpartum hemorrhage. He recommended 5 to 25 drops of tincture twice daily. In addition, he said that *Ustilago* can be used for atony of pelvic structures and is gentler than ergot.

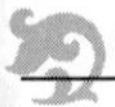

Claviceps purpurea

COMMON NAME ■ Rye ergot

The ergot is obtained from *Secale cornutum. Claviceps* contains a large number of alkaloids of the lysergic acid amide and ergopeptine types. One of the more important alkaloids is ergotamine.

Claviceps is an oxytocic and a hemostatic. It promotes rapid parturition by stimulating contractions of the myometrium. The tincture dose as an oxytocic is 30 drops. *Claviceps* acts on the smooth muscles and sympathetic nerves of the uterus, bladder, blood vessels, heart, and iris. It increases contractile force of the heart, which can cause a slight increase in blood pressure. Dr. Bastyr used *Claviceps* homeopathically for Raynaud's syndrome.

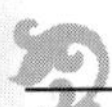

Erigeron canadensis

COMMON NAME ■ Canadian fleabane

Use the whole plant to make medicine. The oil contains limonene, myricene, and a number of other volatile oils. The oil of *Erigeron* is a mild oxytocic. The dose for this purpose is 20 drops.

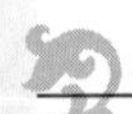

Paeonia officinalis

COMMON NAME ■ Peony

The root is used to make medicine. Besides being a very mild oxytocic, peony is also used for hemorrhoids and other diseases of the rectum. It possesses antispasmodic, diuretic, and sedative qualities and has been used by herbalists to treat bedsores, gout, asthma, and cramps. The dose for each of these conditions is 15 drops of peony tincture four times daily.

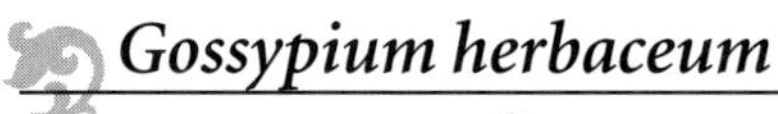

Gossypium herbaceum

COMMON NAME ■ Cotton

The medicine is made from the bark of the root. Dr. Bastyr used this herb to empty the uterus after birth. It is a hemostatic and helps to control hemorrhage in fibroids. Dr. Bastyr commented that *Gossypium* is in a class with *Trillium* as one of the better remedies available for hemorrhage in fibroids. It is an emmenagogue. The tincture is used in very low doses of 1 to 2 drops because it is quite potent. Dr. Bastyr suggested a 2X or 3X homeopathic potency of *Gossypium.*

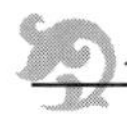

Aristolochia clematitis

COMMON NAME ■ Birthwort

The root and flowering herb are used to make medicine. *Aristolochia* contains aristolochic acid and the isoquinoline alkaloid, corytuberin. *Aristolochia* is a diaphoretic, an emmenagogue, a febrifuge, a stimulant, and an oxytocic. It promotes uterine contractions. For these conditions, herbalists suggest making a standard tea and sipping it as needed up to 2 cups per day. Incidentally, a decoction may be applied externally to wounds and ulcers.

CHAPTER

58

PARASYMPATHETIC DEPRESSANTS

CHAPTER • OUTLINE

Atropa belladonna
Datura fastuosa var. *alba*
Datura metel
Hyoscyamus niger
Duboisia myoporoides

Parasympathetic depressants quiet the activity of the parasympathetic nervous system.

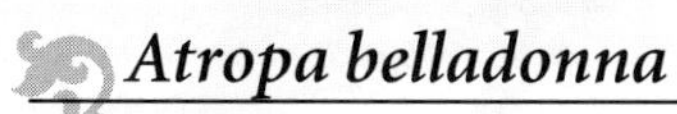

Atropa belladonna

COMMON NAME ■ Deadly nightshade

The roots and leaves are used to make medicine. *CAUTION: A.* belladonna *is a powerful remedy that can be toxic in large doses. A. belladonna* is probably the most famous and widely used parasympathetic depressant in the naturopathic *Materia Medica.* It is used for a temporary anticholinergic effect. *A. belladonna* is used to treat hyperactive bowel situations like spastic colitis. It depresses both peristalsis and secretions of the gastrointestinal tract. I use 10 drops of *A. belladonna* tincture twice daily as a parasympathetic depressant.

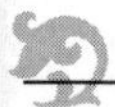

Datura fastuosa var. *alba*

COMMON NAMES ■ Devil's apple, Jimsonweed

Use the leaves and seeds to make medicine. *CAUTION: This plant is a strong hallucinogen.* The scopolamine content of this plant is anticholinergic. Both atropine and scopolamine compete with acetylcholine at the postganglionic synapse of the parasympathetic nervous system. The postganglionic synapse is what is called the muscarinic site.

As a parasympathetic depressant, the dose of scopolamine hydrobromide is 320 μg to 1.1 mg either orally or parenterally. *Datura* is not currently used by naturopathic physicians that I am aware of, nor did Dr. Bastyr use this remedy.

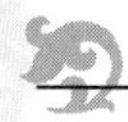

Datura metel

COMMON NAMES ■ Horn of plenty, Downy thorn apple

Datura metel is used in the same way as *Datura fastuosa.* See the preceding discussion; the same rules apply.

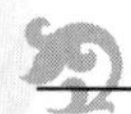

Hyoscyamus niger

COMMON NAME ■ Henbane

Hyoscyamus muticus, or Egyptian henbane, may also be used. Use the whole plant to make medicine. This plant contains scopolamine and hyoscyamine, both of which are anticholinergic. As a parasympathetic depressant, the dose of hyoscyamine hydrobromide is 250 μg to 1 mg. To calm the intestine, Dr. Bastyr used 15 drops of tincture two to three times daily; however, more may be used depending on the tolerance of the patient.

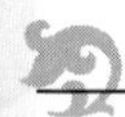

Duboisia myoporoides

COMMON NAME ■ Corkwood tree

One may also use *Duboisia leichhardtii.* The whole plant is used to make medicine. In eclectic literature, a tincture dose of 10 drops twice daily was given to calm the intestinal tract. I have not used this remedy in my practice. This plant is a source of L-hyoscyamine, scopolamine, and other alkaloids.

CHAPTER

59

PESTICIDES

CHAPTER • OUTLINE

Veratrum viride
Cocculus indicus
Cystisus scoparius
Geranium robertianum
Melaleuca leucadendron
Ledum latifolium
Chrysanthemum cinerariaefolium
Urginea maritima
Nicotiana tabacum
Ryania speciosa

Pesticides are agents that kill vermin, especially insects such as flies, lice, and fleas. Many plants are effective insecticides. The use of natural pesticides may become more important as we discover that chemicals currently being used may be too toxic for their use to continue. I encourage readers to contact me with valuable tips. This section needs to be expanded so that farmers might eventually be able to draw upon some of these plants to help them control crop pests.

Veratrum viride

COMMON NAME ■ Green hellebore

Use the root or leaves to make medicine. *CAUTION: Do not use this internally without full knowledge of its medicinal effects.* The tincture of *Veratrum* may be applied to hair to help kill lice and fleas. This plant contains the alkaloids veratramine and jervine, which are similar to those in *Veratrum album.*

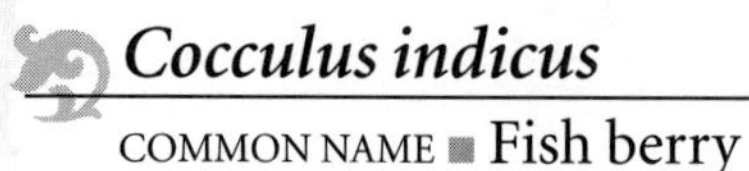

Cocculus indicus

COMMON NAME ■ Fish berry

The berries are used to make medicine. This plant will kill flies when applied externally to the skin. An ointment can be made by mixing 1 ounce of crushed fish berries with 10 ounces of benzoated lard.[28]

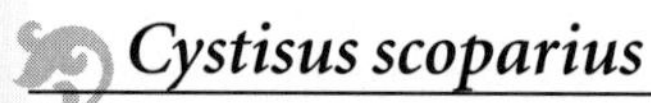

Cystisus scoparius

COMMON NAME ■ Scots broom

The twigs are made into a tea. This can be rubbed into the hair for lice control. *Cystisus* is a famous cardiac remedy. It is also a mild psychotropic, since the flowers and seeds contain lysergic acid.

Geranium robertianum

COMMON NAME ■ Herb robert

This valuable hemostatic has been used in fluid extract or tincture form to remove lice and their eggs. Apply to the hair.

Melaleuca leucadendron

COMMON NAME ■ Cajaput

The oil, which is distilled from the fresh leaves and twigs, is used locally for tinea tonsurans and pediculi. One of the chief ingredients in cajaput oil is cineole.

Ledum latifolium

COMMON NAME ■ Labrador tea

Medicine is made from the leaves and flowering shoots. Labrador tea contains volatile oils, in particular the sesquiterpene ledol.

Dr. Bastyr said that a strong decoction is a delouser when applied topically. I have not tried Labrador tea as a delouser in my practice. A weak infusion is used as a cough remedy at a dose of 1 cup per day.

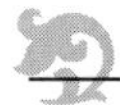

Chrysanthemum cinerariaefolium

COMMON NAME ■ Pyrethrum

The dried flowers are used to make medicine. *Chrysanthemum* is neurotoxic to insects. The berries make birds drunk. This plant contains pyrethrums, which are toxic to scabies and head and to body lice and their nits. Apply the botanical extract of *Chrysanthemum* topically.

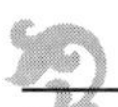

Urginea maritima

COMMON NAME ■ Red squill

The red variety of squill is used as a rat poison. It causes vomiting in humans in large doses and should be used cautiously. It is a heart medicine that acts similarly to digitalis. Dr. Bastyr used this remedy as an expectorant in doses of 5 drops of tincture three times daily.

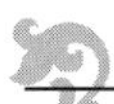

Nicotiana tabacum

COMMON NAME ■ Tobacco leaves

The powder of the leaves has been used on plants as an insecticide. Tobacco juice may be applied to the skin to ward off flies, gnats, and mosquitoes. The patient may not like this application of tobacco, however, since it can irritate sensitive skin.

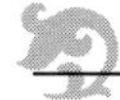

Ryania speciosa

COMMON NAME ■ Ryania

This insecticide is used as a dust made from a 40% extract. It is used to control the sugar cane borer, coddling moth, and European corn borer.

CHAPTER

60

RESPIRATORY SEDATIVES

CHAPTER • OUTLINE

Respiratory sedatives calm the respiratory system. They are given when coughing becomes excessive, causing pain and damage to the intercostal muscles. This category of remedies may also be called antitussives. Antitussives relieve or prevent cough.

Prunus virginiana

COMMON NAME ■ Choke cherry

As I recall, Dr. Bastyr spoke of *Prunus virginiana*; however, choke cherry is also the name given to *Prunus serotina*, which is the name that occurs more often in the literature. The inner bark is used to make medicine. Many of the *Prunus* species contain the isoflavone prunetin. There is also a cyanogenic glycoside in *Prunus serotina* called prunasin.

Prunus is a sedative and an expectorant. It is quite astringent and helps to decrease mucous membrane secretions. It is used for chronic respiratory problems, although Dr. Bastyr taught us to use it for whooping cough. The tincture dose is 15 drops four times daily.

Prunus serotina

COMMON NAME ■ Wild cherry

The bark is used to make medicine. As far as I know, this may be the same plant as *P. virginiana*. At any rate, the usage and action of the plant as medicine are the same. *Prunus* is an antitussive, an expectorant, and an antispasmodic. The active ingredient in wild cherry bark is prunasin, which is a cyanogenetic glycoside. Take about 20 drops three to four times daily to help quiet a painful, harsh cough. I add licorice to *Prunus* to increase cough expectoration and to coat the throat.

The wax of the leaf of *Prunus* contains two novel gamma-tocopherol derivatives, prunasol A and prunasol B.[35] These are both antioxidants. Leaf waxes in general deserve further study.

Myroxylon balsamum

COMMON NAME ■ Tolu balsam

The medicine is made from wood resin from the trunk. *Myroxylon* contains resin esters such as toluresinotannol cinnamate, which is its main active constituent. It also contains quite a bit of free cinnamic acid, which makes up 15% of the volatile oil. *Myroxylon* is a sedative and soothes membranes made sore by short, hacky coughs. The syrup is used in doses of 2 to 6 drams two to three times daily. Dr. Bastyr used doses of 120 drops of the tincture four times daily.

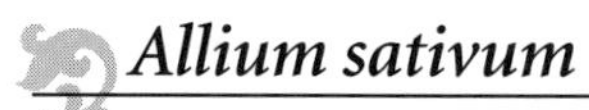

Allium sativum

COMMON NAME ■ Garlic

The bulb is used for medicine. It is an expectorant, an antiviral, an antibiotic, and a vasomotor depressant. Garlic is useful against many staphylococcal infections, streptococcal infections, and tuberculosis. Take garlic for excessive, irritating, and persistent coughs. For all of the listed conditions, garlic may be eaten in foods or given in a tincture dose of 5 to 25 drops three times daily. I prefer to have my patients chop up two cloves of raw garlic and slug them down with water two or three times daily.

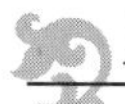

Helianthus petiolaris

COMMON NAME ■ Sunflower

You can also find this plant under the name *Helianthus annuus.* The tincture made from the seeds of the sunflower can be used to treat subacute pulmonary infections, including allergy-related coughs. Dr. Bastyr said that it is good for bronchial coughs in tincture doses of 20 to 30 drops three times daily. Sunflower seed tincture is also a slight diuretic.

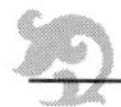

Eriodictyon californicum

COMMON NAME ■ Yerba santa

The leaves are used to make medicine. The tincture and tea are made from the leaves. One of yerba's main active ingredients is a resin called eriodictyol, which is the aglycone of eriodictin. Yerba is both an expectorant and a stomachic. Dr. Bastyr taught its use for irritating, dry, persistent cough. Herbalists have also used it to treat the paroxysmal coughing associated with bronchial asthma and postpneumonia coughing. For all conditions, a dose of 30 drops of the tincture may be used several times daily.

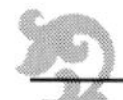

Glycyrrhiza glabra typica

COMMON NAME ■ Licorice root

The root is used to make medicine. This plant has many uses. As a respiratory sedative, Dr. Bastyr suggested combining equal parts of licorice and *Grindelia.* Give 60 drops of the mixture three times daily. The effects of licorice are immediate. Licorice improves energy and increases the ability of the body to manage inflammation by sparing the adrenal hormones. Licorice is a moisturizing expectorant and a sweetening agent. It helps to cure ulcers. Overuse of licorice may result in hypokalemia. Therefore it may be a good idea to use a potassium supplement when using licorice on an ongoing basis. I recommend supplementing with 100 mg of potassium twice daily.

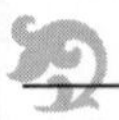

Castanea dentata

COMMON NAME ■ Chestnut

The leaves are used to make medicine. This remedy is a mild respiratory sedative and treats spasmodic coughs. Dr. Bastyr called *Castanea* an antitussive astringent. He taught us to use a dose of 15 to 60 drops of tincture every 3 or 4 hours as a respiratory sedative. Historically, it was used by eclectic physicians to treat pertussis. However, it is rarely used for this today.

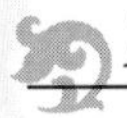

Lippia mexicana

COMMON NAME ■ Verbena

Use the leaves and stalks in tea. Dr. Bastyr was probably referring to *Verbena officinalis*, or vervain. Some people confuse this plant with *Lippia triphyllae.* While I regret the confusion, I have no way to go back and talk to Dr. Bastyr about this. The indications that Dr. Bastyr taught for *Lippia* were whooping cough, asthma, and chronic bronchitis. These are the very same indications that herbalists teach for *Verbena officinalis.* In addition, *Lippia* is used to treat dry, hard, resonant, ringing coughs. A standard cup of tea is sipped throughout the day.

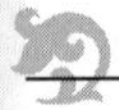

Penthorum sedoides

COMMON NAME ■ Virginia stonecrop

The whole plant is used to make medicine. Herbalists, eclectics, and naturopaths have used *Penthorum* to treat chronic diseases of the fauces, larynx, and pharynx, such as viral or allergic bronchitis. A dose of 10 to 30 drops of tincture is given several times daily. In addition to its use in respiratory problems, this medicine is somewhat astringent. Dr. Bastyr taught us that it is useful in treating gastritis, ileitis, and proctitis and in cases where there is excessive mucous production and discharge.

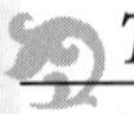

Trillium pendulum

COMMON NAME ■ Bethroot

Also look for this plant under the name *Trillium erectum. Trillium* contains diosgenin and the steroid saponin trillin. The root is used to make medicine.

Dr. Bastyr taught us that *Trillium* could be used to soothe the cough of catarrhal bronchitis and to sedate the thorax. It soothes the cough of incipient phthisis. Dr. Bastyr underscored *Trillium*'s use when there is a possibility of hemorrhage, whether in the gastrointestinal tract or the upper respiratory tract. The dose of the tincture is up to 60 drops several times daily.

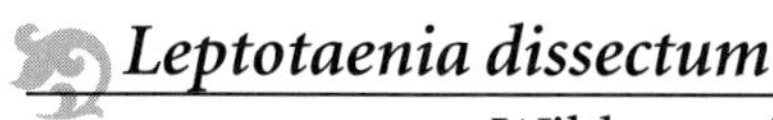

Leptotaenia dissectum

COMMON NAME ■ Wild parsnip

The resin and oil of the root are used to make medicine. This wonderful plant is an antiviral and an antibacterial. *Leptotaenia* is a great upper respiratory flu medicine. It is very useful in viral pneumonia. I always add this plant to my upper respiratory formulas. Dr. Bastyr suggested a dose of 10 drops of tincture three times daily. This plant kills gram-positive and gram-negative bacteria. Incidentally, it is also useful to treat urinary tract infections.

Hyssopus officinalis

COMMON NAME ■ Hyssop

The dried aerial parts are used to make medicine. This plant is a carminative, a diaphoretic, and a sedative. Historically, it has been used for bronchitis and chronic nasal catarrh. Dr. Bastyr used it for allergic rhinitis and the common cold. The tincture dose suggested by eclectics, herbalists, and naturopathic physicians is 60 drops twice daily.

Bryonia alba

COMMON NAME ■ White bryony

CAUTION: This is a toxic plant. Even five or six berries of this plant will cause abdominal distress in children. The stomach should be pumped and activated charcoal given. The root is used to quiet pleurisy, to help stop exudations, and to help absorb inflammatory products of either serous or sanguineous character. Notice the language in the preceding sentence. This language permeates the eclectic literature and Dr. Bastyr's teaching. The dose of *Bryonia* is 1 drop of tincture in a cup of water to be sipped in very small amounts every 15 to 30 minutes. A cup is consumed over the course of the day. The use of *Bryonia* homeopathically is well known. Dr. Bastyr used a 6X remedy most frequently.

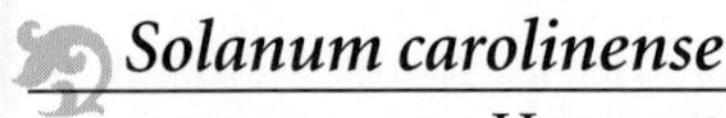

Solanum carolinense

COMMON NAME ■ Horsenettle

Solanum has been used for pertussis to mitigate the spasmodic cough. The whole plant is used in doses of 15 to 30 drops three to four times daily. Dr. Bastyr mentioned that it has even been used to moderate the shaking of Parkinson's disease.

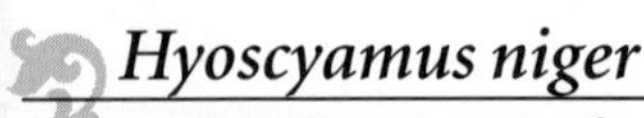

Hyoscyamus niger

COMMON NAME ■ Henbane

The flowering tops and seeds are used to make medicine. The eclectic physicians used it to treat pneumonitis in infants for its sedative effect on cough. Dr. Bastyr taught its use in bronchitis when there is a short, sharp, dry cough. He suggested taking five seeds in the morning and at night. The tincture dose is 5 to 10 drops three times daily.

Symplocarpus foetidus

COMMON NAME ■ Skunk cabbage

The dried root is used to make medicine. *Symplocarpus* is a good lung and upper respiratory remedy. *Symplocarpus* has been used to treat asthma and bronchitis. Dr. Bastyr taught us to use a dose of 3 to 15 drops of the tincture three times daily. For asthma, he combined *Symplocarpus* with equal parts of *Lobelia* and *Capsicum*. He gave 20 drops of the tincture mixture every 2 hours until the asthma symptoms subsided.

Lobelia inflata

COMMON NAME ■ Indian tobacco

The whole plant is used to make medicine. *Lobelia* contains a number of piperidine alkaloids, chief among which is lobeline. Because *Lobelia* relaxes the respiratory apparatus, it is useful in treating spasmodic cough. Eclectics, herbalists, and naturopaths use 5 to 10 drops of tincture three times daily for this purpose. For elderly patients, Dr. Bastyr said to use *Sanguinaria* instead of *Lobelia* for respiratory tightness and upper respiratory disease. *Sanguinaria* is mixed with equal parts of licorice, *Grindelia*, and *Hydrastis* and given in doses of 30 drops of the tincture.

Lobelia contains alkaloids similar to nicotine, and it is used as a nicotine substitute to help people stop smoking. The idea of using *Lobelia* as a tobacco-withdrawing medicine was approved by the Food and Drug Administration some time ago.[33] The dose for a light smoker is 7 drops in a glass of water three times daily. The dose for a heavy smoker is 3 drops in a glass of water eight times daily. The number of doses may be decreased as the urge to smoke decreases.

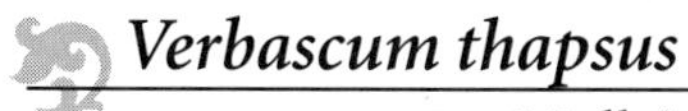

Verbascum thapsus

COMMON NAMES ■ Mullein, Jacob's staff

Also look for this under the name *Verbascum densiflorum*. Mullein is in the snapdragon or figwort family, *Scrophulariaceae*. Medicine is made from the entire plant, including the root. Mullein contains mucilage, saponins, iridoide monoterpenes, and caffeic acid derivatives. It also is rich in iron, magnesium, potassium, sulfur, and calcium phosphate. It contains the oligosaccharide verbascose.

This plant is an excellent antitussive remedy. Herbalists recommend 10 to 40 drops of tincture or a cup of standard tea. For bronchitis or asthma, I combine equal parts of mullein, *Lobelia*, and ephedra tinctures and give 30 drops twice daily.

Curiously, the seeds are narcotic, and when thrown into very slow moving water will cause temporary stupor in fish. In this manner, the seeds have been used to catch fish. Also of note is the field use of mullein. The dried leaves make excellent tinder for starting fires.[36]

Tussilago farfara

COMMON NAME ■ Coltsfoot

The tops of the plant are used to make medicine. *Tussilago* is an expectorant and a very soothing emollient. I frequently include it in my upper respiratory formulas. Dr. Bastyr pointed out that *Tussilago* allays cough caused by irritation of the mucous membranes. It can be used for dry cough, laryngitis, pharyngitis, bronchitis, and asthma. A dose of 30 to 60 drops of the tincture may be taken three times daily. Dr. Bastyr taught us to give *Tussilago* with licorice root as an expectorant.

Trifolium pratense

COMMON NAMES ■ Red clover, Trefoil

The flowers are used to make medicine. Red clover is from the pea family, *Leguminosae*. Dr. Bastyr reported the use of *Trifolium* to treat mild cachexia, the cough of measles, laryngeal congestion, and whooping cough. Herbalists use *Trifolium* to treat whooping cough. It is mixed with *Glycyrrhiza glabra typica* and *Grindelia squarrosa* in equal parts and given in doses of 90 drops of tincture four times daily. In addition, herbalists say that the standard tea made of red clover can be given in wineglass doses frequently throughout the day.

Pinguicula vulgaris

COMMON NAME ■ Butterwort

The whole plant is used to make medicine. This is a carnivorous plant, as is the sundew, *Drosera rotundifolia. Pinguicula* is a member of the butterwort family, *Lentibulariaceae.* Dr. Bastyr used to talk about this plant. Perhaps, like anyone, he just liked to say the word *Pinguicula.* This plant is a respiratory sedative used to treat whooping cough or any other violent cough. I prescribe 30 drops of *Pinguicula* hourly until relief is obtained.

CHAPTER

61

RESPIRATORY STIMULANTS

CHAPTER • OUTLINE

Respiratory stimulants stimulate the respiratory system. Principally, I think the idea is to promote expectoration. Remember that there are a number of immunoglobulins in the mucus that help the body fight infection. A healthy flow of mucus, regularly expectorated, is the goal in treating infections of the upper respiratory tract. Another goal in using respiratory stimulation is to prevent pneumonia by promoting an upward movement of infectious agents so that they are carried out of the body during expectoration. Respiratory stimulation is also achieved by stimulating the nervous system near the respiratory centers.

Atropa belladonna

COMMON NAME ■ Deadly nightshade

Use the root or leaves to make medicine. *CAUTION:* A. belladonna *is a powerful remedy that can be toxic in large doses. It is contraindicated in glaucoma.*

Dr. Bastyr said that *A. belladonna* is useful for patients who complain that they cannot get an adequate breath. The alkaloid atropine stimulates respiration rate. A dose of 0.5 to 1 mg exerts a mild central vagal excitation that subsequently increases the rate and depth of respiration. I suggest using a dose of 5 to 10 drops of tincture twice daily. *A. belladonna* tends to dry the mucous membranes and is a bronchodilator.

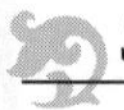

Strychnos nux-vomica

COMMON NAME ■ Quaker buttons

The seeds are used to make medicine. *CAUTION: Use only 1 to 5 drops of the tincture because this plant is poisonous in larger doses.* This remedy stimulates the respiratory tract. *S. nux-vomica* contains the extremely toxic alkaloid strychnine, which is a stimulant to the nervous system and accounts for the respiratory-stimulating effect of the plant. Dr. Bastyr said that this remedy, when used properly, is quite effective to help stimulate the respiratory tract.

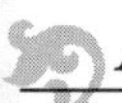

Aspidosperma quebracho-blanco

COMMON NAME ■ Quebracho

The bark is used to make medicine. Quebracho is a respiratory and cardiac stimulant. It is useful in emphysema and bronchial asthma. This plant contains the potent indole alkaloids aspidospermine and yohimbine.

For use in cystic fibrosis to help clear the lungs, Dr. Bastyr taught the use of 25 drops of the tincture two or three times daily. Patients with cystic fibrosis should also take selenium, which is needed to make the hepatic detoxification enzymes. In addition, I make sure that the patient has good pancreatic support. The bioflavonoids may also be helpful for these patients. This remedy works almost identically to *Coryanthe yohimbe.*

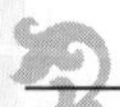

Populus candicans

COMMON NAME ■ Balm of Gilead

The bark and leaves are used to make medicine. Dr. Bastyr said that *Populus* is a fine respiratory stimulant and expectorant. The tincture may be taken in doses of 30 drops three times daily. It is a good cough medicine to make the cough "work better" for the patient—to be more productive. Historically, herbalists have used this plant for the treatment of laryngitis. According to herbalists, *Populus* is a good antiinflammatory for joint or arthritic pains. The ache of rheumatism may also be helped.

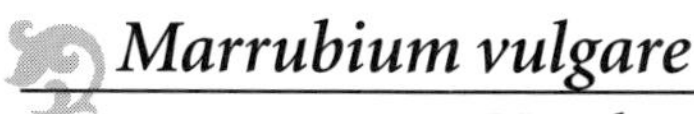

Marrubium vulgare

COMMON NAME ■ Horehound

The dried aerial parts of the plant are used to make medicine. The diterpene marrubiin is a main constituent in horehound. Horehound is a stimulating expectorant. It can be used in doses of 30 drops three times daily to improve the production and flow of mucus. In *King's American Dispensatory*,[133] horehound is described as a stimulant tonic, an expectorant, and a diuretic. I frequently mix a tincture of horehound with equal parts of licorice, *Grindelia*, and *Sanguinaria* to make an active respiratory tonic and stimulant. The dose I recommend is 60 drops three times daily.

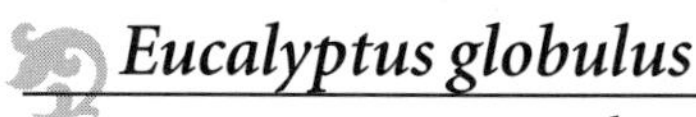

Eucalyptus globulus

COMMON NAME ■ Eucalyptus

The medicine is extracted from the leaves. The chief ingredient in the oil of eucalyptus is eucalyptol, also called cineole. Eucalyptus oil and cajeput oil are similar in usage, probably because they both contain a large amount of their active ingredient, cineole.

Eucalyptus is one botanical that most of us have experienced directly as a chest rub to help our breathing during chest colds and flu. In addition, the tincture of *Eucalyptus* may be used internally. For respiratory problems, use 20 drops of the tincture three times daily to help clear the airways. Eclectics, herbalists, and naturopaths have used *Eucalyptus* to treat a variety of other problems. It can be used for relieving asthma, for bladder infections and catarrh, for whooping cough (it has saved lives here), and as a topical application for suppurative and ulcerative wounds. It is, of course, a great deodorizer.

Ephedra sinica

COMMON NAME ■ Ma Huang

Also look for this under the names *Ephedra viridis* and *Ephedra nevadensis*, or Mormon tea. This plant is in the ephedra family, *Ephedraceae*. One of the active constituents in this plant is the alkaloid ephedrine, which has an action similar to that of adrenaline. It is a sympathomimetic. *Ephedra* is one of the more potent respiratory stimulants. It dilates the bronchioles in the treatment of asthma. For the treatment of asthma, I recommend 20 drops of tincture two to three times daily.

CHAPTER

62

Rubefacients and Vesicants

CHAPTER • OUTLINE

A rubefacient is an agent that produces reddening of the skin. A vesicant is an agent that produces blistering of the skin. In older *Materia Medica*, some of these remedies can be found under counterirritants.

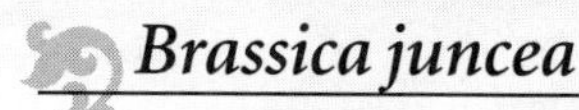

Brassica juncea

COMMON NAME ■ Mustard

The crushed seeds are used to make medicine. To warm the chest, make a mustard pack by using one part dried powdered mustard to three parts flour. Add water and make a paste. Sandwich this between layers of a diaper or cotton cloth. Apply to the body for 10 to 15 minutes, or until the body part becomes pink. *Do not leave this on the skin too long, as it may burn the tissue.*

You can also use mustard in a footbath or pediluvial. For dysmenorrhea, Dr. Bastyr said to use the pediluvial and put a cold compress on the abdomen. He said that the cold compress should be covered with wool. I suggest trying these therapies to appreciate them. Just put 1 teaspoon of dried mustard in some hot water and soak the feet in it for about 5 minutes. You can then experiment with larger doses of mustard or with keeping the feet in the water for longer amounts of time.

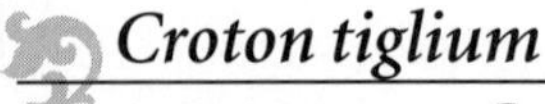

Croton tiglium

COMMON NAME ■ Croton oil

The seeds are used to make medicine. Eclectic physicians used *Croton* locally as a vesicant and a counterirritant. *CAUTION: Internally, this remedy is primarily used homeopathically. Dr. Bastyr told us that internally 1 drop of oil on a sugar cube is a drastic cathartic. Do not use more than 1 drop!*

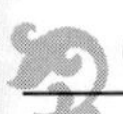

Cantharis vesicatoria

COMMON NAME ■ Spanish fly

The whole insect is used as a vesicant. *Cantharis* blisters the skin. Naturopathic physicians have used a homeopathic preparation for many years to treat urinary tract disorders, especially cystitis and urethritis. I use 1 drop of the tincture with other urinary tract remedies for these conditions.

Cinnamomum camphora

COMMON NAME ■ Camphor

The bark is used to make medicine. Topically, 1 to 5 drops of *Cinnamomum* applied to the skin is a rubefacient and a counterirritant, and as such it is helpful in myalgia caused by overwork. *Cinnamomum* may be applied as a chest pack for bronchitis and pleurisy. For this use, make a poultice by placing 1 ounce of the bark in a pint of boiling water. After cooling slightly, soak a cotton cloth in this mixture to be applied to the chest. Cover the chest with a dry towel. The chest pack should be left on for about 15 minutes, or until redness occurs.

CHAPTER

63

SEDATIVES (ANODYNAL)

CHAPTER • OUTLINE

Hyoscyamus niger
Piscidia erythrina
Betonica officinalis
Primula veris
Anthemis nobilis
Atropa belladonna
Datura stramonium
Symplocarpus foetidus

A sedative is a medicinal agent that reduces nervous energy and excitement. Anodynal sedatives are sedatives that tend to relieve pain. The pain relief decreases anxiety, which contributes to the sedative effect.

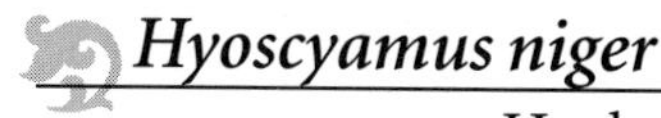

Hyoscyamus niger

COMMON NAME ■ Henbane

The leaves, flowering parts, and seeds are used to make medicine. The alkaloid hyoscyamine is a main active ingredient in *Hyoscyamus.* This plant can induce sleep when the patient has pain or when there is restless agitation. Dr. Bastyr said that it could be used for insomnia of the aged and infants. Eclectic physicians used it for chronic mania, neuralgia with spasm, sphincter spasm, and cerebral congestion with excitement. For all of these conditions, I use 1 drop of tincture in a small amount of water. To achieve close to the same effect as 1 drop of the tincture, you can use *Hyoscyamus* homeopathically in a 3X potency. Herbalists use it as an ingredient for foot-baths. The antidote for *Hyoscyamus* toxicity is pilocarpine. The emergency dose for *Hyoscyamus* poisoning is $\frac{1}{4}$ dram of pilocarpine administered beneath the skin.

Piscidia erythrina

COMMON NAME ■ Jamaican dogwood

The root bark is used to make medicine. *Piscidia* contains a number of isoflavonoids, including jamaicin and ichthynone. This plant is used for insomnia and pain relief. According to Dr. Bastyr, it can be used for pain relief after fractures. He used *Piscidia* for nervous tachycardia, general nervousness, ovarian neuralgia, and facial and sciatic neuralgia. The tincture dose is 60 drops every 3 hours until full relief is attained.

Betonica officinalis

COMMON NAME ■ Betony

The flowering herb is used to make medicine. *Betonica* is a mild bitter, an antineuralgic, and a calmative. The dose of *Betonica* is 30 drops twice daily. Use this great anodynal sedative to treat hysteria and anxiety headaches. For this purpose, I recommend combining it with equal parts of *Scutellaria.* I suggest using 45 drops of this mixture three times daily. *Betonica* is a gentle remedy.

Primula veris

COMMON NAME ■ Cowslip

Look for this plant also under the name *Primula officinalis.* The whole herb, including the root, is used to make medicine. It is calming to the nervous system and, according to Dr. Bastyr, has been used to encourage sleep even when headache is present. To take this remedy, he suggested either using six to eight flower heads in salad or taking 10 to 30 drops of the tincture as needed, up to four times daily. Make a tea from the root to use in chronic bronchitis. Drink 1 cup of this tea twice daily.

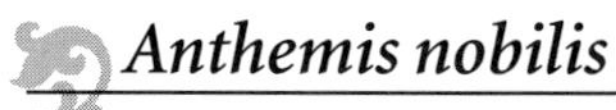

Anthemis nobilis

COMMON NAME ■ Roman chamomile

The flowering tops are used to make medicine. Dr. Bastyr said that *Anthemis* tea should be used for patients who have colds and who are so uncomfortable that they are not sleeping well. Have the patient drink 1 cup of the tea several times daily to calm the body and relieve discomfort. Don't confuse this remedy with German chamomile, *Chamomilla*, which is used in pediatrics. *Chamomilla* 3X homeopathic potency is used to calm and decrease pain and restlessness in children with teething difficulties.

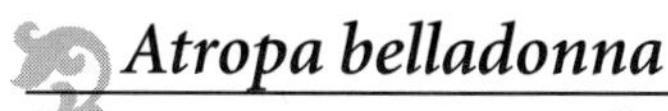

Atropa belladonna

COMMON NAME ■ Deadly nightshade

The root and leaves are used to make medicine. *CAUTION:* A. belladonna *is a powerful remedy that can be toxic in large doses.* To help decrease the pain of duodenal ulcers, *A. belladonna* helps by quieting the gastrointestinal tract and decreasing secretions. Dr. Bastyr said that even a 6X homeopathic potency of *A. belladonna* is highly anodynal. The tincture dose is 10 drops two to three times daily.

Datura stramonium

COMMON NAME ■ Jimsonweed

The leaves and seeds are used to make medicine. *Datura* is a narcotic, an anodyne, an antispasmodic, and a sedative. *Datura* contains potent tropane alkaloids, including hyoscyamine. When using it as an anodynal sedative, Dr. Bastyr suggested using 1 to 8 drops of the tincture twice daily. Naturopaths use *Datura* homeopathically at a 12X potency twice daily for nervousness and anxiety. Dr. Bastyr said that this plant could be used to treat acute mania and delirium, and it is sometimes very effective when pain is present.

Symplocarpus foetidus

COMMON NAME ■ Skunk cabbage

The root is used to make medicine. As an anodynal sedative, I use *Symplocarpus* locally for hemorrhoids and other mucous membrane problems. For hemorrhoids, have the patient make a paste of powdered *Symplocarpus* and olive oil and apply this locally before bedtime.

CHAPTER

64

SEDATIVES (MILD)

CHAPTER • OUTLINE

Passiflora incarnata
Ferula asafoetida
Humulus lupulus
Symplocarpus foetidus
Melissa officinalis
Mimulus lewisii
Reseda lutea
Atropa belladonna
Cypripedium pubescens

Sedatives calm the mind. As medicine, these plants help reduce nervousness, distress, and irritation. They are safe remedies that can be used over a prolonged period.

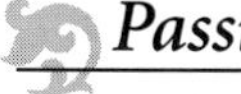

Passiflora incarnata

COMMON NAME ■ Passionflower

The whole plant is used to make medicine. *Passiflora* contains a large number of flavonoids. The dose of *Passiflora* as a mild sedative is 60 drops of the tincture as needed. To assist with sleep, a dose of 150 drops should be taken 1 hour before going to bed. Specifically, Dr. Bastyr taught us that *Passiflora* is useful in helping elderly people sleep, even if their wakefulness is caused by fear. In addition,

Passiflora is useful in cases of nervous excitement with muscular twitching. For this purpose, I would strongly recommend sweetening *Passiflora* tea with 1 teaspoon of glycine. Glycine enhances the ability of the tea to relax twitching muscles. Glycine and *Passiflora* taken together are specific for the uncomfortable muscle twitching seen in multiple sclerosis and amyotrophic lateral sclerosis. I have had a number of these patients who have responded well to the *Passiflora* and glycine combination.

Ferula asafoetida

COMMON NAME ■ Asafoetida

The gum of the root is used to make medicine. The chief component of the volatile oil is sec-propenyl-isobutyl disulfide.[25] As with many remedies that have a rich folk tradition, *Ferula* has quite a collection of uses. It is used for nervous paroxysms, hypochondriasis, whooping cough, bronchitis of the weak or aged, and flatulence. Dr. Bastyr taught us to use *Ferula* primarily for the treatment of coughs. The tincture dose is 30 drops three times daily. Dr. Dirk Powell, a classmate at National College of Naturopathic Medicine, recounted Dr. Bastyr saying that *Ferula* is useful in treating globus hystericus, tympanitis, and hypochondriasis.

Humulus lupulus

COMMON NAME ■ Hops

The dried strobile is used as medicine. *Humulus* contains humulone, lupulone, and colupulone.[25] *Humulus* is a good general mild sedative. It is used to treat anxiety-induced insomnia, nervous dyspepsia, stomach atonia, and delirium tremens (especially effective when used with *Capsicum*). Use up to 90 drops of *Humulus* tincture four times daily. If *Humulus* is being used to aid sleep, have the patient take at least 180 drops in a single dose. Counting the 180 drops may make one sleepy!

Humulus helps to increase the appetite and aids in the digestion of starch. Dr. Bastyr mentioned that an often-overlooked use of *Humulus* tincture is as eardrops for earache. Dr. Powell recalls from his notes that Dr. Bastyr used *Humulus* for patients with sexual dysfunction, including alternating nymphomania and frigidity and impotence.

Symplocarpus foetidus

COMMON NAME ■ Skunk cabbage

The root is used to make medicine. *Symplocarpus* is a mild sedative, a spasmolytic, and a good whooping cough remedy. I have used it to treat bronchitis and asthma. A tincture dose of 30 to 90 drops several times daily is used. The powdered root may be taken in doses of 7 to 15 grains.

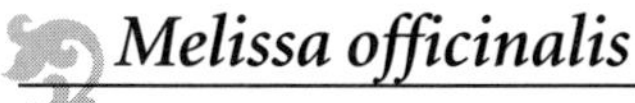

Melissa officinalis

COMMON NAME ■ Lemon balm

The herb and leaves are used to make medicine. *Melissa* is a sedative, an antispasmodic, a diaphoretic, and a mild antacid. Dr. Bastyr said that it is used much like *Mitchella* in female reproductive system complaints. The fresh edible plant may be added to salads, and the dried herb may be used to make tea. I prescribe 60 drops of tincture three times daily as a mild sedative. It can also be used to treat gastric dyspepsia.

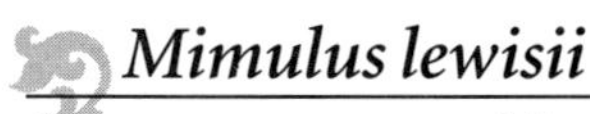

Mimulus lewisii

COMMON NAME ■ Monkey flower

The petal of the flower is used to make medicine. This plant is said to be a useful calmative as a Bach flower remedy. Homeopathic physicians tell us that it has some specific use as an antifear remedy. I have prescribed this remedy many times. One drop of the remedy on the tongue is my usual recommendation. I have fond memories of *Mimulus lewisii* because it is one of the plants that we studied on our hikes with Dr. Joe Boucher in British Columbia. Dr. Boucher was a contemporary of Dr. Bastyr. We frequently came across this plant growing at high elevations along mountain streams. We would pick a petal of the flower and rest it on our tongues as we hiked along.

Reseda lutea

COMMON NAME ■ Mignonette

Herbalists teach us to stuff pillows with the dried aerial parts of this plant to help induce a tranquil sleep. As a tea, it is sedative. The dose is 3 tablespoons of the standard tea three times daily.

Atropa belladonna

COMMON NAME ■ Deadly nightshade

The root and leaves are used to make medicine. *CAUTION:* A. belladonna *is a powerful remedy that can be toxic in large doses.* I have found that small doses of *A. belladonna* tincture can calm a nervous patient to some degree. Homeopathically, a 6X to 200X potency is used to relieve delirium.

Cypripedium pubescens

COMMON NAME ■ Lady's slipper

The root is used as medicine. *CAUTION:* Cypripedium *is toxic in large doses. Cypripedium* is a sedative and a mild spasmolytic. Herbalists have used it to induce sleep in cases of restless insomnia. Use 30 drops of the tincture as needed. The standard tea makes a good remedy for nervous headache. I do not recommend taking more than 1 cup per day. *Cypripedium* is an endangered plant. I ask you to use other sedatives, such as *Valeriana* or *Scutellaria*, to help save this plant.

CHAPTER

65

SEDATIVES (STRONG)

CHAPTER • OUTLINE

Strong sedatives are sedatives that produce a powerful relaxing effect on the body or the mind. Given their strength, they require a more cautious application.

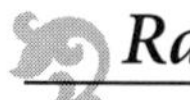

Rauwolfia serpentina

COMMON NAMES ■ Snakeroot, Rauwolfia

The root is used to make medicine. *CAUTION:* Rauwolfia *crosses the placental barrier and also enters breast milk.* Rauwolfia must be used respectfully. Overuse can result in severe depression in sensitive individuals. It is important that the patient be informed about rauwolfia's potential side effects. It may cause depression and electrolyte depletion. Patients who are taking rauwolfia should be given a well-balanced mineral supplement at dinnertime. This helps to maintain electrolyte balance. In all my years of using rauwolfia, I have never run into any problems with it. Rauwolfia contains many alkaloids, namely reserpine. When using it as a sedative, Dr. Bastyr said that 5 drops of rauwolfia tincture should be taken in combination with other sedatives. Rauwolfia has been used for hyperactivity associated with psychoneurosis.

Valeriana officinalis

COMMON NAME ■ Valerian

The root is used to make medicine. Dr. Dirk Powell recalls Dr. Bastyr saying that valerian was contraindicated in patients with pruritus caused by nervousness. Valerian's sedative action is caused in part by the valepotriates, such as isovaltrate. Valerian also contains isovaleric acid. The valepotriates and valeric acid in valerian bind to benzodiazepam receptors, also called GABA receptors, and exert a calming effect. Two examples of GABA receptors are valtrate and dihydrovaltrate. These account for some of the mental effects of valerian such as sedation and sleep induction.

Valerian is a nervine, an antispasmodic, and a sedative. Dr. Bastyr often prescribed valerian as a sedative when the patient had paleness of the face and coolness of the skin. I have noticed that eclectic physicians frequently use this kind of language in differentiating remedies. I prescribe 90 drops of tincture three times daily as a sedative. Nervous sleeplessness can frequently be alleviated by valerian. Valerian relaxes the mind, without interfering with clear thought. Therefore it may not work for patients with insomnia. On the other hand, some patients do very well on valerian to help with sleep. I have given patients valerian capsules to treat insomnia. I have varied the dose greatly because I have observed that some patients do well on two 350-mg capsules before bed and others require up to eight capsules.

Valerian is a mild hypotensive, and therefore hypertension exacerbated by anxiety may indicate valerian. Dr. Bastyr mentioned that a large dose of valerian increases the heart action. I am unclear as to what he meant by "action." Eclectic physicians have suggested its use for treating hysteria and to stimulate circulation to the stomach, mouth, and intestines. Valerian tends to increase peristalsis.

I have rubbed valerian on sore muscles when hiking to good effect. It is interesting to read the Native American usage of the plant. The Cree Indians used a chewed poultice of valerian applied topically for earache. They also used the poultice externally to treat seizures in babies.[156] This makes sense when one considers the antispasmodic effects of valerian.

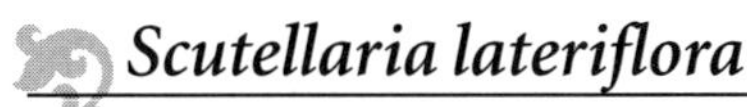

Scutellaria lateriflora

COMMON NAMES ■ Madweed, Skullcap

The entire plant is used to make medicine. *Scutellaria* contains a number of monoterpenes and flavonoids, including scutellarein, which has an action similar to quercetin. Both scutellarein and quercetin are flavones that decrease mast cell activity. Scutellarein is the active nervine in *Scutellaria.*

This plant has been used historically by eclectic physicians to treat hysteria, delirium, insomnia, irregular muscular actions, and postillness nervousness associated with mental and physical exhaustion. According to Dr. Bastyr, one of the main uses of *Scutellaria* is for nervousness when the muscles or heart are affected. Even the choreas can be helped. For hysteria and mania, *Scutellaria* may be used with other botanicals such as *Pulsatilla, Cimicifuga,* and *Avena.* I would recommend 180 drops of *Scutellaria* tincture at night to aid sleep. Although this dose may seem high, it is not. In fact, I have used as much as 300 drops for patients with insomnia. More may be used depending on the tolerance of the patient. Teething discomfort can be helped with *Scutellaria.* The tincture dose is 10 to 30 drops twice daily; however, I have used doses as high as 50 drops twice daily.

Dr. Dirk Powell, in his notes from Dr. Bastyr's lectures, said that Dr. Bastyr used *Scutellaria* for drug addiction and epilepsy. Dr. Bastyr said that the action in epilepsy is slow in developing, but the medicinal effects will last a few days.

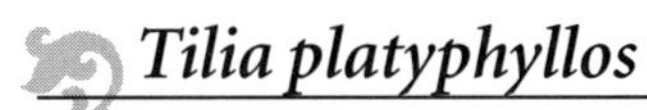

Tilia platyphyllos

COMMON NAME ■ Lime flowers

The flowers are used to make medicine. Make the tincture from the dried flowers. I prescribe 90 drops of *Tilia* tincture three times daily as a sedative. This dose may be taken more frequently if needed.

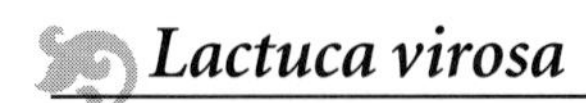

Lactuca virosa

COMMON NAME ■ Wild lettuce

The juice of the stem is used for medicine. *Lactuca* contains a sesquiterpene lactone, lactucin, which probably accounts for the sedative action of this herb.

Lactuca decreases the activity of the parasympathetic nervous system. Dr. Bastyr taught its use as a sedative that allows gentle sleep. The dose that I prescribe as a sedative is higher than you will see in most other herbals. I start at 120 drops of tincture at bedtime to induce sleep.

In addition to its use as a sedative, Dr. Bastyr taught that *Lactuca* could be used for an overactive thyroid. It can also help mild diabetes. Even so, I strongly suggest other supportive remedies for treating the early stages of diabetes. The berry anthocyanins are especially effective for this purpose.

Piper methysticum

COMMON NAME ■ Kavakava

The rhizome is used to make medicine. Kavakava contains kava lactones, also termed kava pyrones. One of the chief active kava lactones is kawain, also called kavain. Also present and significant are dihydromethysticin and yangonin.[157] This plant is a fairly strong sedative and an anxiolytic. When using kavakava as a general sedative, I suggest using 30 drops of tincture twice daily. The results are generally felt within 10 minutes. Thankfully, kavakava seems to be free of side effects.

Kavakava is a good acute medicine in anxiety states. It is a great plant to prevent impending anxiety attacks. I use it to calm the mind and relax skeletal muscles. I recommend a single dose of 30 drops as a mental relaxant. The dose for helping to relax skeletal muscles is 30 drops of tincture three times daily.

In large doses, kavakava will stimulate skeletal muscles. I took 150 drops of the tincture one evening and found that my muscles had an uncomfortable desire to be stretched. The only relief was to take a walk. If kava dosen't work in lower doses (below 50 drops), then other medications should be used.

Tryptophan

This amino acid is included here simply to spotlight a natural medicinal material that, for some, may be useful as a sedative. I suggest giving 200 to 300 mg of 5-hydroxytryptophan at bedtime as a sleep aid. Many patients have told me that this simple amino acid is their miracle hypnotic.

Glycine and gamma-amino-benzoic acid (GABA) combination

In combination, these amino acids produce sedation. Depending on the dose, glycine and GABA can be classified as moderate sedatives. For a nontoxic and gently calming or anxiolytic effect, I have patients take 1 teaspoon of glycine powder and 500 mg of GABA together when needed. Limit this dose schedule to twice daily. If more is used, the sedative effect is stronger.

CHAPTER

66

SKIN REMEDIES

CHAPTER • OUTLINE

Pilocarpus jaborandi
Aristolochia serpentaria
Argentum nitrate
Cantharis vesicatoria
Adeps or *Adeps lanae*
Beeswax
Scrophularia nodosa
Impatiens capensis
Fumaria officinalis
Aconitum napellus
Veratrum virde
Vaccinium oxycoccus
Cocculus indicus
Sanguinaria canadensis
Grindelia squarrosa
Aloe communis
Safflower oil
Juglans cinerea
Iris versicolor
Berberis aquifolium
Arctium lappa
Rumex crispus
Citrus limon
Thuja occidentalis
Anagallis arvensis

Galanthus nivalis
Chlorophyll
Kalmia angustifolia
Citrus bergamia
Smilax species
Ammi majus
Melaleuca alternifolia
Fragaria virginiana

Skin remedies are a group of agents used to fight diseases of the skin and mucous membranes. Some of these remedies improve the health of the skin by improving the function of internal organs.

Pilocarpus jaborandi

COMMON NAME ■ Jaborandi

The dried leaves are used to make medicine. This remedy is a very powerful diaphoretic. The active constituent is the imidazole alkaloid pilocarpine.

Pilocarpus is a cholinergic and a mitotic. Its historical use among naturopaths was to bring out the rash in exanthematous diseases. In other words, it was used to speed up the disease process. The dose is 2 drops of the tincture twice daily. The eclectic physicians suggested that small doses of *Pilocarpus* be given internally to treat eczema and pruritus. Dr. Bastyr highly recommended this remedy to increase salivation. I use *Pilocarpus* for patients with dry mouth, including the dry mouth that patients often experience when they are undergoing chemotherapy.

Aristolochia serpentaria

COMMON NAME ■ Virginia snakeroot

The root is used to make medicine. *Aristolochia* is hard to find, or at least I have had trouble finding it. I have an old bottle of it, and when it's gone I'm out of luck. I don't use this remedy often because my supply is limited. I will be sad when it is gone. *Aristolochia* is a diaphoretic and a diuretic. It has been used to produce sweating in the early stage of skin eruptions. It stimulates the appetite and tonifies the digestive tract. It is the perfect remedy to help with internal cleansing, which in turn improves the tone and health of the skin. The dose is 5 to 10 drops of the tincture twice daily.

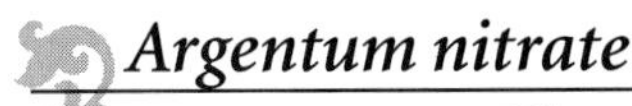

Argentum nitrate

COMMON NAME ■ Silver nitrate

I include this remedy because it was discussed in Dr. Bastyr's class. He did not recommend this treatment. For many years, physicians put a 1% solution of silver nitrate in the eyes of newborns to kill organisms such as syphilis and gonorrhea. The old-time naturopaths preferred argenol because it is less corrosive. Dr. Bastyr said that argenol temporarily stains the eyes brown. An herbalist/midwife once told me that chlorophyll could be put in the eye for this purpose. Sadly, I cannot remember her name. Dr. Bastyr did not recommend any of these remedies; instead, he would have the mother put colostrum in the baby's eyes.

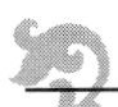

Cantharis vesicatoria

COMMON NAME ■ Spanish fly

Cantharis is both a vesicant and a rubefacient. As a skin remedy, *Cantharis* is a counterirritant. I have no personal experience using *Cantharis* as a rubefacient. I have included it here for historical purposes because Dr. Bastyr discussed it as a skin remedy.

Adeps or *Adeps lanae*

COMMON NAMES ■ Hog's fat, Lamb's wool fat

This is an important naturopathic remedy because naturopaths frequently compound ointments. They use *Adeps lanae* as a base.

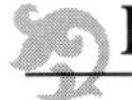

Beeswax

Beeswax is slightly antiseptic. Herbalists who compound their own ointments often use beeswax with cocoa butter as an ointment base.

Scrophularia nodosa

COMMON NAME ■ Figwort

The entire plant is used as medicine. *Scrophularia* contains the flavonoid diosmin. *Scrophularia* is a diuretic and an anodyne. When taken internally, it is also a blood purifier that is excellent for skin eruptions. It helps to expedite the rash. *Scrophularia* may be added to ointments and applied topically on skin eruptions, minor wounds, swellings, and glandular inflammations.

Scrophularia was used by Dr. Bastyr to treat eczema, psoriasis, and pruritus. For all of these conditions, he recommended 20 to 30 drops of tincture twice daily.

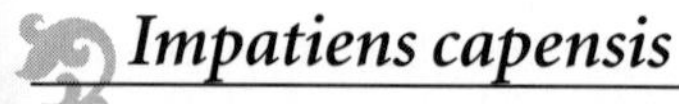

Impatiens capensis

COMMON NAME ■ Jewelweed

The whole fresh plant is used to make medicine. *Impatiens* contains the naphthoquinone lawsone. Use the fresh plant or ice cubes of the tea made from the fresh plant directly on poison ivy or poison oak.

Fumaria officinalis

COMMON NAME ■ Fumitory

The flowering herb is used to make medicine. This medicine is a depurative, an antispasmodic, a hypotensive, and a diuretic. At least 22 alkaloids have been found in fumitory thanks to the work of many fine researchers, especially the French chemist Forgacs.[158,159] Three of the alkaloids in fumitory are protopine, fumaritene, and a berberine-like alkaloid called aurotensine. Fumitory also contains the flavonoids quercetin and rutin.

Naturopaths and herbalists use fumitory internally and externally for skin diseases. Herbalists have suggested using a topical application of fumitory on scabies. When treating eczema or acne, use 30 drops of the tincture three times daily. The juice of the herb may be used as an eyewash. Fumitory helps to alleviate chronic constipation. By improving intestinal emptying, fumitory decreases the toxic load on the body, thereby improving the health of the skin.

Fumaria is a cholagogue. The resulting increase in the emulsification of fatty acids caused by increased bile and the cleansing of the liver caused by the flow of bile from the gallbladder help to improve the condition of the skin.

Aconitum napellus

COMMON NAME ■ Monkshood

The root is used to make medicine. This remedy has been used in liniments and ointments as an antibacterial and an anodyne. It is bacteriocidal against most staphylococcal and streptococcal microorganisms. It is important to prevent staphylococcal infections in skin lesions. Mix 1 tablespoon of *Aconitum* root powder in a 1-pound jar of ointment base. Apply this mixture twice daily to the affected area.

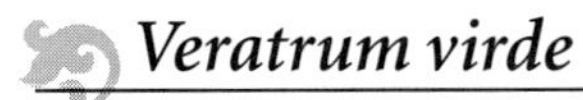

Veratrum virde

COMMON NAME ■ Green hellebore

The root and leaves are used to make medicine. *CAUTION: Do not use this remedy internally without full knowledge of its medicinal effects.* Externally, use *Veratrum* tincture on furunculosis, carbuncles, acneiform lesions, and erysipelas. I personally have no experience using this plant for these afflictions. Dr. Bastyr taught us to use *Veratrum* externally and internally for cellulitis to ease pain and facilitate resolution. The dose of the tincture for internal use is 1 to 5 drops twice daily. Externally, rub several drops into the skin one to two times daily.

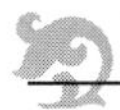

Vaccinium oxycoccus

COMMON NAME ■ Cranberry

Use the crushed berries to make medicine. Dr. Bastyr told us to apply fresh, crushed cranberries topically for severe dermatitis of the scalp. The treatment is a little messy but useful. When Dr. Bastyr talked about this remedy, he also mentioned using unsweetened cranberry tea to treat cystitis, whether caused by bacteria or yeast. He said to drink 1 cup of juice four times daily.

Cocculus indicus

COMMON NAME ■ Fishberry

CAUTION: This remedy is for external use only. The berries are used to make medicine, which is used topically for parasitic and fungal skin diseases. An ointment can be made by mixing 1 ounce of the crushed berries with 10 ounces of benzoinated lard. Apply to the skin twice daily. In telling us about the use of this botanical, Dr. Bastyr read to us from the eclectic herbals. I am not sure whether he used the remedy on any of his patients.

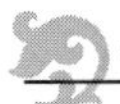

Sanguinaria canadensis

COMMON NAME ■ Bloodroot

The rhizome is used to make medicine. *Sanguinaria* is escharotic, meaning that it sloughs dead tissue from wounds. Dr. Bastyr taught its use for treating cervical erosion. Apply about 3 drops of the tincture to the cervix for this purpose. I have used *Sanguinaria* successfully in a number of patients who had cervical erosion. The root juice is antiseptic. Dr. Bastyr taught us to use *Sanguinaria* as a gargle for sore throat. He suggested 10 drops of tincture in a mouthful of water.

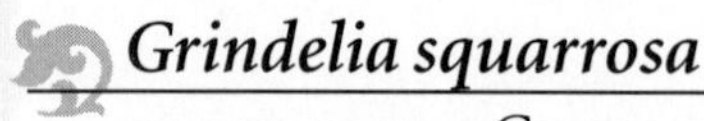

Grindelia squarrosa

COMMON NAME ■ Gumweed

The flowers and terminal leaves are used for medicine. *Grindelia* tincture may be applied to poison ivy or poison oak. I dispense 1 ounce of tincture and ask the patient to simply drip it on the lesion. When applied topically several times daily, *Grindelia* is a good fungicide. I have frequently relied on this tincture to treat nail fungus.

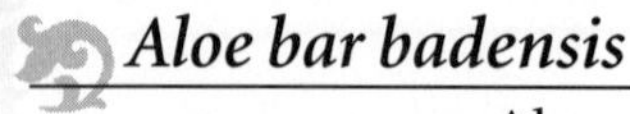

Aloe bar badensis

COMMON NAME ■ Aloe

The juice of the leaf is used to make medicine. *Aloe* juice is well known as a great topical vulnerary. *Aloe* is an excellent remedy for patients who have burns caused by sun or radiation therapy.[160] Dr. Bastyr taught us to apply the juice of the leaf directly on the skin. Herbalists commonly use *Aloe* in this way. Many herbalists that I have talked to have stories about the effectiveness of *Aloe* on radiation burns. *Aloe* may be applied to herpes blisters as an emollient to speed healing. *Aloe* is one of the best underarm deodorants available.[36] In addition, *Aloe* juice is effective when taken internally to soothe colitis. I have prescribed this remedy many times for this purpose. I suggest using about $\frac{1}{4}$ cup of the juice daily.

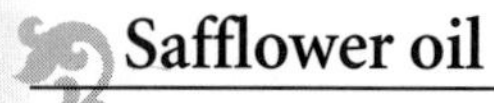

Safflower oil

COMMON NAME ■ Safflower

For sunburn, I add cod liver oil and vitamin E to 1 tablespoon of safflower oil and apply it daily to the burned area. It works wonderfully. It is healing and protective and decreases the duration of the pain from 3 or 4 days to 1. In addition to relieving pain, it helps to reduce damage caused by the sun.

Juglans cinerea

COMMON NAME ■ Butternut

The root is used to make medicine. To treat eczema, herpes, impetigo, pruritus, pemphigus, and chronic scaly skin, make a fresh infusion of *Juglans* and apply it locally. Eclectics, naturopaths, and herbalists also use *Juglans* internally as a liver medicine. Naturopathic physicians believe that helping the liver improves the quality of the blood. This in turn improves the health of the skin. The dose is 1 to 20 drops of the tincture three times daily.

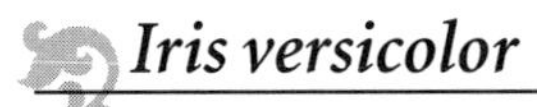

Iris versicolor

COMMON NAME ■ Iris

The root is used to make medicine. *Iris* is one of the ingredients in Dr. Fox's skin cancer liniment. His formula is a mixture of 2 ounces of *Iris* and 1 ounce each of the tinctures of *Trifolium* and *Sanguinaria*. Apply to the affected area. Cover with plastic wrap to retain moisture. This can be left on for up to 4 hours. I apologize for the obscurity of Dr. Fox; for the life of me I cannot remember who he is.

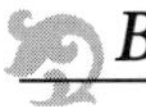

Berberis aquifolium

COMMON NAME ■ Oregon grape

The root is used to make medicine. I use a tincture of *Berberis* for treating acne and other skin lesions. I suggest a dose of 30 drops of the tincture three times daily.

In addition to using *Berberis*, I modify the diet and supplement with zinc. *Berberis* works by clearing and cleaning the intestine. Patients tell me that they have more bowel movements when taking *Berberis*. Improving and encouraging intestinal emptying decreases the toxic load on the body, thereby improving the health of the skin. This remedy is also used to treat psoriasis. Psoriasis is difficult to treat. There seems to be no single-remedy answer. *Berberis* is not the answer to psoriasis, but it is a helpful tool.

Arctium lappa

COMMON NAME ■ Burdock

The root is used to make medicine. To help resolve boils and abscesses, macerate and apply *Arctium* topically. Dr. Bastyr said that *Arctium* is one of the better medicines to treat dermatitis of the dry variety, where the skin may be scaly or there may be dry, cracked eczema. He suggested 40 drops twice daily. In addition, *Arctium* can be used to treat psoriasis. I mix *Arctium* and *Momordica charantia* for the treatment of psoriasis. The *Momordica* blocks guanylate cyclase, which helps to decrease the production of hyperproliferative cyclic nucleotides. This sounds good in theory, but in practice, *Momordica* is not as effective as I would like.

Arctium helps improve digestion. Eclectics and herbalists have frequently used it as an alterative in skin diseases and for rheumatism and gout. The dose is 20 to 40 drops of tincture several times daily. A poultice of *Arctium* can be put on cradle cap. Olive oil also often works for cradle cap. Apply topically.

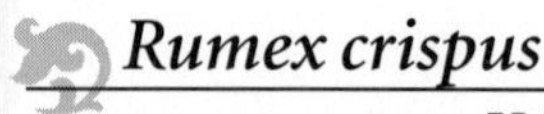

Rumex crispus

COMMON NAME ■ Yellow dock

The leaves are used for medicine. *Rumex* contains anthraquinone glycosides. Naturopaths and herbalists use *Rumex* for both acute and chronic skin problems. *Rumex* is beneficial to the liver, through which it has a positive influence on the skin. I use *Rumex* tincture in combination with other remedies to treat eczema. Herbalists apply the crushed leaves of *Rumex* topically to allay the discomfort of stinging nettle exposure. This is probably the most famous use for *Rumex*. For the treatment of ulcerative stomatitis, have the patient chew a piece of the leaf into a wet bolus and apply it to the mouth sore. For patients with pruritus, I have used 60 drops of *Rumex* tincture twice daily. I like to use the dried herb in 500-mg capsules twice daily to treat anemia.

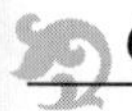

Citrus limon

COMMON NAME ■ Lemon

Use the juice of the fruit to make medicine. Dr. Bastyr commented that lemon juice can be used as a mouthwash three times daily for Vincent's angina. A pulpy mass of whole lemon may be applied to warts and held on with a bandage at night during sleep. This is an old folk remedy.

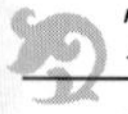

Thuja occidentalis

COMMON NAME ■ Yellow cedar

I have instructed patients to use the oil of *Thuja* on verrucae. Dr. Bastyr taught us to use homeopathic *Thuja* to treat genital condylomata. He suggested a 200X potency taken once weekly. *Thuja* is one of the ingredients in the uterine-depleting pack because it is effective against bacteria, viruses, and yeast. The depleting pack is a tampon that is soaked in a premixed solution of glycerine, Epsom salts, *Thuja* oil, bitter orange oil, and an eschloretic called VM 120. The tampon is then inserted vaginally against the cervix. It can be used to treat cervicitis and vaginitis. I have used this pack successfully for many patients with abnormal Papanicolaou tests. I recommend using one uterine pack weekly for 8 weeks.

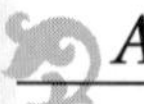

Anagallis arvensis

COMMON NAME ■ Scarlet pimpernel

Herbalists recommend using *Anagallis* for soothing nettle and poison ivy rash. Apply the tincture topically three times daily, or as needed. The tea is a diuretic. The dose is a standard cup of tea daily. For melancholy, use the tea in combination with large doses of B complex and an additional 50 mg of vitamin B_6.

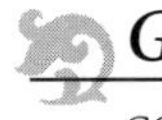

Galanthus nivalis

COMMON NAME ■ Snowdrop

Externally, this medicine is applied as a poultice to treat frostbite and chilblains. The medicine is made from 3 to 4 crushed bulbs per $\frac{1}{2}$ pint of water and applied topically.

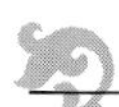

Chlorophyll

Liquid solutions of chlorophyll can be used to treat pyorrhea, nasal inflammations, throat infections, periodontal problems, external ulcers, and decubitus ulcers. Dr. Bastyr recommended a douche of chlorophyll and vinegar for yeast infections and vaginitis. He said to add 5 tablespoons of chlorophyll and 1 tablespoon of vinegar to 1 cup of water. Chlorophyll may be used as a toothpaste, mixing it with avocado. The avocado contains lectins that help prevent tooth decay.

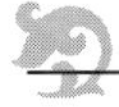

Kalmia angustifolia

COMMON NAME ■ Sheep laurel

Kalmia may be applied locally for pest infestation and/or itching dermatitis. Dr. Bastyr said, "It smarts, but it cures well." Internally, the tincture may be taken in doses of 5 drops to allay myalgia and bursitis.

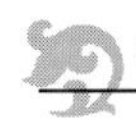

Citrus bergamia

COMMON NAME ■ Bergamot orange

The oil is used in Earl Grey tea. Bergamot oil was included in my original notes from Dr. Bastyr's lectures. I assume that the following application for psoriasis was a treatment that he used. The oil may be applied to psoriasis and followed with $\frac{1}{2}$-hour exposure to the sun or to a sunlamp. Bergamot orange tends to sensitize the skin and is very effective against psoriasis. Beware of sunburn caused by photosensitization.

Smilax species

COMMON NAME ■ Sarsaparilla

The root is used to make medicine. *Smilax* is useful in treating psoriasis[161] and eczema. However, don't bet the farm on the effectiveness of *Smilax* in the treatment of psoriasis. *Momordica* and *Smilax* are useful plants in the treatment of psoriatic eczema, but these medicinals need to be used in conjunction with a total program of gut and liver tonification and hygiene and, as Dr. Bastyr would tell you, plenty of water.

Smilax contains about 2% steroid saponins, which tend to bind to endotoxins in the alimentary canal.[162] This decreases general complement levels, which lowers the inflammatory milieu in the body as a whole. *Smilax* contains the steroid sapogenin, sarsasapogenin. In the 19th century, herbalists used *Smilax* to treat arthritis and gout. The French physician Monardes wrote about the use of *Smilax* for syphilis, as did the Chinese.[163] I personally have never used *Smilax* for this purpose. It is possible that the steroids serve as precursors to some of the hormones and in so doing serve as a tonic to the endocrine system. The dose of *Smilax* extract is 150 drops three times daily. *Smilax* has also been touted as a fertility and steroid enhancer. The sarsasapogenin saponin may be converted to other steroid molecules in the body, but as far as I know, this has not been proven.

Ammi majus

COMMON NAME ■ Bishop's weed

The ancient Egyptians used this plant to treat what we now call vitiligo. The Egyptian method was to give 4 to 6 grams of powdered *Ammi majus* per day. The fluid preparation, or tincture, was applied locally. This was reported to be effective. Given the difficulty of treating this problem, it is worth trying. I have no experience with this plant as yet.

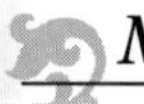

Melaleuca alternifolia

COMMON NAME ■ Tea tree

The leaves are used to make medicine. I have found that tea tree is nothing short of amazing when applied topically to burns. It is fabulous for this purpose. Also, tea tree is useful in the treatment of eczema of the hands. I suggest that the patient apply the ointment at bedtime. An improvement is often noticeable by morning.

Fragaria virginiana

COMMON NAME ■ Wild strawberry

The whole plant is used to make medicine. *Fragaria* has been used for eczema and acne both as an internal and an external medicine. For patients with acne, I combine equal parts of the tinctures of *Frageria* and *Berberis aquifolium* and give 30 drops of this mixture four times daily. I also give the patient 50 to 100 mg of zinc per day.

CHAPTER

67

SPLEEN REMEDIES

CHAPTER • OUTLINE

This group of remedies benefits the spleen. These remedies are used especially when there is splenic congestion or enlargement.

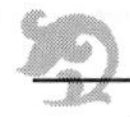

Iris versicolor

COMMON NAME ■ Blue flag, Iris

The dried rhizome is used to make medicine. *Iris* contains several triterpenoids including iriversical, which is the chief constituent of the plant.[164,165] Dr. Bastyr pointed out that *Iris* acts similarly to *Phytolacca* in treating congestion and fullness of the lymphatics and spleen. *Iris* is also a good liver remedy. I use 1 to 20 drops of tincture three times daily for congestion of the lymphatics and spleen. The powdered dose is 3 to 15 grains twice daily.

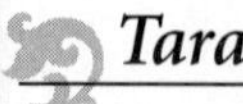

Taraxacum officinale

COMMON NAME ■ Dandelion

The root is used to make medicine. Dandelion contains a number of terpenes such as stigmasterol, beta-sitosterol, and cycloartenol. It also contains the coumarins scopoletin and esculetin.[20,166]

This plant is used to treat enlargement of both the liver and the spleen. Dr. Bastyr emphasized its use as an alterative in chronic splenomegaly. He probably combined it with *Ceanothus,* which was his favorite spleen remedy. For this purpose, combine equal parts of each and give 30 drops of the mixture two to three times daily.

Polymnia uvedalia

COMMON NAME ■ Bearsfoot

The root is used to make medicine. This medicine is an alterative and a lymphatic stimulant. Dr. Bastyr used *Polymnia* to treat organomegaly, especially of the spleen. In spleen disorders, use *Polymnia* internally at a dose of 10 drops of tincture three times daily. For splenomegaly, Dr. Bastyr told us that either a tincture or an infusion of *Polymnia* could be used on a cotton cloth to create a pack. This pack is then placed over the spleen. He also suggested combining equal parts of *Polymnia* with *Ceanothus* for splenomegaly. I have used this combination in my practice and have been very impressed with the results. I prescribe 60 drops of the tincture combination twice daily for splenomegaly.

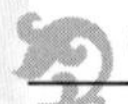

Ceanothus americanus

COMMON NAME ■ New Jersey tea

The bark of the root is used to make medicine. *Ceanothus* does not have a strong flavor; however, the astringency of this plant is immediately apparent when you put the tincture on your tongue. *Ceanothus* contains ceanothic acid, also called emmolic acid, some cyclic alkaloids, and a number of triterpenes.

Use *Ceanothus* for pain in the liver or spleen. *Ceanothus* is an excellent remedy for splenomegaly. I have been astounded by its effectiveness in treating this condition. Dr. Bastyr mentioned its use in splenomegaly associated with hemolytic anemia. I have also used it to good effect for treating splenomegaly associated with lymphatic cancers. It is impressive in treatment of lymphatic leukemia. Dr. Bastyr used it to treat mononucleosis when the patient had splenic tenderness. He and other naturopaths have used 30 drops of the tincture three times daily in a glass of water. If bacterial infection is present, I combine *Ceanothus* with *Hydrastis.* I use 20 drops of *Ceanothus* and 30 drops of *Hydrastis* together four times daily.

Phyllitis scolopendrium

COMMON NAME ■ Hart's tongue fern

The dried leaves are used to make medicine. Naturopaths and herbalists use *Phyllitis* to treat mucous colitis, disorders of the spleen, and splenomegaly in blood dyscrasia. Blood dyscrasia refers to any disorder of the blood. Disorders of the blood can mean pooling of the blood in various tissues, bruising, or frank septicemia. The dose of *Phyllitis* is 30 drops of tincture twice daily. In cases of septicemia, I also use 40 drops of *Echinacea* tincture per hour.

Berberis vulgaris

COMMON NAME ■ Barberry

The dried root is used to make medicine. When Dr. Bastyr talked about *Berberis*, he said that it is tonic to the spleen, causing splenic contractions. I've never been exactly sure what he meant by splenic contractions. This information is presented because Dr. Bastyr mentioned it. *Berberis* is useful in treating gallstones. Historically, eclectic physicians used *Berberis* to treat tuberculosis. The dose for all of these conditions is 30 drops four times daily.

Quercus alba

COMMON NAME ■ White oak

The acorn kernels are used to make medicine. The distilled tincture of white oak acorn kernels has been used by herbalists for chronic spleen affections and spleen dropsy. Use 10 drops of the tincture four times daily. We also use a 2X or 3X homeopathic potency. *Quercus* is astringent. It contains a number of tannins consisting of gallic, ellagic, and catechin tannins.[167] Dr. Bastyr taught us to crush acorn kernels that have been soaked in water overnight. The resulting solution was to be strained and the liquid portion used as a douche in atony of the uterus and vagina with recurrent vaginitis. This is great herbalism and should be thought of even in modern medicine as an adjunctive therapy to antibiotics for recurrent vaginitis.

CHAPTER

68

STIMULANTS (MILD)

CHAPTER • OUTLINE

Capsicum frutescens
Zanthoxylum americanum
Avena sativa
Theobroma cacao
Cinnamomum camphora
Commiphora molmol
Sassafras albidum
Panax quinquefolius
Zingiber officinale
Centella asiatica

Mild stimulants excite or quicken the activity of physiologic processes. Many physicians think of stimulants as working through the central nervous system. Naturopaths think differently. We believe that stimulating any of the major body functions will have an effect on the mind. For example, stimulating liver function will improve overall digestion. With improvement in digestion, the mind and body are less sluggish because they no longer have to deal with heavy, poorly digested meals. The mind can then function better. Hippocrates covered this concept in his tract *Ancient Medicine.* This kind of integrative thinking is the heart and soul of the naturopathic philosophy.

Capsicum frutescens

COMMON NAME ■ Red pepper

The fruit is used to make medicine. Think of *Capsicum* as an excellent systemic stimulant. If the patient is unable to tolerate the tincture, *Capsicum* capsules may be used as a general systemic stimulant. *Capsicum* combines well with most other stimulants and may have a synergistic effect. Many of the early naturopaths spoke of plants that were frequently added to remedies as synergists. *Capsicum* was one of the plants commonly mentioned for this purpose. I remember William Turska talking about this plant as a synergist. He also spoke about aconite, *Bryonia, Gelsemium*, and *Phytolacca* as what he called endocrinologic synergists.

Capsicum tends to produce vasodilation. It has been used after strokes. Dr. Bastyr also used *Capsicum* for atonic dyspepsia. The dose he suggested was 1 to 60 drops of tincture. It has been used historically to treat lethargy, alopecia, muscle spasms, and cold feet. Dr. Bastyr recommended putting *Capsicum* powder in the socks of patients complaining of cold feet to help keep their feet warm at night. For chilblains, use it locally.

Capsicum depletes substance P, which decreases pain if it is used daily for 2 weeks or longer. For example, it can decrease pain in the treatment of mouth sores resulting from chemotherapy. *Capsicum* contains carotenes that have antioxidant properties. The pungent principle in *Capsicum* is capsaicin, which is found in many species of *Capsicum*.

Zanthoxylum americanum

COMMON NAME ■ Northern prickly ash

The bark and fruit are used to make medicine. Prickly ash is a stimulant tonic. It increases cardiac action, stimulates digestive juices, increases salivation, and decreases tympanitis. Dr. Bastyr recommended a dose of 10 to 30 drops of tincture four times daily. To stimulate salivation, I mix 20 parts of prickly ash tincture with one part pilocarpine tincture. The dose is 40 drops of the tincture mixture twice daily. Dr. Bastyr said that this plant helps to overcome constipation by stimulating the alimentary tract. It is also restorative after diarrhea.

Avena sativa

COMMON NAME ■ Oats

The green head of the oat is used to make medicine. *Avena* treats neurasthenia and aids in convalescence. It contains a number of steroid saponins and sterols. I can't help but think that these compounds are somehow involved in *Avena*'s medicinal actions.

Dr. Bastyr told us to use *Avena.* He suggested that we give it to patients to help them kick habitual drug use. For this purpose, you may use *Avena* alone or combine it with equal parts of *Eleutherococcus.* The dose I recommend of the combined remedy is 60 drops of tincture four times daily. If you are using *Avena* only, use the same dose.

Dr. Bastyr taught us that *Avena* serves well in the treatment of wasting disease from nerve paralysis. The dose for this purpose is two 400-mg capsules of powdered *Avena* three times daily. For a footbath for tired feet, put $\frac{1}{2}$ cup of oats in 2 gallons of hot water and soak. Oats is also used as a local wash for skin diseases. Mix 90 drops of *Avena* tincture in $\frac{1}{8}$ cup water and dab the solution onto the diseased skin.

Theobroma cacao

COMMON NAME ■ Chocolate

The seed is used. This plant contains theobromine and caffeine. Dr. Bastyr taught that chocolate is a mild nervous system stimulant because of its caffeine content. The flavonoid content in chocolate is actually fairly high. Small amounts of chocolate as a stimulant and antioxidant can be prescribed safely. In my opinion, semisweet dark chocolate is the best.

Cinnamomum camphora

COMMON NAME ■ Camphor

The oil extracted from the tree is used to make medicine. Camphor is a rubefacient and a stimulant. Eclectics and herbalists have suggested using 1 teaspoon of camphor in 1 pint of water to be taken internally in doses of 1 dram as a stimulating diaphoretic and expectorant in the treatment of asthma and bronchitis to control hypersecretion. Rub the oil in locally to treat sore muscles. Camphorated oil can be rubbed on the chest to help with bronchial congestion. The inhalation of camphor and eucalyptus clears the sinuses.

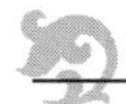

Commiphora molmol

COMMON NAME ■ Myrrh

The gum resin is used. Myrrh contains a number of furanosesquiterpenes. Furanoeudesma-1,3-diene is one of many furanogermacranes. Their derivatives have also been identified, including 2-methoxyfuranodiene.[20,168,169] Myrrh is a mild stimulant to the nervous system. According to Dr. Bastyr, myrrh increases the rate and power of the heartbeat. Internally, a dose of 10 to 30 drops of tincture can be taken twice daily.

This plant provides an astringent for use in mouthwashes. Herbalists back to the ancient Egyptians used myrrh to treat stomatitis, pharyngitis, tonsillitis, and toothache. The gum resin can be applied locally. For mastoiditis, use 4 drops each of myrrh, *Echinacea*, and mullein inserted with a syringe.

Sassafras albidum

COMMON NAME ■ Red sassafras

The bark is used to make medicine. This is a stimulant, a diaphoretic, and an estrogen precursor. I use *Sassafras* in respiratory formulas as a respiratory stimulant. If using *Sassafras* alone, I suggest 10 to 20 drops of the tincture three times daily for up to 2 weeks. Dr. Bastyr used it as a diaphoretic. His dose was 60 drops in 1 cup of hot water. One of its constituents, safrole, shows evidence of being carcinogenic in large doses.[170] When the plant is used for a short period of time for a specific problem, we have always believed that it was safe.

Panax quinquefolius

COMMON NAME ■ American ginseng

One may also find this under the name *Panax ginseng*. The root is used to make medicine. The active constituents in ginseng include the steroids panaxadiol and panaxatriol.[42]

Ginseng is a reliable mild stimulant. The standard tea may be taken on alternate days, interspersing the schedule with other stimulants. The reason it is used on alternate days is that back when Dr. Bastyr was teaching us about this remedy, he told us that he had heard that Chinese medicine texts recommended that ginseng not be used continuously. I use 90 drops a day for 2 weeks at a time for adrenal tonification. I mix equal parts of ginseng and licorice root as a stimulant. The dose I suggest is 90 drops of the combination per day at lunchtime for 2 weeks. Rest for 1 week, and then repeat this dose.

Zingiber officinale

COMMON NAME ■ Ginger

The root is used for medicine. *Zingiber* is a systemic stimulant. It warms the stomach and stimulates digestion. It is positively inotropic, meaning that it increases the strength of muscular contraction.[25] I suggest two capsules per meal as a mild digestive stimulant. *Zingiber* also stimulates the bowel. Dr. Bastyr taught that the tea benefits a hypotonic bowel. Take 30 drops of *Zingiber* root three times daily. It has been used in marasmus as a stimulator of appetite. Similarly, it is useful in anorexia.

Although *Zingiber* is a stimulant, it does not produce hyperactivity or frenzied activity. It is a good anxiolytic that acts like Valium (diazepam). I use it to wean patients from Valium. Like Valium, it acts on the benzodiazepam receptor sites. Dr. Ellingwood makes an interesting comment in his discussion of *Zingiber*. He says that if *Zingiber* is given at the beginning of a hysterical attack, it will often abort the attack. *Zingiber*'s action on benzodiazepam receptors is its probable modus operandi in this case. For hysteria, excessive anxiety, and panic attacks, have the patient take three capsules three times daily. Once the condition is stable, the dose should be decreased.

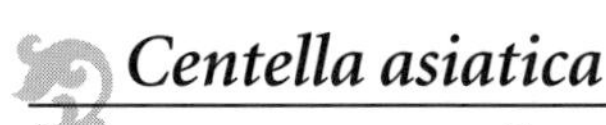

Centella asiatica

COMMON NAME ■ Gotu kola

The aerial parts are used to make medicine. Gotu kola is a mental stimulant. For thousands of years Buddhist monks have used this plant to improve their ability to attain cosmic information during their meditations. You can feel the activity of gotu kola in the brain. When I meditate, I take 10 drops of tincture.

In the 1970s, researchers in an article in the *Indian Journal of Psychiatry* noted that disabled children who were given gotu kola showed improved mental abilities.[171] I often use gotu kola alone or in combination with *Ginkgo*.

CHAPTER

69

STIMULANTS (STRONG)

CHAPTER • OUTLINE

Strychnos nux-vomica
Strychnos ignatii
Cocculus indicus
Erythroxylon coca
Coffea arabica
Physostigma venenosum
Abrus precatorius
Amyl nitrite
Phoradendron flavescens
Cicuta maculata
Yerba mate

The strong stimulants stimulate the nervous system more aggressively than the mild stimulants. One must pay close attention to the dose of these remedies because some of them are toxic if used too liberally.

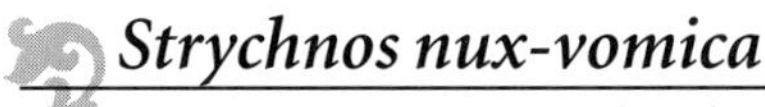

Strychnos nux-vomica

COMMON NAMES ■ Quaker buttons, Poison nut

The nut of the plant is used to make medicine. *CAUTION:* S. nux-vomica *is extremely toxic. No more than 1 or 2 drops should be given in a single dose.* This plant stimulates the smooth muscles of the gastrointestinal tract. Dr. Bastyr taught us to use either 1 drop of tincture or *S. nux-vomica* 2X to 3X twice daily. It is a bitter tonic and stimulant to digestion. To treat the effects of overindulgence of food or alcohol, use a 3X or 6X. In problems of paralysis or partial paralysis, it is a stimulant to the nervous system.

I talked to Dr. William Turska about using this plant as a synergist with other nervous system and digestive system stimulants. Dr. Turska agreed that this is a good use for it. I sometimes add 25 drops of *S. nux-vomica* tincture to a 1-ounce dropper bottle of either ginger root tincture, eleutherococcus, or ginseng, among many other possibilities, to increase the force of action of these other remedies.

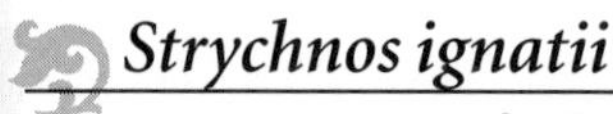

Strychnos ignatii

COMMON NAME ■ St. Ignatius bean

Medicine is made from the seeds and the dried root bark. *Strychnos* is a neuromuscular tonic and stimulant. It is similar in action to *S. nux-vomica,* only it is milder. Like *S. nux-vomica, Strychnos* contains indole alkaloids, chiefly strychnine. Dr. Bastyr used *Strychnos* homeopathically for globus hystericus. In addition, *Strychnos* increases the fatigue threshold and increases auditory acuity. It temporarily improves cardiac action and intestinal peristalsis. The dose of the powder is $\frac{1}{2}$ to 1 grain daily. The dose of the tincture is 5 to 10 drops daily.

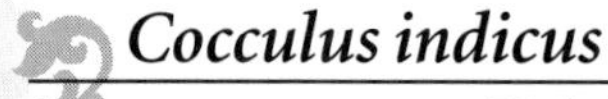

Cocculus indicus

COMMON NAME ■ Fish berry

Also look for this remedy under the name *Amanita occulus.* The seeds, which contain picrotoxin, are used to make medicine. Dr. Bastyr commented that *Cocculus* is a long-lasting respiratory stimulant and diaphoretic. It tends to stimulate secretions and is eliminated through the kidneys and the skin. Dr. Bastyr suggested a tincture dose of 1 to 10 drops twice daily. For headaches use *Cocculus* as a homeopathic. For debility of the nervous system, use it internally.

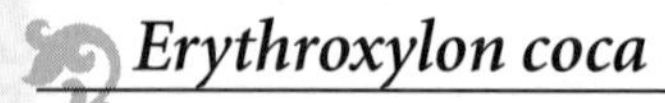

Erythroxylon coca

COMMON NAME ■ Cocaine

One may also use *Erythroxylon truxillense.* The leaves are used to make medicine. A small dose of cocaine is a cerebral, cardiac, and respiratory stimulant. Dr. Bastyr taught that we could use 2X. Peruvian Indians chew cocaine to sustain themselves during hard physical work. As a local anesthetic, a 2% to 4% solution is used topically. When using cocaine as an anesthetic, the dose is not to exceed 0.03 gram, or $\frac{1}{2}$ grain, of cocaine hydrochloride. Cocaine reduces hunger. Historically, a 5% solution of cocaine has been found helpful when applied to poison ivy. I wonder whether anyone having a 5% solution of coca would ever use it on poison ivy. Because cocaine is currently illegal, it must not be used. However, historically it was used by eclectic physicians.

Coffea arabica

COMMON NAME ■ Coffee

The bean is used to make medicine. Coffee contains the alkaloid caffeine. It is a general neural stimulant and diuretic. For many decades naturopaths have used coffee enemas to detoxify the liver. Coffee is also an adrenal stimulant. I prescribe 1 cup of coffee, about 100 to 150 mg of caffeine, as a stimulant as needed. It is very easy to abuse the use of coffee as a source of false energy. I advise against the overuse of coffee. In cases where neck pain is associated with tight neck muscles, particularly the levator scapulae, and in cases where there is low back pain, elimination of coffee is particularly effective.

Coffee is an antidote to central nervous system depressant poisons. The caffeine content of a cup of coffee generally ranges from 100 to 150 mg per cup. It reaches peak plasma level in about 1 hour. It should be cautioned that coffee contributes to an imbalance of insulin and is a mild hyperglycemic. It might be wise to help diabetics wean off of coffee. Coffee is mildly addicting and can disturb the electrolyte balance, creating cardiac dysrhythmia.

Physostigma venenosum

COMMON NAMES ■ Calabar bean, Ordeal bean

The medicine comes from the seeds. The principal ingredient of calabar bean is the indole alkaloid, physostigmine, which is a parasympathomimetic.

In small doses, *Physostigma* stimulates the intestinal and bladder musculature. This medicine accelerates intestinal secretions by stimulating the nervous system. The dose is 1 to 5 drops of the tincture twice daily. It may be used for elderly patients at a 3X potency to tone the bladder. Dr. Bastyr recommended a 6X to 12X potency in the treatment of myasthenia gravis. In the annals of medical history, a 0.25% ointment has been used medically to treat glaucoma.

Abrus precatorius

COMMON NAME ■ Jequirty

The seeds are used to make medicine. *CAUTION: One seed can kill a child, two seeds can kill an adult. This plant is always used in potency.* This plant contains abrin, which is a toxic lectin and hemagglutinin. Dr. Bastyr used a 3X homeopathic preparation as a gastrointestinal stimulant. Dr. Bastyr taught us that a dilute fluid may be used in the eye for conjunctivitis. I have never tried this so I cannot comment about its effectiveness.

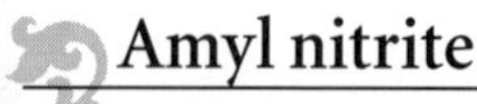

Amyl nitrite

COMMON NAME ■ Smelling salts

This compound dilates the coronary arteries either as smelling salts or internally at a dose of 3 to 5 drops. It can be used to rouse a person who has fainted. Dr. Bastyr used a 6X homeopathic remedy for climacteric flushes.

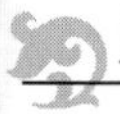

Phoradendron flavescens

COMMON NAME ■ American mistletoe

The whole aerial part of the plant is used to make medicine. This is a powerful smooth muscle stimulant. It increases the blood pressure and increases intestinal peristalsis. Dr. Bastyr taught its use as a uterine stimulant. It has been used to treat amenorrhea. The tincture dose he recommended is 2 drops four times daily.

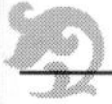

Cicuta maculata

COMMON NAME ■ Water hemlock

The root is used. *CAUTION: This is a powerful central nervous system stimulant. Eating even a small portion of the root of this plant can result in convulsions and, frequently, death.* As a central nervous system stimulant, Dr. Bastyr used 2X sublingually four times daily.

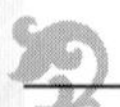

Yerba mate

The leaves are used to make medicine. The tea is a stimulant. I recommend 1 cup of the standard tea daily.

CHAPTER

70

STOMACH REMEDIES

CHAPTER • OUTLINE

Anthemis nobiles
Angelica archangelica

This list includes remedies that affect the stomach in particular. It includes remedies that stimulate digestion, reduce hyperactivity, and tonify and nourish the tissues that line the stomach. In some cases, these remedies also affect the nervous supply to the stomach or the stomach musculature. Several of these remedies also influence appetite.

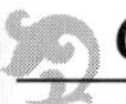

Collinsonia canadensis

COMMON NAME ■ Stone root

The whole plant is used. This remedy is a stomachic and is astringent to mucous membranes. *Collinsonia* stimulates gastric secretions and tonifies venous walls. At a dose of 15 to 20 drops of the tincture, *Collinsonia* is actively tonic to the stomach. I combine *Collinsonia* with *Taraxacum* to stimulate stomach secretions in geriatric patients.

Dr. Bastyr used *Collinsonia* for clergyman's throat. It was mentioned in my notes from Dr. Bastyr's lectures that *Collinsonia* is useful in treating contorted uterine veins. I have not used *Collinsonia* in this way. Nevertheless, it is an interesting therapy that was probably used long ago.

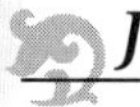

Jateorrhiza palmata

COMMON NAME ■ Columbo root

The root is used to make medicine. Columbo root contains the isoquinoline alkaloid jateorrhizine. It is a stomachic and a bitter tonic.

Columbo root increases salivary and gastric secretions. I prescribe 20 drops of the tincture twice daily at meal times to stimulate stomach secretions. Eclectics and herbalists use columbo root to treat both the morning sickness of pregnancy and seasickness. For these conditions, a standard tea should be sipped. Dr. Bastyr said that a cold infusion should be the preparation method of choice.

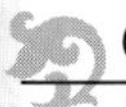

Gentiana lutea

COMMON NAME ■ Yellow gentian

The root is used to make medicine. This remedy is an antiperiodic and is a substitute for quinine. *Gentiana* is our most valuable bitter tonic. Dr. Bastyr touted *Gentiana* to increase the stomach's secretion of hydrochloric acid. For this purpose, it may also be combined with wormwood. Two double-ought capsules of *Gentiana* and wormwood are used in combination before meals. This remedy helps to control gout by decreasing uric acid levels.

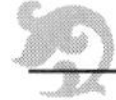

Eupatorium perfoliatum

COMMON NAME ■ Boneset

The flowering tops and leaves are used to make medicine. *CAUTION: Large doses of* Eupatorium *are emetic. Eupatorium* tincture is a stomachic at a dose of 5 to 60 drops.

Eupatorium is a stimulating tonic. Eclectics and herbalists have used a cold tea twice daily or 10 drops of tincture in 1 cup of cold water for this purpose. Dr. Bastyr mentioned that this tea is helpful for people who regurgitate all of their food. I cannot recall the details of this discussion or how to use *Eupatorium* for this purpose, but it is included for historical purposes. *Eupatorium* may be used for dyspepsia and is antibacterial against *Staphylococcus aureus* and *Escherichia coli.*

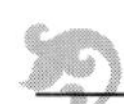

Lycopodium clavatum

COMMON NAME ■ Club moss

The dried stigma is used to make medicine. Club moss contains the alkaloid lycopodine.[172] Dr. Bastyr used this plant for dyspepsia caused by fermentation in the stomach. He used doses of 5 drops of the tincture twice daily for this purpose. In addition, Dr. Bastyr taught that powdered *Lycopodium* could be used as a hemostatic in nosebleeds.

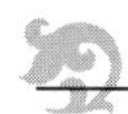

Crocus sativa

COMMON NAME ■ Autumn crocus

The dried stigmata are used to make medicine. This is a very mild antiinflammatory to the stomach. I recommend 15 drops of tincture per meal. In eclectic literature, *Crocus* evidently checks mild cases of uterine hemorrhage, but I have no experience with this particular usage of *Crocus.*

Quassia excelsa

COMMON NAME ■ Quassia

One may also use *Quassia amara.* The wood and bark are used to make medicine. This medicine is a very bitter tonic and a stomachic. The bitter principle is quassin. Take 10 drops twice daily as a bitter tonic.

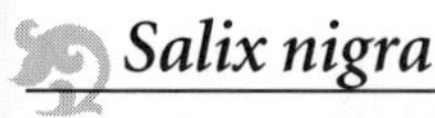

Salix nigra

COMMON NAME ■ Black willow

The bark is used to make medicine. This medicine is an astringent, a stomachic, an antiperiodic, and an antirheumatic. Although some of the old eclectics considered *Salix* a stomachic, the presence of salicylates in this plant may contraindicate it for some, especially those with a history of ulcers. I use *Salix* frequently and have yet to see any ulcer problems result. The dose I use is 30 drops of tincture twice daily. Dr. Bastyr recommended 30 drops of the tincture twice daily as an antirheumatic. In addition, he treated proctitis by using a tea as an enema. Herbalists have used it in a douche to treat infections caused by *Trichomonas.*

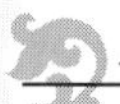

Rhus glabra

COMMON NAME ■ Smooth sumac

The whole plant is used to make medicine. Eclectic physicians and herbalists described *Rhus* as an astringent, an antiseptic, and an antidiarrheal. It has been used to treat mucous colitis, prolonged diarrhea, and stomatitis and has been used as a gargle to treat pharyngitis. The dose of the tincture is 10 to 30 drops. I remember Dr. Bastyr talking about *Rhus* for prolonged diarrhea. His dose recommendation of the tincture was 30 drops twice daily.

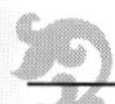

Cornus florida

COMMON NAME ■ Flowering dogwood

The bark of the root is used to make medicine. *Cornus* contains a number of steroid saponins, including sarsapogenin.

Cornus increases appetite and assists in the removal of catabolic wastes, especially in combination with other alteratives. This plant medicine is a mild alterative and an antiperiodic. Using it as an antiperiodic, Dr. Bastyr taught that it is a substitute for quinine. His dose recommendation was 30 drops of the tincture three times daily. In class, we discussed taking *Cornus* prophylactically during trips to the tropics. Dr. Bastyr thought that was a fine idea.

Frasera canadensis

COMMON NAME ■ American columbo

The root is used to make medicine. This plant is a bitter stomachic, a laxative, an astringent, and an antidiarrheal. Dr. Bastyr used *Frasera* to treat dysentery and catarrhal gastritis. He mentioned that a curious symptom that may respond to *Frasera* is a sense of fullness in the stomach even though little food has been consumed. The dose is variable. I recommend trying 10 drops of the tincture several times daily.

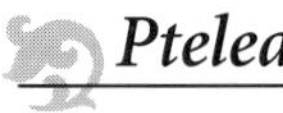

Ptelea trifoliata

COMMON NAME ■ Shrubby trefoil

The bark and root are used to make medicine. *Ptelea* contains a number of furoquinoline alkaloids and furocoumarins. Evidently, the alkaloid ptelea-tinium chloride is effective against *Mycobacterium tuberculosis.*[25] Eclectics used *Ptelea* in dyspepsia. They also used this plant medicine as a diaphoretic, an astringent, and a mild tonic to promote appetite. The tincture is used in doses of 1 to 30 drops.

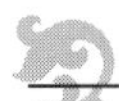

Piper nigrum

COMMON NAME ■ Black pepper

Use the unripe berries for medicine. *Piper* is a mild stomachic, an irritant, a stimulant, and a condiment. It is also a liver medicine with a potency about half as efficient as milkthistle. It may be sprinkled on food to stimulate gastric secretions. I suggest using $\frac{1}{4}$ teaspoon per meal.

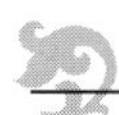

Alnus serrulata

COMMON NAME ■ Tag alder

The leaves and bark are used to make medicine. This is a tonic, an emollient, and an astringent. It can be used for excess mucous secretions of the stomach and gastrointestinal tract. The dose is 1 cup of standard tea twice daily. Dr. Bastyr told us to have our patients put the leaves of *Alnus* in their shoes to relieve sore, aching feet. A standard tea can be used as a gargle for sore throat.

Asarum canadensis

COMMON NAME ■ Wild ginger

Use the root for medicine. Wild ginger is a good mild stimulant and a carminative and may be used for bloating. Take 60 drops of the tincture twice daily to improve digestion. To treat colitis, Dr. Bastyr recommended a combination of equal parts of wild ginger, *Hydrastis*, and *Geranium*.

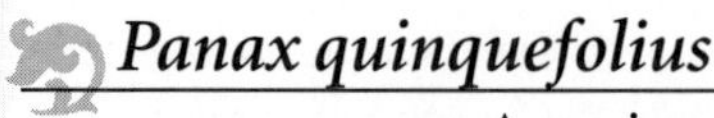

Panax quinquefolius

COMMON NAME ■ American ginseng

The root is used to make medicine. This is a stomachic and a stimulant. It is used to treat debility, polyuria, poor memory, fatigue, orthostatic hypotension, and the inability to handle stress. Dr. Bastyr underscored its importance in the treatment of orthostatic hypotension. It may help to increase sperm count. For all of these conditions, Dr. Bastyr taught a dose of 30 drops of tincture twice daily.

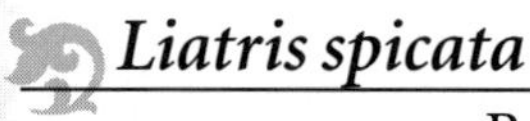

Liatris spicata

COMMON NAME ■ Button snake root

The rhizome is used to make medicine. *Liatris* contains coumarin. The eclectics used *Liatris* as a stimulant bitter tonic and as an antispasmodic for the muscles of the intestines. It seems to me that this is a curious and seemingly contradictory action. On the one hand, we have a stimulant bitter tonic, and on the other hand, we have an antispasmodic. Perhaps *Liatris* is a modulator.

Dr. Bastyr taught that *Liatris* is useful in treating diarrhea. He suggested that the tincture be used in doses of 15 drops twice daily. The powder is taken in doses of $\frac{1}{2}$ teaspoon six times daily.

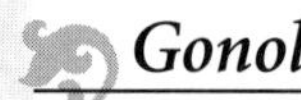

Gonolobus cundurango

COMMON NAME ■ Eagle vine

The bark is used to make medicine. This is a stomachic and an alterative. Dr. Bastyr taught its use to treat gastric ulcers and to relieve the distress of stomach cancer. His dose was 15 drops of tincture three times daily. I have no experience to share with this plant.

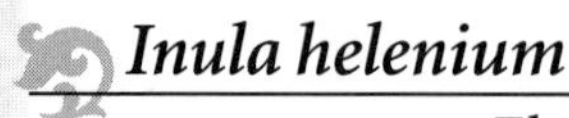

Inula helenium

COMMON NAME ■ Elecampane

The root is used to make medicine. This is a digestive aid, a stomachic, a tonic, and an antibacterial. When it is used as a stomachic, the dose is 40 drops of tincture three times daily.

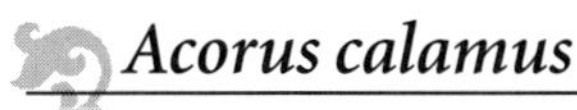

Acorus calamus

COMMON NAME ■ Sweet flag

The rhizome is used to make medicine. Dr. Bastyr taught that this plant is used to treat flatulent colic. Herbalists have used *Acorus* to treat a variety of problems, including anorexia, gastritis, gastric ulcers, and hyperacidity. Dr. Bastyr suggested a dose of 40 to 60 drops three times daily. He also mentioned that the patient could chew the dried root to help stop smoking.

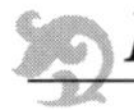

Mentha species

COMMON NAME ■ Mint

The leaves are used to make medicine. *Mentha* is a carminative, a condiment, and a nervine, as well as a fair circulatory stimulant. Dr. Bastyr talked about using *Mentha* to treat dyspepsia of neurogenic origin. He used 1 to 15 drops of the oil or 6 to 60 drops of the tincture for this purpose. Classically, peppermint tea has been used in colic and gastrodynia, and it is soothing to the stomach. For diarrhea, take 15 drops of the essence of peppermint in 1 cup of hot water every 3 hours until the diarrhea stops.

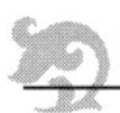

Chrysanthemum parthenium

COMMON NAME ■ Feverfew

Look for this also under the name *Tanacetum parthenium*. The dried aerial parts are used to make medicine. This medicine is tonic to the mucous membranes. Dr. Bastyr taught us to use *Chrysanthemum* to treat colic and flatulence. The tincture dose is 20 drops three times daily. In hot water, *Chrysanthemum* is a diaphoretic.

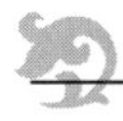

Pimento officinalis

COMMON NAME ■ Pimento

The berries are used to make medicine. The volatile oil extracted from the pimento berries contains eugenol, chavicol, and limonene. Dr. Bastyr taught that *Pimento* is a stomachic and a carminative that stimulates gastric secretions. He said that the round brown fruits should be powdered and given in a dose of 10 to 30 grains twice daily.

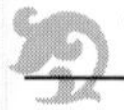

Trigonella foenum-graecum

COMMON NAME ■ Fenugreek

The seeds are used to make medicine. This plant contains steroid saponins, specifically trigofoenosides A to G.[25] It is a general tonic and a stomach remedy. Dr. Bastyr used fenugreek as a nervine to help stimulate the appetite. The seeds provide a strong, emollient mucilage. Use 1 ounce of seeds to 1 pint of water and drink 1 cup twice daily after meals.

Coriandrum sativum

COMMON NAME ■ Coriander

The dried fruit is used to make medicine. Coriander is rich in constituents. It contains hydroxycoumarins, among which are umbelliferone and scopoletin and a volatile oil composed of linalool, borneol, camphor, limonene, alpha-pinenes, and geraniol.

Coriander is a good stomachic and a carminative. Dr. Bastyr pointed out that coriander helps to overcome the disturbing action on the stomach of medicines such as rhubarb, *Gentiana*, aspirin, quassia, and senna. Herbalists and naturopaths have suggested taking 60 drops of tincture four times daily or 6 to 20 grains of powder three times daily. Herbalists have also recommended 2 teaspoons of the whole dried seeds added to 1 cup of water and taken in a dose of 1 cup daily.

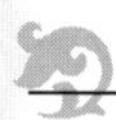

Anthemis nobiles

COMMON NAME ■ Roman chamomile

Anthemis is a member of the daisy family, *Compositae.* The flower is used to make medicine. As a stomach remedy, *Anthemis* has at least five potential uses. It kills bacteria, acts as an antispasmodic, relieves flatulence, decreases inflammation, and has an antiulcer effect. The antiulcer effect is caused by alpha-bisabolol. Rats given alpha-bisabolol in laboratory trials were protected from developing ulcers brought on by the irritants alcohol, methacin, and acetic acid.[173]

For the treatment of ulcers, I give two 300- to 500-mg capsules of freeze-dried chamomile three times daily. Alpha-bisabolol is lipid soluble, as is azulene, another important antiinflammatory in chamomile. Chamomile flowers can be chopped up and added to olive oil and put on rice or salads. Making medicinal oil preparations from herbs is a tradition that has a long history in herbal medicine.

For general stomachache, herbalists say to drink hot chamomile tea as needed up to three or four times daily. Make a strong infusion using 2 teaspoons of chamomile per cup of water. I use chamomile for chronic stomach problems as well. Some of these problems are caused by spasms in various parts of the stomach and some are caused by atrophy of the gastric lining and resulting tissue hypersensitivity.

A final use of chamomile that must not be missed is as a poultice made of dried, nearly powdered chamomile flowers and water. Put the chamomile mush on decubitus ulcers and any open, chronic ulcers on the skin, including peripheral necrotic ulcers seen in diabetic patients.

Angelica archangelica

COMMON NAME ■ Angelica

The seeds are used to make the medicine. A little known but effective treatment for the pain of gastric ulceration is the use of a decoction of angelica seeds. Use $\frac{1}{2}$ teaspoon of the seeds boiled in 1 cup of water.[112] Drink up to 2 cups daily.

CHAPTER

71

UTERINE SEDATIVES

CHAPTER • OUTLINE

Uterine sedatives decrease uterine cramping. These remedies were developed before the discovery of prostaglandins.

Viburnum prunifolium

COMMON NAME ■ Blackhaw

You may also use *Viburnum opulus, Viburnum carlcephalum*, and *Viburnum chenaulti*. The bark is used to make medicine. *Viburnum* contains coumarin and salicin, as well as flavonoids and triterpenes. These triterpenes include ursolic acid, hydroxycoumarins, caffeic acid derivatives, phenolcarboxylic acids, and tannins. Ursolic acid, incidentally, occurs in the waxy coating of many leaves and fruits such as uva-ursi.

Viburnum is an antispasmodic, a nervine, and a tonic. It can be used for cramplike pain. Dr. Bastyr recommended *Viburnum* as a uterine relaxant that helps to prevent threatened miscarriage. It is a remedy to consider for treating habitual abortion. Dr. Bastyr would give a woman who was bleeding and might miscarry 30 drops of *Viburnum* every 30 minutes until the bleeding stopped. Dr. Bastyr also suggested sabina, a homeopathic remedy prepared from the tops of *Juniperus sabina,* an evergreen shrub, in a 3X homeopathic potency four times daily for this purpose. After treatment with sabina, I have seen many pregnancies go to term.

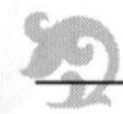

Scutellaria lateriflora

COMMON NAME ■ Skullcap

The whole herb is used to make medicine. Skullcap contains the flavonoid scutellarein, which works like quercetin as a modifier of eicosanoids. Dr. Bastyr said to use 30 drops of the tincture three times daily to depress uterine activity.

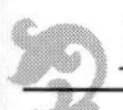

Piscidia erythrina

COMMON NAME ■ Jamaican dogwood

The medicine is made from the bark. *Piscidia* contains isoflavonoids, which may account for this plant's uterine sedative effect. Some of the isoflavonoids are jamaicin, ichthynone, and millettone.[25] *Piscidia* works wonders to quiet the uterus. I use *Piscidia* to relieve the pain of menstrual cramps. The dose is 1000 mg of *Piscidia* every 2 hours until the cramps are relieved. Usually the first dose does it. Another 500 mg may be taken if the cramps seem to be returning. *Piscidia* is safe and effective and absolutely reliable.

CHAPTER

72

UTERINE TONICS

CHAPTER • OUTLINE

These remedies improve uterine health by improving the venous and nervous system traffic to the myometrium.

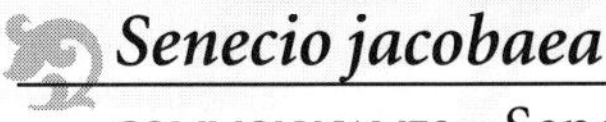

Senecio jacobaea

COMMON NAMES ■ Senecio, Ragwort

Senecio aureus and *S. vulgaris* may also be used. Herbalists have used this remedy to treat amenorrhea, dysmenorrhea, metrorrhagia, and menorrhagia. Dr. Bastyr taught that *Senecio* is especially useful in engorged atonic conditions. He recommended a tincture dose of 20 drops three times daily. Consider this remedy for women who have uterine atony as the result of childbearing.

Helonias opulus

COMMON NAME ■ False unicorn

The root is used to make medicine. It is used for uterine prolapse and can be used in menopause when patients are experiencing frequent urination. Dr. Bastyr pointed out that this remedy could also be useful in prostatitis in which the patient feels as though he was sitting on a ball. The general dose for all of the above conditions is 10 to 60 drops of tincture three times daily, or 20 to 40 grains of powder twice daily. *Helonias* is shown as mainly a female remedy in the literature. I think it is especially apropos that Dr. Bastyr used this remedy for men.

Mitchella repens

COMMON NAMES ■ Partridgeberry, Squaw vine

The whole plant is used to make medicine. *Mitchella* is used for most menstrual problems. It is a main ingredient in many of the partus preparatus formulas. In fact, Dr. Bastyr thought that it was the most important ingredient in these formulas. *Mitchella* helps to prevent miscarriage in the last trimester. Dr. Bastyr said, "Use it with *Viburnum* and *Caulophyllum* during pregnancy for no tears and easy deliveries." Doses of 20 drops of tincture may be taken twice daily. *Mitchella* may be used during the entire lactation period. The powder is used in doses of 30 grains for treating metrorrhagia. It helps to regulate dysmenorrhea at the menarche.

Aletris farinosa

COMMON NAMES ■ Blazing star, True unicorn root

Use the roots for medicine. *Aletris* contains volatile oils and saponins. This plant tones the uterus after childbearing. It is used for uterine anteversion, hypoovarianism, habitual abortion, and poor ovarian function. Dr. Bastyr mentioned that this plant was especially helpful during the third month. I don't have any more information on this fragment from Dr. Bastyr. I include it for historical purposes and hope that it might mean something to someone. It helps to increase appetite in patients who have nausea and uterine reflexes. The tincture is taken in doses of 20 to 40 drops several times daily.

Leonurus cardiaca

COMMON NAME ■ Motherwort

This plant belongs to the *Labiatae* family. Use the whole plant for medicine. *Leonurus* contains several alkaloids, among which are lachydrine and leonuride.

It also contains diterpenoids, triterpenes, ursolic acid, and flavonoids, especially the polyhydroxal flavonoids such as quercetin, kaempferol, and genkwanin.[20,174,175]

Leonurus is a tonic and a laxative. Dr. Bastyr used it for dysmenorrhea with anxiety or hysteria. The tincture is taken in doses of 20 to 40 drops and the powder in doses of 5 to 45 grains. Dr. Bastyr told us to think of this remedy primarily to help start delayed or scanty menstruation, especially when it is associated with anxiety. I do not limit the use of this remedy to menstrual problems; I also use it for patients with general nervous tension.

Angelica sinensis

COMMON NAME ■ Dong quai

A similar plant, *Angelica acutiloba*, or Japanese angelica, may also be used. The root is used to make medicine. *Angelica* contains volatile oils and the furocoumarins bergapten, xanthotoxin, scopoletin, and umbelliferone. It also contains safrole, carvacrol, and isosafrole. Carvacrol is an antiinfective and an anthelminthic for nematodes.

The water extract of *Angelica* causes uterine contractions. The tincture causes uterine relaxation. This remedy is primarily used for menstrual problems like dysmenorrhea, amenorrhea, menorrhagia, and metrorrhagia. It may be taken in a standard tea or in tincture form depending on its intended use.

Angelica is a diuretic and has been used to treat menopausal symptoms including hot flushes. It is a phytoestrogen and is useful as a hormone replacement therapy, especially when combined with *Vitex* and *Cimicifuga*. *Angelica sinensis* may be used to treat either hyperestrogen or hypoestrogen problems. Because of this wide range of applications, it is considered to be an estrogenic alterative. Equal parts of the three plants are given in doses of 30 drops twice daily.

CHAPTER

73

VULNERARIES

CHAPTER • OUTLINE

Hamamelis virginiana
Calendula officinalis
Aesculus hippocastanum
Gibberella fujikuroi
Arnica montana
Plantago major
Hypericum perforatum
Stellaria media
Symphytum officinale
Nymphaea odorata
Populus tremuloides
Lavandula vera
Centella asiatica

Vulneraries soothe tissue and assist healing. Vulneraries are applied to wounds or to inflamed mucous membranes as needed.

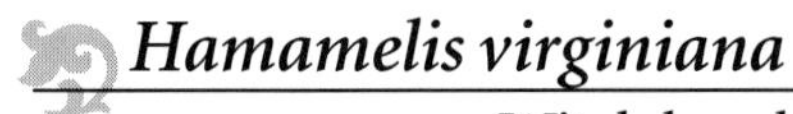

Hamamelis virginiana

COMMON NAME ■ Witch hazel

The bark and leaves are used to make medicine. This plant is an astringent and a hemostatic. It is used to treat muscle aches, pains, and strains. Dr. Bastyr said that it could be used to treat mucous membranes with venous stasis. It is useful in uterine prolapse where vaginal walls are redundant. For varicosities, apply the fluid extract of witch hazel topically and leave it on overnight. For bags under the eyes, apply cotton swabs to the area and have the patient lie down for 15 minutes. Dr. Bastyr said that a standard tea of *Hamamelis* makes a good enema for hemorrhoids. The dose of the tincture is 20 to 30 drops twice daily.

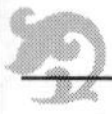

Calendula officinalis

COMMON NAME ■ Marigold

The flowers are used to make medicine. Use *Calendula* on open wounds. It helps prevent keloids when used locally. When treating keloids, use vitamin E internally. *Calendula* cream is available for skin irritations. Dr. Bastyr always applied *Calendula* to the umbilicus of newborns. It was his favorite remedy for this. As a vaginal wash, he put tincture of *Calendula* in a small amount of water and swabbed the vagina. In addition, *Calendula* is a good gargle for sore throats.

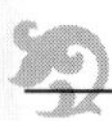

Aesculus hippocastanum

COMMON NAME ■ Chestnut

The fruit and bark are used to make medicine. Its active ingredient is aescin. *Aesculus* is a useful astringent tonic. It is a classic remedy for hemorrhoids and is often used in suppository form. For esophageal varices, I recommend using the tincture internally in doses of 20 to 40 drops.

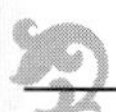

Gibberella fujikuroi

This is a type of fungus. A tincture of *Gibberella* is applied directly on the skin in ulcerative skin conditions.

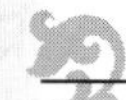

Arnica montana

COMMON NAME ■ Arnica

Look for this under the name *Arnica alpina* as well. *Arnica* is a member of the sunflower family, *Compositae*. The flower heads are used for medicine. Salves made with *Arnica* can be applied to sprains and strains to help reduce swelling and speed recovery. Dr. Bastyr used small doses of *Arnica* tincture to stimulate the respiratory center. His dose was 3 drops twice daily. *Arnica* is a premier remedy for soft tissue injury. A 6X or a 30X homeopathic potency works amazingly well to speed recovery from sprains, strains, and the soreness of overwork. I also suggest this remedy to treat soreness after tooth extraction.

A little-used application of *Arnica* is for the tonification of the heart. Seven drops of tincture may be taken daily for this. It has a fast stimulating action on the heart.

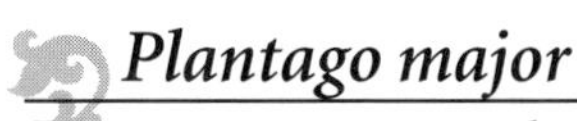

Plantago major

COMMON NAME ■ Plantain

This plant may also be found under the name *Plantago ovata* or *Plantago lanceolata.* It is a member of the plantain family, *Plantaginaceae.* The leaves and roots are used to make medicine. Use bruised leaves as a poultice on skin problems. This remedy can be applied to hemorrhoids and can also be used in dysuria and hematuria. Internally, it is also useful for inflammations of the gastrointestinal tract. The tincture dose is 5 to 10 drops twice daily.

For conjunctivitis or pinkeye, apply a plantain poultice to the closed infected eye. A warm sterile infusion using distilled water is also applicable as an eyewash. For this purpose, use a preparation of chickweed or yellow dock mixed with plantain. For added antibacterial effect, use a very small amount of goldenseal in the eyewash.

Dr. Bastyr used *Plantago* together with *Echinacea* to treat blood poisoning. He would have used equal parts of these two remedies at a dose of 30 drops six times daily. I would use a lot more than that; I would use 60 drops every hour for 3 days.

Hypericum perforatum

COMMON NAME ■ St. John's wort

This remedy has gained popularity as treatment for depression when taken in doses of 300 mg three times daily over an extended time. Classically, *Hypericum* is to the nerves what *Arnica* is to the soft tissues. Dr. Bastyr used this remedy for spinal tenderness. It is an excellent local anodyne. In acute neuritis, use a 3X potency preparation every hour. In bedwetting, when all else fails, try 20 drops of *Hypericum* tincture twice daily.

Stellaria media

COMMON NAME ■ Chickweed

The dried flowering herb is used to make medicine. This plant contains rutin. Dr. Bastyr told us that his mother saved his life by applying a chickweed poultice to his suppurative appendicitis wound. The greens are edible. The leaves may be bruised and applied locally to wounds. The tincture may be used internally for rheumatic pains that tend to shift from place to place. The dose is 30 drops three times daily.

Symphytum officinale

COMMON NAMES ■ Comfrey, Knitbone

The leaves or root may be used to make medicine. Comfrey is rich in vitamins and minerals, especially thiamin, riboflavin, vitamin B_{12}, ascorbic acid, vitamin E, pantothenic acid, manganese, and calcium.

This plant can be used to treat chronic inflammations of the gastrointestinal mucosa and chronic catarrh of the respiratory and renal structures. Gargle the decoction for throat inflammations and for bleeding gums. A hot comfrey pack may be applied for bronchitis, pleurisy, and muscle strains. It is an excellent tea for convalescence. The tincture dose is 10 to 30 drops.

Comfrey is famous for its results as a poultice on sprained knees. It helps broken bones to knit faster. Dr. Bastyr suggested giving a cup of comfrey tea daily for people with broken bones. *Symphytum* is derived from the Greek word *sympho*, which means to unite. Notice that one of the common names for comfrey is knitbone. Its use as a vulnerary is in part because of its ability to reduce swelling in the fractured area when it is applied as a poultice. Comfrey poultices were frequently suggested by Dr. Bastyr for fractures or swellings of the joints.

Nymphaea odorata

COMMON NAME ■ White pond lily

The root is used to make medicine. This makes a good gargle for sore throats and also has been used as an eyewash. Herbalists have told me that *Nymphea* is a useful antiseptic for a vaginal douche. It has also been used as a softening agent in skin lotion.

Populus tremuloides

COMMON NAME ■ Poplar

The bark and leaves are used to make medicine. This plant restores digestive disturbances. It is a good alterative. Dr. Bastyr said that for urinary tract problems, we should combine poplar with uva-ursi and give our patients 30 drops of the formula in 1 cup of water four times daily.

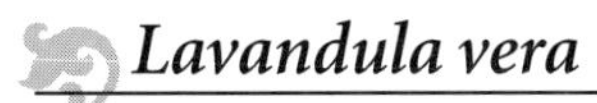

Lavandula vera

COMMON NAME ■ Lavender

Also look for this under the name *Lavandula angustifolia.* The flowers are used to make medicine. The essential oil is extracted from the flowers. I have frequently heard that *Lavandula* has been used for scabies by applying the oil to the lesions. I have not tried this therapy. Dr. Bastyr used *Lavandula* tea for nervous dyspepsia. His dose was $\frac{1}{2}$ ounce of the tea made from the flowers.

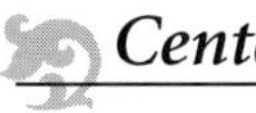

Centella asiatica

COMMON NAME ■ Gotu kola

The dried aerial parts of the plants are used to make medicine. Dr. Bastyr did not lecture on this remedy, I have added it to this list. This plant has been used for many hundreds of years as a vulnerary. The principal active ingredient of *Centella* as a vulnerary is asiaticoside. It has been used to heal wounds and even to assuage the lesions of leprosy.[176] Use 30 drops of the tincture internally several times daily to speed wound healing. A mash of the plant can also be applied topically.

Centella has been used on burns and probably works for a number of reasons. It contains flavonoids and sterols, and it tends to increase the revascularization of connective tissue.[177] *Centella*'s fibrinolytic ability has been demonstrated in its use in scleroderma, which results in a lessening of joint pain and finger motility. Use 30 drops of tincture twice daily. Capsules may also be used.

Centella is the plant that I add to my 7-Chakra tea to stimulate the connection to the 7th Chakra. It has long been used by Tibetan monks to improve their meditation skills.

REFERENCES

1. Bohn B, Nebe CT, Birr C: Flow-cytometric studies with eleutherococcus senticosus extract as an immunomodulating agent. *Arzneim Forsch* 37(10):1193-1196, 1987.
2. Dorling E: Do ginsenosides influence performance? *Notabena Medici* 10(5):241-246, 1980.
3. Gutnikove LI, Vorobyeva PO, Gupronow NI: The Institute of Biologically Active Compounds.
4. Willard T: *Textbook of modern herbology*. Calgary, Alberta, 1988, CW Progressive Publ. Inc.
5. Lectures of Dr. Jeffrey Bland, National College of Naturopathic Medicine, 1975.
6. Lectures of Ed Madison, Bastyr University, Seattle, WA, 1984.
7. Krause, Mahan: *Food, nutrition and diet therapy*. Philadelphia, 1984, WB Saunders Co.
8. Kutsky: *Handbook of vitamins and hormones*. 1973, Van Nostrand Reinhold Co.
9. Srivastava R, Dikshit M, Srimal RC, Dhawan BN: Anti-thrombotic effect of curcumin. *Thromb Res Suppl* 40(3):413-417, 1985.
10. Polasa K, Rughuram TC, Krishna JP, Krishnaswamy K: *Mutagenesis* 7(2):107-109, 1992.
11. Subbarao D, Chandrasekhara N, Satyanarayana MN, Srinivasan, MJ: *Nutrition* 100:1307-1315, 1970.
12. Huang M-T, Smart RC, Wang C-Q, Conney AH: *Cancer Res* 48: 5941-5946, 1998.
13. Weiss RF: *Herbal medicine*, ed 2, New York, 2000, Thieme Medical Pub.
14. Meanier MT, Duroux E, Bastide P: Free radical scavenger activity of procyanidolic oligomers and anthocyanosides with respect to superoxide anion and lipid peroxidation, *Plant Med Phytother* 4: 267-274, 1989.
15. Hertog MG, et al.: Dietary antioxidant flavonoids and risk of coronary heart disease: the zutphen elderly study, *Lancet* 342: 1007-1011, 1993.
16. Ho C, et al.: Antioxidant effect of polyphenol extract prepared from various Chinese teas, *Prevent Med* 21:520-525, 1992.
17. Khan SG, et al.: Enhancement of antioxidant and phase II enzymes by oral feeding of green tea polyphenols in drinking water to SKH-1 hairless mice: possible role in Ca chem prevention, *Cancer Res* 52:4050-4052, 1992.
18. Baver R, Wagner H: Echinacea species as potential immunostimulatory drugs, *Econ Med Plant Res* 5:253-321, 1991.
19. Pizzorno JE, Murray MT: *Textbook of natural medicine*, ed 2, London, 1999, Churchill Livingstone.

20. Bradley PR: *British herbal compendium, vol 2, A handbook of scientific information on widely used plants,* Bournemouth, UK, 1992, British Herbal Medicine Association.
21. *Merck Index,* ed 13, Rahway, NJ, 2001, Merck Publishing Group.
22. Bradbury, White J: *Chem Soc,* 1951, p. 3447.
23. Bate-Smith, Swain: Chem and Ind, London, 1953, p. 1127.
24. Clymer R: *Nature's healing agents,* Pittsburgh, PA, 1963, Dorrance Publishing.
25. Gruenwald J: *Physician's desk reference for herbal medicines,* ed 2, Montvale, NJ, 2000, Medical Economics Co.
26. Bruneton J: *Pharmacognosy: phytochemistry, and medicinal plants,* ed 2, Andover, UK, 1999, Intercept Ltd.
27. Head KA: Ipriflavone: an important bone-building isoflavone, *Altern Med Rev* 4(1):10-22, 1999.
28. Kuts-Cheraux AW: *Naturae medicina and naturopathic dispensatory,* Des Moines, IA, 1953, American Naturopathic Physicians and Surgeons Association.
29. Hostettmann K, Marston A: *Phytochemistry of plants used in traditional medicine: proceedings of the Phytochemical Society of Europe, No 37,* Oxford, UK, 1995, Clarendon Press.
30. Wagner H, Seagert K, Gupta MP, et al.: Cardiotone Wirkstoffe aus Spigelia anthelmia, *Planta Medica* 5:378-380, 1986.
31. Grieve M: *A modern herbal,* vol 1, New York, 1971, Dover Publications, Inc.
32. Wren RC: *Potter's new cyclopaedia of medicinal herbs and preparations,* New York, 1972, Harper & Row.
33. Tyler VE, Brady LR, Robbers JE: *Pharmacognosy,* ed 9, Philadelphia, 1987, Lea & Febiger.
34. Osawa T, Kawakishi S, Namiki M: In Kuroda Y, Shankel DM, Waters MD, editors: *Antimutagenesis and anticarcinogenesis mechanics II,* New York, 1990, Plenum.
35. Osawa T, Kumazawa S, Kawakishi S: Prunusols A and B, novel antioxidative tocopherol derivatives isolated from the leaf wax of *Prunus grayana* Maxim, *Agric Biol Chem* 55(7):1727-1731, 1991.
36. Barlow M: *From the shepherd's purse: the identification, preparation, and the use of medicinal plants,* McCammon, ID, 1979, Spice West.
37. Skvortsov et al.
38. Sun D, Courtney HS, Beachey EH: Berberine sulfate blocks adherence of *Streptococcus pyogenes* to epithelial cells, fibronectin, and hexadecane, *Antimicrob Agents Chemother* 32:1370-1374, 1988.
39. Mohan M, et al.: Berberine in trachoma, *Indian J Ophthalmol* 30:69-75, 1982.
40. Roser V, Valenzuela L, Bello H, et al.: Composition and antimicrobial activity of the essential oil of peumus boldus leaves, *Planta Medica* 65:178-179, 1999.
41. Motimitsu Y, Kawakishi S: Inhibitors of platelet aggregation from onion, *Phytochemistry* 29:3453-3439, 1990.
42. Evans WC: *Trease and Evan's pharmacognosy,* ed 15, Philadelphia, 2002, WB Saunders.
43. Institute of Microbiology II, University of Cagliari, Italy, 1979.
44. Voaden D, Jacobson M: Tumor inhibitors. 3. Identification and synthesis of an oncolytic hydrocarbon from American Coneflower

roots, *J Med Chem* 15:619-623, 1972.

45. Harkrader RJ, et al.: The history, chemistry, and pharmacokinetics of *Sanguinaria* extract, *J Can Dent Assoc* 56(7 suppl.):7-12, 1990.
46. Hoffmann D: Therapeutic herbalism: a correspondence course in phytotherapy.
47. Jaeger T (food scientist with Northwest Naturals): Personal communication.
48. Fujita Y, et al.: Inhibitory effect of (-)-epigallocatechin gallate on carcinogenesis with N-ethyl-N′-nitro-N-nitrosoguanidine in mouse duodenum, *Jpn J Cancer Res* 80(6):503-505, 1989.
49. Chung F-L, et al.: In Huang M-T, Ho C-T, Lee CY, editors: *Phenolic compounds in food and their effects on health II: antioxidants and cancer prevention, ACS Symposium Series No. 507,* Washington, DC, 1992, American Chemical Society.
50. Wang ZY, Hong J-Y, et al.: Inhibition of N-nitrosodiethylamine- and 4-(methylnitrosamino)-1-(3-pyridyl)-1-butanone-induced tumorigenesis in A/J mice by green tea and black tea, *Cancer Res* 52(7):1943-1947, 1992.
51. Wang ZY, Cheng SJ, Zhou ZC, et al.: Antimutagenic activity of green tea polyphenols, *Mutat Res* 223(3):273- 285, 1989.
52. Wang ZY, Agarwal R, Bickers DR, Mukhtar H: Protection against ultraviolet B radiation-induced photocarcinogenesis in hairless mice by green tea polyphenols, *Carcinogenesis* 12(8):1527-1530, 1991.
53. Wang Z, Huang M-T, Ferraro T, et al.: Inhibitory effect of green tea in the drinking water on tumorigenesis by ultraviolet light and 12-O-tetradecanoylphorbol-13-acetate in the skin of SKH-1 mice, *Cancer Res* 52(5):1162-1170, 1992.
54. Ho C-T, Osawa T, Huang M-T, Rosen RT: *Food phytochemicals for cancer prevention II: teas, spices, and herbs, ACS Symposium series 547,* Washington, DC, 1994, American Chemical Society.
55. Kim M, Hagiwara N, et al.: Preventive effect of green tea polyphenols on colon carcinogenesis. In Ho C-T, Osawa T, Huang M-T, Rosen RT: *Food phytochemicals for cancer prevention II: teas, spices, and herbs, ACS Symposium series 547,* Washington, DC, 1994, American Chemical Society.
56. Matsuzaki T, Hara Y: *Nippon Nogeikagaku Kaishi* 59:129-134, 1985.
57. Schwarz K, Ternes WZ: Antioxidative constituents of Rosmarinus officinalis and Salvia officinalis. II. Isolation of carnosic acid and formation of other phenolic diterpenes, *Z Lebensm Unters Forsch* 195(2):99-103, 1992.
58. Huang M-T, Ho C-T, Wang ZY, et al.: Proc Am Assoc, *Cancer Res* 33:165, 1992 (abstract).
59. Huang M-T, Ho C-T, Wang ZY, et al.: Tumour initiation: the significance of endogenous biotransformation. In Waldron K, Johnson IT, Fenwich GR: *Food and cancer prevention: chemical and biological aspects,* Cambridge, UK, 1993, Royal Society of Chemistry.
60. Huang M-T, Ho C-T, Wang ZY, et al.: Inhibition of skin tumorigenesis by rosemary and its constituents carnosol and ursolic acid, *Cancer Res* 54(3):701-708, 1994.
61. Ohigashi H, Murakami A, Koshimizu K: Antitumor promoters from edible plants. In Ho C-T, Osawa T, Huang M-T, Rosen RT:

Food phytochemicals for cancer prevention II: teas, spices, and herbs, ACS Symposium series 547, Washington, DC, 1994, American Chemical Society.
62. Noro T, Sekiya T, Katoh M, et al.: *Chem Pharm Bull* 36:244-248, 1988.
63. Reiners JJ, Pence BC, Barcus CS, Cantu AR: 12-O-tetradecanoylphorbol-13-acetate-dependent induction of xanthine dehydrogenase and conversion to xanthine oxidase in murine epidermis, *Cancer Res* 47(7):1775-1779, 1987.
64. Wang ZY, Agarwal R, Zhou ZC, et al.: Protection against ultraviolet B radiation-induced photocarcinogenesis in hairless mice by green tea polyphenols, *Carcinogenesis* 12(8):1527-1530, 1991.
65. Hajto T, Lanzrein C: Natural killer and antibody-dependent cell-mediated cytotoxicity activities and large granular lymphocyte frequencies in Viscum album treated breast cancer treated patients, *Oncology* 43(2):93-97, 1986.
66. Zhang W, Law RE, Hinton DR, et al.: Growth inhibition and apoptosis in human neuroblastoma SK-N-SH cells induced by hypericin, a potent inhibitor of protein, C *Cancer Lett* 96(1):31-35, 1995.
67. Hamilton HB, Hinton DR, Law RE, et al.: Inhibition of cellular growth and induction of apoptosis in pituitary adenoma cell lines by the protein kinase C inhibitor hypericin. Potential therapeutic applications, *J Neurosurgery* 85(2):329-334, 1996.
68. Thiede HM, Walper A: Inhibition of MAO and COMT by Hypericum extracts and hypericin, *J Geriatr Psychiatry Neurol* 7(suppl 1):S54-S56, 1994.
69. Perovic S, Muller WEG: Pharmacological profile of Hypericum extract: Effect on serotonin uptake by postsynaptic receptors, *Arzneim Forsch* 45(11):1145-1148, 1995.
70. Lloyd KG, Zivkovic B, Scatton B, et al.: The gabaergic hypothesis of depression, *Prog Neuro-psychopharmacol Biol Psychiatry* 13:341-351, 1989.
71. Mowrey D, Clayson D: Motion sickness, ginger, and psychophysics, *Lancet* 1:655-657, 1982.
72. Wright J: *Dr. Wright's book of nutritional therapy*, Emmaus, PA, 1979, Rodale Press.
73. Wegrowski J, Robert AM, Moczar M: The effect of procyanidolic oligomers on the composition of normal and hypercholesterolemic rabbit aortas, *Biochemic Pharmacol* 33(21): 3491-3497, 1984.
74. Patacchini R, Maggi CA, Meli A: Capsaicin-like activity of some natural pungent substances on peripheral endings of visceral primary afferents, *Arch Pharmacol* 342:72-77, 1990.
75. Seligman B: Oral bromelains as adjuncts in the treatment of acute thrombophlebitis, *Angiology* 20(1):22-26, 1969.
76. Hatano T, Fukuda T, Liu Y-Z, Noro T: Phenolic constituents of licorice. IV. Correlation of phenolic constituents and licorice specimens from various sources, and inhibitory effects of licorice extracts on xanthine oxidase and monoamine oxidase, *Yakugaka Zasshi* 111(6):311-321, 1991.
77. Kastner Y, Hussain AS, Koch HH: Pharmacokinetics and bioavailability of beta-sitosterol in the beagle dog, *Arzneimittelforschung* 40(4):463-468, 1990.

78. Lamson D: Lectures at the 1997 AANP Convention.
79. Nielsen HK, Loliger J, Hurrell RF: Reactions of proteins with oxidizing lipids. 1. Analytical measurements of lipid oxidation and of amino acid losses in a whey protein-methyl linolenate model system, *Br J Nutr* 53(1):61-73, 1985.
80. Shibamoto T, Hagiwara Y, Hagiwara H, Osawa T: Flavonoid with strong antioxidative activity isolated from young green barley leaves. In Ho C-T, Osawa T, Huang M-T, Rosen RT: *Food phytochemicals for cancer prevention II: teas, spices, and herbs, ACS Symposium series 547,* Washington, DC, 1994, American Chemical Society.
81. Kikuzaki H, Kawasake Y, Nakatane N: Structure of antioxidative compounds in ginger. In Ho C-T, Osawa T, Huang M-T, Rosen RT: *Food phytochemicals for cancer prevention II: teas, spices, and herbs, ACS Symposium series 547,* Washington, DC, 1994, American Chemical Society.
82. Kawakishi S, Morimitsu Y, Osawa T: Chemistry of ginger compounds and inhibitory factors of the arachidonic acid cascade. In Ho C-T, Osawa T, Huang M-T, Rosen RT: *Food phytochemicals for cancer prevention II: teas, spices, and herbs, ACS Symposium series 547,* Washington, DC, 1994, American Chemical Society.
83. Puri RN, Colman RW: Inhibition of ADP-induced platelet shape change and aggregation by o-phthalaldehyde: evidence for covalent modification of cysteine and lysine residues, *Arch Biochem Biophys* 286(2):419-427, 1991.
84. Fukuda Y, Osawa T, Namiki M: *Nippon Shokuhin Kogyo Gakkaishi* 28:461-464, 1981.
85. Budowski P, Menezes FGT, Dollear FG: *J Am Oil Chem Soc* 27: 377-380, 1950.
86. *Dorland's Illustrated Medical Dictionary,* ed 29, Philadelphia, 2000, WB Saunders.
87. Winship KA: Toxicity of comfrey, *Adverse Drug React Toxicol Rev* 10(1):47-59, 1991.
88. Witte L, Ernst L, Adam H, Hartman T: Chemotypes of two pyrrolizidine alkaloid-containing senecio species, *Phytochemistry* 31:559-565, 1992.
89. Junior P: Recent developments in the isolation and structure elucidation of naturally occurring iridoid compounds, *Planta Medica* 56:1-13, 1990.
90. Lanhers MC, Fleurentin J, Mortier F, et al.: Anti-inflammatory and analgesic effects of an aqueous extract of harpogophytum procumbens, *Planta Medica* 58(2): 117-123, 1992.
91. Dr. Sarkar: Mitchell's lecture at the SW College of Naturopathic Med and Nat. Health Sciences, 1999, A comment from Dr. Sarkar, a visiting teacher and doctor from India.
92. Murray MT, Pizzorno JE: *Encyclopedia of natural medicine,* ed 2, Roseville, CA, 1998, Prima Publishing.
93. Burnett AR, Thomson RH: Naturally occurring quinones. X. The quinoid constituents of Tabebuia avellandar (Bignoniaceae), *J Chem Soc* (C):2100-2104, 1967.
94. Lagrota M, et al.: Antiviral activity of Lapachol, *Rev Latinoam Microbiol* 14(1):21-26, 1983.
95. Selway JWT: Antiviral activity of flavones and flavins. In Cody V, Middleton E, Harborne JB: *Plant flavonoids in biology and medicine: biochemical, pharmacological, and*

structure-activity relationships, New York, 1986, Wiley-Liss.

96. Steve McDougal, CDC, Atlanta, GA.
97. Robinson T: *The organic constituents of higher plants: their chemistry and interrelationships,* 1991, Cordus Press.
98. Tucker AO: Frankincense and myrrh, *Econ Bot* 40:425-433, 1986.
99. Hattori M, Kusumoto IT, Namba T, et al.: Effect of tea polyphenols on glucan synthesis by glucosyltransferase from *Streptococcus mutans, Chem Pharm Bull (Tokyo)* 38(3):717-720, 1990.
100. Burchell HB: The countryside of William Withering, *Postgrad Med* 26:228, 1959.
101. Arora RB, et al.: Effect of some lipid fractions of *Commiphora mukul* on various serum lipid levels in hypercholesterolemic chicks and their effectiveness in myocardial infarction in rats, *Indian J Exp Biol* 11(3):166-168, 1973.
102. Satyavati GV, Dwarakanath C, Tripathi SN: Experimental studies of the hypocholesterolemic effect of *Commiphora mukul, Indian J Med Res* 57(10):1950-1962, 1969.
103. Satyavate GV: Gugulipid: a promising hypolipidaemic agent from gum guggul *(Commiphora wightii), Econ Med Plant Res* 5:47-82, 1991.
104. Tripathi YB, et al.: Thyroid stimulatory action of (Z)-guggulsterone: mechanism of action, *Planta Medica* 54(4):271-272, 1988.
105. Montini M, Levoni P, Angoro A, Pagani G: Controlled trial of cynarin in the treatment of the hyperlipemic syndrome: observations in 60 cases, *Arzneim-Forsch* 25(8): 1311-1314, 1975.
106. Orekhov AN, et al.: Direct antiatherosclerosis-related effects of garlic, *Ann Med* 27(1):63-65, 1995.
107. Mikus P, Polak O, Ochsenreither AM: Clinical and electroencephalo graphic results of a double-blind test with vincamine (Pervincamine) in advanced cerebral sclerosis, *Pharmakopsychiatr Neuropsychoph armakol* 6(1):39-49, 1973.
108. DeFeudis FV: *Ginkgo biloba Extract (Egb 761): pharmacological activities and clinical applications,* Paris, 1991, Elsevier Science.
109. Sikora R, et al.: *Ginkgo biloba* extract in the therapy of erectile dysfunction, *J Urol* 141:188A, 1989.
110. Murray MT: *The healing power of herbs,* ed 2, Roseville, CA, 1995, Prima Publishing.
111. Giffard P-L: Les Gommiers: *Acacia senegal* Willd: *Acacia laeta, R Br Bois Forets Trop* 105:21-28, 1966.
112. Brown T: *Tom Brown's guide to wild edible and medicinal plants,* New York, 1995, Berkley Pub Group.
113. Karrer P, Benz P, Morf, et al.: Konstitution des Safranfarbstoffes Crocetin, Synthese des Perhydrobixinathylesters and Perhydronorbixins, vorlaufige Mittdilung, *Helv Chim Acta* 15:1218-1219, 1932.
114. Karrer P, Salomon H: Uber Pflanzenfarbstoffe IV. Uber die Safranfarbstoffe II, *Helv Chim Acta* 11:513-525, 1928.
115. Ghosal S, Singh SK, Battacharya SK: Mangicrocin, an adaptogenic xanthone carotenoid glycosidic conjugate from saffron, *J Chem Res Synop* 70-71, 1989.
116. Gainer JL, Chisolm GM III: Oxygen diffusion and atherosclerosis,

Atherosclerosis 19(1): 135-138, 1974.
117. Lindner E, Dohadwalla AN, Bhattacharya BK: Positive inotropic and blood pressure lowering activity of a diterpene derivative isolated from *Coleus forskohlii:* Forskolin, *Arzneimittel-Forsh* 28(2):284-289, 1978.
118. Felter HW: *The eclectic materia medica, pharmacology, and therapeutics*, Prod. by John K Scudder, 1922.
119. Pieters LA, Vlietinck AJ: Spartioidine and usaramine, two pyrrolizidine alkaloids from *Senecio vulgaris, Planta Medica* 54:178-179, 1988.
120. Altman PM: Australian tea tree, *Aust J Pharm* 69:276-278, 1988.
121. Pena EF: *Melaleuca alternifolia* oil, *Obstet Gynecol* 19:793-795, 1962.
122. Sourgens H, et al.: Antihormonal effects of plant extracts. TSH- and prolactin-suppressing properties of *Lithospermum officinale* and other plants, *Planta Medica* 45(2):78-86, 1982.
123. Svendsen AB, Karlsen J: *Planta Medica* 14:376, 1966.
124. Haraguchi H, et al.: Antiperoxidative components in *Thymus vulgaris, Planta Medica* 62(3): 217-221, 1996.
125. Marguardt P, et al.: *Planta Medica* 30:68, 1976.
126. Huang ZJ, Kinghorn AD, Farnsworth NR: Studies on herbal remedies I: Analysis of herbal smoking preparations alleged to contain lettuce *(Lactuca sativa* L.) and other natural products, *J Pharm Sci* 71(2):270-271, 1982.
127. Schreiber K, Pufahl K, Brauninger H: Liebigs, *Ann Chem* 671:142, 1964.
128. Leung AY, Foster S: *Encyclopedia of common natural ingredients used in food, drugs and cosmetics,* ed 2, New York, 1995, Wiley-Interscience.
129. Cheney G, Waxler SH, Miller IJ: Vitamin U therapy of peptic ulcer, *California Med* 84(1):39-42, 1956.
130. Kaiser R, et al.: *J Agric Food Chemistry* 23:943-950, 1975.
131. Didry N, Pinkas M: Plant medicine, *Phytotherapy* 16(4):249, 1982.
132. Swiatek L, Komorowski T: Occurrence of monotropein and of asperuloside in some species of the families Ericaceae, Empetraceae and Rubiaceae, *Herba Pol* 18(2):168-173 [Polish], 1972; through *Chem Abstr,* 1973, 78, 1979.
133. Felter HW, Lloyd JU: *King's American dispensatory,* ed 18, Sandy, OR, 1898, Eclectic Medical Publications: 1983.
134. Guha et al.: *J Nat Prod* 42:1, 1979.
135. Obrowski L: *Wiener Med Wschr* 108:396, 1958.
136. Kang SS, Woo WS: Triterpenes from the berries of *Phytolacca americana, J Nat Prod* 43(4): 510-513, 1980.
137. John M, Gumbinger HG, Winterhoff H: The oxidation of caffeic acid derivatives as model reaction for the formation of potent gonadotrophin inhibitors in plant extracts, *Planta Medica* 59(3):195-199, 1993.
138. Kraus R, Spiteller G: Phenolic compounds from the roots of *Urtica dioica, Phytochemistry* 29:1653-1659, 1990.
139. Chaurasia N, Wichtl M: Flavonol glycosides from *Urtica dioica, Planta Medica* 53:432-433, 1987.
140. Chandler RF, Hooper SN, Harvey MJ: Ethnobotany and phytochemistry of yarrow, *Achillea millefolium,* Compositae, *Econ Botany* 36:203-223, 1982.

141. Piscopo G: Kava kava: gift of the islands, *Alt Med Rev* 2(5):355-364, 1997.
142. Inouye H, et al.: Purgative activities of iridoid glucosides, *Planta Medica* 25(3):285-288, 1974.
143. Hara Y, Honda M: *Agric Biol Chem* 54:1339-1345, 1990.
144. Spinella G: Natural anthocyanosides in treatment of peripheral venous insufficiency, *Arch Med Int* 37:21-29, 1985.
145. Foust CM: *Rhubarb, the wondrous drug*, Princeton, NJ, 1992, Princeton University Press.
146. McDaniel HR, et al.: Extended survival and prognostic criteria for acemannan (ACE-M) treated HIV-1 patients, *Antiviral Res Suppl* 1:117, 1990.
147. McDaniel HR, et al.: An increase in circulating monocyte/macrophage (MM) is induced by oral acemanan (ACE-M) in HIV-1 patients, *Am Clin Pathol* 94:516-517, 1990.
148. Westendorf J: Anthranoid derivatives—general discussion. In De Smet PAGM, Keller K, Hansel R, Chandler RF: *Adverse effects of herbal drugs, vol. 2*, Berlin, 1993, Springer-Verlag.
149. Gracza L, Koch H, Loffler E: Biochemical-pharmacologic studies of medicinal plants. 1. Isolation of rosmarinic acid from *Symphytum officinale* L. and its anti-inflammatory activity in an in vitro model, *Arch Pharm (Weinheim)* 318(12):1090-1095, 1985.
150. Fujita Y, Uehara I, Morimoto Y, et al.: Studies on inhibition mechanism of autoxidation by tannins and flavonoids. II. Inhibition mechanism of caffeetannins isolated from leaves of *Artemisia* species on lipoxygenase dependent lipid peroxidation, *Yakugaku Zasshi* 108(2):129-135, 1988.
151. Kimura Y, Okuda H, Okuda T, Arichi S: Studies on the activities of tannins and related compounds. VIII. Effects of geraniin, corilagin, and ellagic acid isolated from *Geranii herba* on arachidonate metabolism in leukocytes, *Planta Medica* (4):337-338, 1986.
152. Weber G, Galle K: The liver, a therapeutic target in dermatoses, *Med Welt* 34(4):108-111, 1983.
153. Valenzuela A, Aspillaga M, Vial S, Guerra R: Selectivity of silymarin on the increase of the glutathione in different tissues of the rat, *Planta Medica* 55(5):420-422, 1989.
154. Madison E: Lectures at the Bastyr University (1984).
155. Roder E: Pyrrolizidinhaltige arzneipflanzen, *DAZ* 132(45): 2427-2435, 1992.
156. Moerman DE: *Native American ethnobotany*, Portland, OR, 1998, Timber Press.
157. Singh YN: Kava: an overview, *J Ethnopharmacol* 37(1):13-45, 1992.
158. Forgacs P, Jehanno A, Provost J, et al.: Alcaloides des Papaveracees II: Composition Chimique de Dix-Sept Especes de Fumaria, *Plantes Med Phytother* 20:64-81, 1986.
159. Forgacs P, Buffard G, Jehanno H, et al.: Composition Chimique de Fumariacees. Alkaloides de Quatorze Especes de Fumaria, *Plantes Med Phytother* 16:99-115, 1982.
160. Lushbough CC, Hale DB: Experimental acute radiodermatitis following beta radiation v. histopathological study of the mode of action of therapy with Aloe vera, *Cancer* 6:690-698, 1953.

161. Duke JA: *Handbook of medicinal herbs*, Boca Raton, FL, 1985, CRC Press.
162. Thurman FM: The treatment of psoriasis with sarsaparilla compounds, *N Engl J Med* 227: 128-133, 1942.
163. Bensky D, Gamble A: *Chinese herbal medicine*, London, 1981, Jill Norman & Hobhouse.
164. Krick W, Marner F-J, Jaenicke L: Isolation and structural determination of a new methylated triterpenoid in rhizomes of iris versicolor L, Z *Naturforsch* 38c:689-692, 1983.
165. Marner FJ, Longerich I: Isolation and structure determination of new iridals from *Iris sibirica* and *Iris versicolor, Liebigs Ann Chem* 269-272, 1992.
166. Komissarenko NF, Derkach AI: *Taraxacum officinale* coumarins, *Khim Prir Soedin* (4):519, 1981.
167. Konig M, et al.: Ellagitannins and complex tannins from *Quercus pertaea* Bark, *J Nat Product* 57(10):1411-1415, 1994.
168. Maradufu A: Furanosesquiterpenoids of *Commiphora erythraea* and *C. myrrh, Phytochemistry* 21:677-680, 1982.
169. Brieskorn CH, Noble P: Constituents of the essential oil of myrrh II: sesquiterpenes and furanosesquiterpenes, *Planta Medica* 44:87-90, 1982.
170. *Fourth Annual Report on Carcinogens*, Research Triangle Park, NC, 1985, National Toxicology Program.
171. Appa Rao MVR, Srinivasan K, Koteswara RTL: The effect of *Centella asiatica* on the general mental ability of mentally retarded children, *Indian J Psychiatry* 19:54-59, 1977.
172. Pelletier SW: *Alkaloids: chemical and biological perspectives, vol 5*, New York, 1985, John Wiley.
173. Isaac O: *Physikal Med U Rehab* 16:223, 1975.
174. Gulubov AZ, Chervenkova VB: Structure of alkaloids from *leonurus cardiaca,* Nauch Tr Vissh Pedagog Inst, Plovdiv, *Mat Fiz Khim Biol* 8:129-132, 1970.
175. Schultz OE, Alhyane M: Enhaltsstoffe von leonurus cardiaca, *L Sci Pharm* 41:149-155, 1973.
176. Kartnig T: Clinical applications of *Centella asiatica* (L) Urb. In Craker LE, Simon JE: *Herbs, spices, and medicinal plants: recent advances in botany, horticulture, and pharmacology, vol 3*, Phoenix, AZ, 1986, Oryx Press.
177. Barletta S, Borgioli A, Corsi C: Results with *Centella asiatica* in chronic venous insufficiency, *Gaz Med Ital* 140:33-35, 1981.

Glossary of Medicinal Effects

Abortifacient: Agent that induces abortion

Absorbent: Medicine or dressing that promotes the collection and removal of diseased tissue or morbid matter

Abstergent: This term is not used any longer but meant detergent

Acetum: Solution of substances in vinegar

Acrid: Pungent biting taste that usually causes minor irritation

Adjuvant: Agent added to a mixture to aid the effect of the principal ingredient

Adsorbent: Acid, alkaline, or amphoteric substance with a large molecular surface area that attracts and holds to its surface gases or other substances in solution

Alkalizer: Agent that causes something to be less acid

Alterative: An old term used for agents that favorably altered unhealthy conditions of the body and helped to restore normal function

Amylolytic: Agent that improves starch digestion

Analeptic: Central nervous system stimulant; a restorative medicine

Analgesic: Drug that relieves or diminishes pain

Anaphrodisiac: Agent that reduces sexual drive

Anesthetic: Agent that deadens sensation

Anhydrotic: Agent that decreases the amount of water or perspiration

Anodyne: Agent that soothes or relieves pain

Antacid: Medicine used to neutralize or reduce acid in the stomach or intestines

Anthelminthic: Agent that is destructive to worms infesting the human body

Antiarteriosclerotic: Agent that prevents plaque formation on the blood vessel walls

Antiarthritic: Medicine for the relief of inflammatory joint pain and gout

Antibilious: Agent that decreases bile secretion

Antibiotic: Agent that destroys or arrests the growth of microorganisms

Anticatarrhal: Agent that relieves the overproduction of mucus

Anticoagulant: Agent that prevents clotting in a fluid, especially blood

Antiemetic: Agent that relieves nausea and vomiting

Antihemorrhagic: Agent that stops bleeding

Antihydraulic: Agent that checks perspiration by reducing the action of sweat glands

Antilithic: Agent that reduces urinary calculi (stones)

Antiluetic: Antisyphilitic agent

Antimalarial: Agent effective against malaria

Antiperiodic: Agent that prevents the return of certain diseases; it counteracts periodic or intermittent diseases

Antiphlogistic: Agent that counteracts inflammation and fever
Antiphthisic: Agent that eliminates or lessens asthma
Antipruritic: Medicine that relieves or prevents itching
Antipyretic: Agent that controls fever
Antirachitic: Agent that is therapeutically effective against rickets
Antirheumatic: Agent that relieves or prevents rheumatism
Antiscrofulous: Agent that counteracts scrofula (tuberculosis of the lymphatic glands)
Antiseptic: Agent that destroys or inhibits pathogenic or putrefactive bacteria
Antispasmodic: Agent that relieves cramps or spasms
Antisudorific: Agent that prevents or relieves excessive perspiration
Antithrombotic: Agent that prevents thrombus or clots
Antitussive: Agent that relieves coughing
Aperient: Agent that produces natural movement of the bowels
Aphrodisiac: Agent that provokes sexual interest and excitation
Appetizer: Agent that stimulates the appetite or stimulates interest in food
Aromatic: Something that has agreeable odor
Aromatic bitter: Herb with the properties of aromatics and bitters
Astringent: Agent that causes contraction of tissue
Balsamic: Of the nature of a balsam. Usually this applies to substances that contain resins and benzoic acid, which are soothing or healing agents obtained from the exudations of various trees
Base: Nonacid part of a salt; the opposite of acid
Bitter: Agent characterized by a bitter taste that stimulates the appetite
Bronchodilator: Agent that dilates the bronchioles
Calefacient: Agent used externally to cause a sense of warmth
Calmative: Agent that produces a sedative or tranquilizing effect
Cardiac: Product that has an effect on the heart
Cardiant: Drug or agent that stimulates the heart
Carminative: Medicine that relieves gas or flatulence
Catarrh: Mucous secretion and congestion
Cathartic: Agent that empties the bowels
Caustic: Corrosive substance capable of burning away or eating tissues
Cholagogue: Agent that increases the flow of bile
Choleretic: Agent that stimulates the production of bile by the liver
Coagulant: Agent that induces clotting
Condiment: Spice
Constrigent: Obsolete term meaning astringent
Convulsant: Agent that causes convulsions
Cordial: Invigorating and stimulating medicine
Corrigent: Agent that renders a medicine less harsh or improves the flavor
Counterirritant: Agent that produces irritation in one part of the body to offset or counteract irritation in another part of the body
Cycloplegic: Agent that paralyzes the ciliary muscle
Decoction: Liquid preparation made by boiling a medicinal plant with water (about one part plant to twenty parts water by volume)
Demulcent: Soothing medicinal liquid that soothes irritated tissue, particularly the mucous membrane
Deobstruent: Agent that assists in clearing away obstructions by opening the natural passages of the body

Deodorant: Agent that inhibits or masks unwanted odors
Depilatory: Substance used to remove hair
Depressant: Agent that lessens nervous activity or functional activity of the tissue
Depurative: Agent that cleanses and purifies the system, particularly the blood
Dermatic: Term applied to drug that acts on the skin
Detergent: Agent that cleanses wounds and sores
Diaphoretic: Agent that promotes perspiration or fluid loss
Digestant: Agent that promotes or aids digestion
Digestive: Agent that promotes or aids digestion
Diluent: Substance that dilutes secretions and excretions
Discutient: Remedy that causes the disappearance of something or a scattering
Disinfectant: Agent that cleanses by destroying or inhibiting the activity of disease-producing microorganisms
Diuretic: Agent that increases the secretion and expulsion of urine
Drastic: Purgative that can cause a lot of irritation
Dusting powder: Medicine dusted on the surface
Ebolic: Drug that accelerates uterine contractions; primarily used to facilitate delivery
Eccoprotic: Term that is no longer used meaning laxative
Elixir: Sweetened aromatic preparation, about 25% alcohol, used as a vehicle for medicinal substances
Embrocation: Liniment
Emetic: Something that causes vomiting
Emetocathartic: Agent that causes vomiting
Emmenagogue: Agent that induces menstruation
Emollient: Agent used externally to soften and soothe
Emulsifier: Agent used to produce an emulsion; it disperses fats and oils
Emulsion: Preparation of one substance (usually a liquid) suspended in a second substance such as the oil and egg in mayonnaise
Epispastic: Blistering agent
Errhine: Agent that promotes nasal discharge, sneezing
Escharotic: Caustic
Essence: Alcohol or alcohol-water solution of medicinal substances
Euphoriant: Agent that induces an abnormal sense of vigor and buoyancy
Euphorigen: Agent that induces an abnormal sense of vigor and buoyancy
Evacuant: Remedy that evacuates the bowels, usually a purgative
Excitant: Agent that excites
Expectorant: Agent that expels mucus from the respiratory tract
Extract: Solution representing four to six times the strength of a crude drug
Febrifuge: Medicine that reduces fever; an antipyretic
Fixative: Substance added to a perfume to prevent the more volatile ingredients from evaporating too quickly
Flavoring agent: Agent that improves the taste of medicines
Fungicide: Agent that kills fungi
Galactagogue: Agent that encourages or increases the flow of milk
Glandular: Medicine made of gland tissue from cows, pigs, or sheep given to support the human glandular system; also plants that promote glandular function
Germicide: Agent that kills germs
Hallucinogen: Agent that induces hallucinations
Hemostatic: Agent that stops bleeding

Hepatic: Drug that acts on the liver
Hydrogogue: Agent that causes watery evacuations
Hypnotic: Agent that produces sleep
Infusion: Extraction of the active properties of a substance
Irritant: Something that causes inflammation or abnormal sensitivity in living tissue
Laxative: Agent that promotes evacuation of the bowels
Lenitive: Agent that soothes
Liniment: Medicinal substance, thinner than an ointment, that is gently rubbed into the skin for relief from pain, bruises, and aches
Liquor: Solution of medicinal substances in water
Local anesthetic: Locally applied herb that decreases sensation
Lotion: Solution of medicinal substances or skin softeners and cleaners applied to the skin
Lozenge: Medicated disk, usually to relieve sore throat
Lubricant: Agent applied to a surface to reduce friction between moving parts
Miotic: Medicine that contracts the pupil
Motor-excitant: Agent that increases activity in neuromuscular systems
Motor-inhibitor: Agent that decreases activity in the neuromuscular system
Mydriatic: Substance that dilates the pupil of the eye
Myotic: Medicine that contracts the pupil
Narcotic: Substance applied to drugs producing stupor or insensibility
Nauseant: Agent that produces the inclination to vomit
Nephritic: Agent that acts on the kidneys
Nervine: Agent that has a calming or soothing effect; these medicines build the integrity of the nervous system
Neuroleptic: Agent that affects cognition and behavior; it produces a state of apathy and limited range of emotion, helping to reduce confusion and agitation of psychomotor activity
Neurotic: Something that acts on the nervous system
Oxytocic: Drug that stimulates contraction of the uterus, thereby speeding up childbirth
Parasiticide: Agent that destroys parasites
Partus preparator: Agent that prepares a woman for childbirth
Pectoral: Remedy for pulmonary or chest diseases
Peristaltic: Agent used to increase peristalsis
Poison: Substance that has harmful effects on the tissue
Prophylactic: Substance that prevents disease
Protective: Agent that affords defense against a deleterious influence; for example, a medicine applied to protect against the effects of the sun's rays
Proteolytic enzymes: Enzymes that digest proteins
Ptyalagogue: Sialogogue
Purgative: Agent that induces emptying of the bowels
Pustulant: Agent that causes the formation of pustules
Refrigerant: Agent that lowers abnormal body heat
Relaxant: Medicine that relaxes the mind and/or body
Respiratory stimulant: Medicine that stimulates breathing
Respiratory vasoconstrictor: Agent that constricts the blood vessels in the lungs
Resolvent: Agent applied to reduce swelling
Restorative: Agent used to bring a person back to consciousness or back to normal vigor

Revulsant: Agent that draws blood from one part of the body to another
Rubefacient: Local irritant that produces reddening of the skin
Secretory depressant: Agent that reduces secretions
Sedative: Agent that soothes and reduces nervousness, distress, or irritation
Sialogogue: Agent that stimulates secretion of saliva
Somnifacient: Soporific
Soporific: Drug that produces sleep
Sorbefacient: Substance that increases absorption
Specific: Agent that cures or alleviates a particular condition or disease
Spirit: Alcohol or alcohol-water solution of medicinal substances
Sternutatory: Agent producing sneezing by irritating the mucous membranes
Stimulant: Agent that excites or quickens the activity of physiologic processes
Stomachic: Agent that strengthens, stimulates, or tones the stomach
Styptic: Astringent, especially one that stops bleeding by contracting blood vessels
Sudorific: Agent that promotes or increases perspiration
Synergist: Agent that increases the effectiveness of another agent working
Taeniafuge: Agent that expels tapeworms
Taeniacide: Agent that kills tapeworms
Tincture: Alcohol or hydroalcohol preparation of an herb or medicinal plant
Tisane: Infusion of flowers
Tonic: Agent that strengthens or invigorates organs or the entire organism
Unguent: Fatty medicinal preparation for external use that liquefies when applied to the skin
Vascular sedative: Agent that lowers the blood pressure and relaxes the walls of veins and arteries
Vasoconstrictor: Agent that narrows blood vessels, thereby elevating blood pressure
Vasodilator: Agent that widens the blood vessels
Vehicle: Substance that confers a suitable consistency to a drug
Vermifuge: Agent that expels worms
Vesicant: Agent that produces blisters
Vulnerary: Healing application for wounds

Index

E

F

G

S

X

Y

Z